Remediation in Medical Education

Adina Kalet · Calvin L. Chou

Editors

Remediation in Medical Education

A Mid-Course Correction

Second Edition

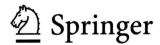 Springer

Editors
Adina Kalet
Robert D. and Patricia E. Kern Institute
for the Transformation of Medical
Education
Medical College of Wisconsin
Milwaukee, WI, USA

Calvin L. Chou
Veterans Affairs Health Care System
University of California, San Francisco
San Francisco, CA, USA

ISBN 978-3-031-32403-1   ISBN 978-3-031-32404-8   (eBook)
https://doi.org/10.1007/978-3-031-32404-8

This Springer imprint is published by the registered company Springer Nature Switzerland AG
The registered company address is: Gewerbestrasse 11, 6330 Cham, Switzerland

Foreword

And then a mighty roar
  Will start the sky to cryin'
  But not even light'ning
  Will be frightening my lion
  And with no fear inside
  No need to run
  No need to hide
  You're standing strong and tall
  You're the bravest of them all
  If on courage you must call
  Then just keep on tryin'
  And tryin', and tryin'
  You're a lion
  In your own way, be a lion...
  Come on. . . be a lion.
  – from *The Wiz*

A colleague reached out to me and said, "I am putting someone on your team. This person has great potential. Great, great, great potential."

Rut roh.

"*But?*" I said.

"But," my colleague repeated with a gentle chuckle.

"I'm ready for it. Hit me."

"Well. It's not so much of a bombshell to drop on you. I mean, not really. I think. . .I guess . . .I don't know. This person has just been. . .I think. . .misunderstood, maybe? I don't know. I think, yeah. I think that's it."

"Misunderstood like how?" I wanted to know.

"Some not so great evaluations. Non-stellar. But it's totally in them to do well. Which is kind of frustrating, you know?"

"Okay. So *what* is it then?"

"It's hard to say."

I squinted. "Well, I don't get it then. What's the disconnect?"

"This is what I'm hoping you can help with."

I thought on what my colleague said for a few moments and then spoke back. "If you have faith in this person, then I am very excited to work with them. And I assure you that if this person is competent, hardworking, kind, and eager to do well, then they *will*. In fact, they will do more than well. This person will do great. Let's just *claim* it." And since both of us had worked at Grady Hospital for some time, we both knew what "claiming it" meant.

My colleague just looked at me and smiled from ear to ear. I did the same. Because we both knew that together we were claiming a victory in advance—and that meant that it was going to be good.

A few weeks later, I joined the team and met this person. One of the first things I did was tell them, along with the other junior learners on the team, what—based upon my years of working with learners—were the features of an exceptional intern or medical student on the clinical service. I was very detailed and said, "I don't want it to be a mystery." And this person carefully took notes.

They sure did.

I observed them carefully for a couple of days, and a few things were very clear. This learner was super earnest. They were super kind and super eager. And mostly just super enthusiastic about taking excellent care of our patients.

I watched for those 48 h and cannot say I unlocked every mystery, but I did make a few observations. The biggest one was simple: This person was somewhat socially awkward. A little nervous sometimes, too. Just enough to make well-intentioned things veer a little too far off to the left. The kind of turns that garner snickers under breath and jokes that you are not in on. Which just makes awkwardness more awkward and nervousness more nervous. So that was mostly it. Nothing else I observed at all was noteworthy or even remotely bad in any way.

Nope.

I sat down with this person and chatted with them. I decided to be honest. Fortunately, they had insight. Before I could say much more, they mentioned their tendency to be awkward in most social situations—particularly when feeling nervous or insecure. I laughed and said, "Feeling nervous and insecure is a given as a student on the hospital service." They looked relieved. Next, I suggested that we would find some ways to work around that. Or better yet work *with it*. I am glad this person was open to the challenge and appreciative of my candor. Together, we strategized ways to tackle what had become a bit of an interpersonal speed breaker.

Here was one of our conversations:

"If I trip and fall in front of everyone, it's not as much fun to make fun of me if I laugh first. Kind of like when my husband and kids catch me dancing like Beyoncé in the bathroom mirror."

"Wow. Beyoncé?" they asked.

"I'm talking *full on* Beyoncé. Every head snap and dance move, too. It's *super* ridiculous. And *ultra*-awkward." I shrugged and smiled. "But I just own the awkward. So, after a while, it's no fun to make fun of me."

"You 'own the awkward.' Hmmm."

"You know what else? I counter a lot of my awkward things by working hard at the high-stakes things, you know? Like hugging my kids and reading them books and making my partner a hot turkey sandwich on the stove instead of a cold one from the fridge."

"Wait. Huh?"

"I guess I'm saying that when you nail the basics--like really nail them--people won't make as big a deal about the bumpy parts."

We both sat in silence and let that resonate. I could tell that their wheels were turning. What would that mean professionally? What would "nailing the basics" even look like? We explored that together. We did.

So, the two of us decided that, on the hospital service, that meant things like advocating for patients and communicating about them to other providers in clear, concise, and fluid language. It meant having a management plan that was evidence-based and that you could fully explain. That would require preparation, yes. And some practice, too. It would mean getting every detail of the history and physical down pat. And knowing as much as you can about the medical problems affecting your patients. We agreed that if these things became the focus, the other awkward quirks would matter far less.

So, here is the other main thing that happened during our time together: I looked at that person like they were a *superstar*. Like they could and would do great work and like they were *number one* in their class of learners. I asked who they wanted me to see. And I promised to work with *that* person—not the one tainted by what had been fed forward by others. I first learned of this concept in Benjamin and Rosamund Zander's book *The Art of Possibility* [1]. Specifically, it was a chapter in that book called "Giving an A"—where the authors push us to harness the power of helping people rise to their loftiest self-expectations. So, armed with this concept, I treated that student "like a winner and not a chicken dinner" (as the kids used to say in my neighborhood growing up). And let me just tell you something—it made *all* the difference.

At the end of our time together, it was easy to write that evaluation. No, not just "so-so." No, not just "good." This student performed at an exceptional level.

While this book will underscore many aspects of remediation in medical education, I cannot help but center on this example. I thought about this colleague of mine who thought enough to fight to help this person to have an optimal learning environment. I wondered: what could or would have happened had this colleague poisoned me with the opposite of what I was told? What if I had been told that this student was a "problem child," and that is it? What if this colleague did not feed forward some hopeful charge like the one I received? How would I have dealt with this learner? Would they have done as well?

Here is the other thing I am thinking about:

It is in our power to be a mirror to those around us. It is. We can, through our reflection of what we see in not only learners but also every person around us, feed them this idea of who they are—good, bad, or indifferent. Our listening ears can say, "Your voice is worth hearing." Our eyes and expressions can affirm, "Your ideas are worth sharing." Which is critical when you are doing this kind of work.

At the end of that time together, I received a note that included these words:

I will always be grateful for what you have taught me, and how much effort you put in to get to know me. I knew that there were aspects about my person-

ality that others might have not understood, but you explained them in a way that I can use it as a strength and not feel judged or embarrassed.

And that? That broke me all the way down and made me cry the ugly cry. It made me want to go harder, be more intentional, listen more carefully, and just . . .try. Our patients got better care because of it. I became a better teacher and attending physician that month. And best of all, someone felt understood and empowered.

No. This was not a hypothetical or made-up story. This was a true account of one pivotal moment in my career as a clinician-educator. I remain grateful to this day—both for the lesson learned and for their willingness to allow me to share this story for the benefit of others.

My suspicion is that there are probably far more "exceptionals" hidden inside of the "so-so" and "very good" ones than we realize. They also lurk beneath the surface of the "marginal" learners. The challenge is just helping to bring them out. The best part? Once the *exceptional* is out, there is no turning back. This I know for sure.

Reference

1. Zander RS, Zander B. *The Art of Possibility*. Boston: Harvard Business School Press, 2000.

Department of Medicine,   Kimberly Manning
Emory University School of Medicine,
Atlanta, GA, USA

Foreword

One of the many insights from this book is the importance of a team that is experienced and trained in remediation to help trainees effect a midcourse correction. Usually, this ideal is not achieved, and remediation is left to front-line teachers who make individual efforts that are generous and often heroic but sometimes lacking a strategy. This characterized our earliest attempts at remediation, which had limited success. Recently, we have uncovered tactics based on relationships and trust that helped us reframe remediation as one of the most rewarding aspects of being a medical educator.

During the time when we co-directed an internal medicine clerkship rotation, we were periodically contacted by supervisors who had concerns about a student's knowledge, skill attainment, or professionalism development. This familiar starting point to the remediation process was bypassed, however, when one student, TM, came to us himself, a week into his rotation, feeling like he was "doing poorly overall." Since we had no data from his team, we had no information to triangulate and instead took the time to get to know him. In this initial meeting, we chatted as if sitting across from each other at a coffee shop. What was his medical school journey to the present moment? What did he enjoy outside of medicine?

It felt odd to not get down to business (e.g., reviewing the gap between where he was and the expectations of his supervisors) at an initial meeting. But this initial investment in getting to know him established safety, which we had underestimated as a bedrock of a successful remediation. When he recognized that we cared about him—not his grade—it allowed him to be vulnerable and honest. This early rapport also allowed him to answer an unspoken question: Could he trust us to help him? We learned that it would take more than one conversation for him to answer "yes."

As we shifted the focus of our conversations to daily growth ("How can you do better tomorrow?"), we perceived that TM gravitated to the pragmatic concern of whether he was on track to pass the rotation. Assurances that our primary focus was coaching, not grading, only went so far, and it became clear that TM did not fully believe them to be separate. Nor did we. We had to admit to ourselves that one person could not perform both roles impartially.

Since there were two of us, we decided to experiment with separating these two tasks: one of us (R.G.) as coach and the other (G.D.) as summative evaluator. The coach checked in daily with TM, got updates on presentations and performance from his supervisors, and provided guidance on improvement and established short-term goals. The evaluator checked in periodically, provided reminders of competency benchmarks, and sparingly outlined the requirements to pass the rotation. Separating these roles allowed the student to speak freely about daily growth with the coach who had no influence on the final grading decision.

We reached out to his team, who felt that TM needed more guidance on structuring his presentations and developing a persuasive diagnostic argument. It was a common situation where the team sensed a problem but was concerned about the grading implications if they elevated it to the clerkship leadership. Their initial plan was to try their best to help TM, although the entire team (intern, resident, and attending) candidly shared that they lacked a structured way to do so. Perhaps this gap between aspiration and skills is what leaves most educators adrift when asked to provide remediation. We realized that we needed to coach the team in parallel to coaching the student.

We met with the resident frequently and the attending less often. We started with the advice that all parties needed direct observational data—not gestalt impressions—to enhance their student's presentation and demonstration of his reasoning. This one guiding principle helped the team provide TM with specific, actionable feedback daily. They also adopted the "take it from the top approach," where they provided TM feedback and had him deliver a revised presentation (usually just focused on the assessment) in the same session. TM would repeat this process until he had fully cemented the crux of their feedback.

As the team adopted tight feedback loops with TM, the coach was able to take a step back. We provided clarifications of the team feedback to TM but shifted to spending most of the time reflecting on the incremental growth he was making. The triangulation of the student, team, and clerkship coach kept frequent, focused, and actionable growth steps flowing throughout the rotation, which TM successfully navigated.

A few months later, we had the opportunity to try this relationship-based process again. A team notified us about a student, AK, who was struggling with his oral presentations, which focused on the plan of action. It was not clear to him why assessments of the diagnostic and therapeutic decision-making were necessary or helpful. We tried to replicate our model from TM, but it was ineffective. Get-to-know-you discussions devolved to a grading debate. Feedback was given but not accepted. The triangulation process was perceived as secretive rather than supportive. AK failed the rotation, but we also know that we failed him.

Though TM's journey in our remediation pathway was complete, it was just the beginning of our reflections and growth, which continued as we worked with more students like AK. We realized that remediation is a high-touch enterprise and that trust and relationship-building, which are at the core of successful remediation, take time and cannot be scaled. We learned how much faculty and residents appreciated guidance in their effort to support their trainees who required help. Above all else, we accepted that our trial-and-error approach to discovering effective strategies was good—but not good enough. To achieve a level of skill in remediation that elevates most learners, we knew that we had to learn from the educators and scholars who have thought deeply about this topic. This book is now our guide—and marks the beginning of our own midcourse correction.

Department of Medicine, University of California,   Gurpreet Dhaliwal
San Francisco, CA, USA   Rabih Geha

Veterans Affairs Healthcare System,
San Francisco, CA, USA

Preface

Much has happened in the field of remediation in health professions education since the first edition of this book was published in early 2014. The remediation literature has grown extensively since then, and our book has had thousands of readers. Due to this burgeoning interest, our understanding of remediation in medical education has deepened and become more complex. We each have had the privilege of speaking with health professions educators far and wide on the topic. So, in 2019, we met in Adina's Brooklyn kitchen to discuss a second edition, which would extend the scope of the work beyond the education of American medical students to include postgraduate, international, and interprofessional perspectives. We dusted off our original documents, culled through our respective Rolodexes, and made plans.

Then the COVID-19 pandemic hit. Health professions education precipitously shifted to a virtual space, bringing with it heightened challenges for learners who struggle. [We deliberately adopt this moniker to replace the label "the struggling learner," as we wish to focus on behaviors rather than taking the risk of creating another subjugated identity.] The social reckoning that followed, and heightening awareness of racism, sexism, and political polarization, further complicated the way we teach, learn, and interact in our professional and personal lives. It has been a dynamic couple of years. Even as we try to resume a semblance of normal life, we are still amidst turmoil and uncertainty about the future.

While the second edition of this book will not resolve all our problems, we hope to provide context, structure, inspiration, and stimulus for continual improvement in our educational work. We have sought to incorporate the many important advances in the field into this new edition. We have endeavored to honor the experience and expertise of an expanding group of committed educators and scholars even when strong research evidence is not yet available. And ultimately, we have tried to identify and reinforce an optimal set of practices that support all learners, not merely the ones who struggle.

As with the last edition, the list of authors includes mostly physicians; however, we have worked to expand the perspectives represented. Contributing authors include physicians from a range of disciplines including internal medicine, emergency medicine, family medicine, obstetrics and gynecology, pediatrics, psychiatry, surgery, and urology; social, behavioral, and educational science researchers; and an array of health professionals including dentists, nurses, pharmacists, physical therapists, and physician assistants. All told, the 73 authors hail from 33 different institutions, representing four continents and seven countries; from the United States, we have authors from 16 states plus the District of Columbia. Though we have increased the diversity of perspectives compared with the last edition, there is clearly more work to do in this area. As before, with deep humility, we know that we should have done more to give voice to the ongoing experiences of learners. There are also numerous viewpoints we have unwittingly excluded due to our own blind spots. We promise to work on these limitations moving forward.

We have structured this edition to highlight emerging lenses on remediation. Chapters 1–6 encompass broad topics that provide the context for remediation work, including institutional systems; diversity and equity; the Master Adaptive Learner framework; and the emerging field of learners' experiences of remediation. This section concludes with a framework for remediation practices (Chap. 6) that provides structure for the second section of the book, Chaps. 7–16, which walks through core clinical competencies as organized by the Accreditation Council for Graduate Medical Education: knowledge, patient care, interpersonal communication, professionalism, practice-based learning, and systems-based practice. Wholly new chapters in this section include those on remediating learners who struggle with procedures; organization, efficiency, and time management; and practice-based learning and systems-based practice. In addition, the coverage of professionalism remediation has been substantially expanded. To incorporate this fount of information, we have heavily edited valuable first edition chapters and incorporated the information into the new structure. For example, material on autism spectrum conditions has been condensed and incorporated into the chapter on interpersonal communication. The third section contains special topics: learning differences and disabilities, well-being and resilience, and faculty development. The fourth and fifth sections zoom out (but not on Zoom™) to address viewpoints from the medical school dean's office and the office of the Designated Institutional Official, respectively, with commentaries from interprofessional and international perspectives. The sixth section focuses on what to do to prepare for the rare instance when a trainee must be dismissed. Finally, as with the prior edition, the Epilogue was written by a medical student who describes his experience of struggle during his journey to becoming a physician.

Incorporating and respecting all the authors' voices and perspectives means that there are differences in tone from chapter to chapter. Some of these differences are intentional. For example, the words "learner" and "trainee," less specific than "student" or "resident," are used interchangeably throughout the book. In addition, we have attempted to avoid judgmental language, framing learner/trainee issues as "struggles" rather than "deficits" or "weaknesses." However, in the sections where difficult judgments must be made, for example, when competency committees or educational leaders determine that the learner is not meeting expectations, we use clear and specific language identifying learner's deficits and weaknesses. As a manifestation of our intention to be inclusive and true to the uneven literature, some chapters take a scholarly tone and are more richly referenced and others more pragmatic. We have worked to provide a unified reader's experience where possible.

Health professions educators and learners have much in common; we are all engaged in the high-stakes work of ensuring a healthcare workforce to serve the public. We all must ensure clinical competence in highly complex, emotionally, intellectually, and physically challenging environments. One merely needs to recall the recent images of healthcare professionals both saving lives and caring for the dying, all while wearing personal protective equipment (or garbage bags early on), to understand what the COVID-19 pandemic has once again demonstrated: healthcare professionals around the world will honor their commitments and serve with dignity even at the risk of their own health. We are trusted by our learners and society to provide education that ensures excellence, readiness to serve, and accountability. Remediation practice is one important aspect of this obligation.

On the other hand, there are many ways in which the health professions differ. There are clear differences between the life experiences of our students. Some have just completed secondary school, and others have robust educational and work experiences before entering training. The differences in individual development require different approaches at both the program and individual levels. Additionally, cultural differences between health professions and in different international contexts cannot be overlooked. We reiterate that we are merely at the beginning of a fuller understanding of remediation practices across health professions and throughout the world—as the saying goes, if you know one institution, you know one institution. Honoring our current and future colleagues who may stumble along their journey to becoming a healthcare professional, we offer this work as an incremental step forward to help.

Milwaukee, WI, USA   Adina Kalet
San Francisco, CA, USA   Calvin L. Chou

Acknowledgments

This book is about educating those who stumble while on the path to becoming health professionals. Since the first edition 9 years ago, the threats to our professions have mounted and the challenges of the modern era have grown ominous. A global pandemic, the impact of climate change, and the noxious aspects of the increasing commercialization of our healthcare system have heightened the need to and importance of recommitting to caring for individual patients, communities, and ourselves with character and excellence.

It is in this context that I am especially appreciative and grateful for the people and institutions who have made this work possible, deeply satisfying, and joyful.

This book is a rare, true collaboration. Calvin Chou has done the yeoman's job on this edition; he has taken the time and applied considerable creativity to leading this effort. First, he gently coaxed me into considering important changes. Then, he spent the time identifying those who could add new perspectives. And finally, he nurtured, cajoled, and curated his way to this final product. No small task with nearly 75 authors. Together, we melded the old and the new, respectfully discussing and debating. Such an intellectual partnership is a precious thing. It is a unique set of skills he has, to write, read, edit, and collate such a complex set of voices. I bow to his orchestration and throw bouquets in honor of his accomplished conducting of this symphony. As I have said before, the single most important thing I did to create this project—oh, so long ago—was to convince Calvin Chou to join me. Without him, it would not have happened.

Much has changed in my life since we published the first edition of this book.

In 2019, after 32 years at the New York University School of Medicine, I took on the Directorship of the Robert D. and Patricia E. Kern Institute for the Transformation of Medical Education at the Medical College of Wisconsin. This has been a remarkable gift and an adventure thanks to many people. First, I thank those who welcomed me with warm hands and hearts: Joseph E. Kerschner, MD, Provost, Executive Vice President, and Dean; John R. Raymond, Sr., MD, President and CEO; and Cheryl A. Maurana, PhD, Senior Vice President for Strategic Academic Partnerships and Founding Director Kern National Network for Caring and Character in Medicine of the Medical College of Wisconsin. These three inspiring leaders are exemplars of integrity, humility, and creativity.

Thank-you to our benefactors at the Kern Family Foundation, starting with Mr. Robert E. Kern, whose passing this year has been a great loss to me personally. Foundation President Mr. Jim Rahn and his colleagues Beth Purvis EdD, Christopher Stawski, PhD, and Stasia Zwisler have been the generous coaches and guides who have "put wind in our sails." Thank-you to all my colleagues at the Kern Institute. To name only a few, to the uniquely talented and dedicated Tavinder K. Ark, PhD; to Ms. Venus Coates who runs a tight ship with heart and soul; to Catherine (Cassie) Ferguson, MD, our Associate Institute Director whose deep intelligence, grace, and courage anchor us; and to our "editor in chief," Bruce Campbell, MD. We all have accomplished much, and there is still much to be done.

In writing the first edition of this book, I was generously supported by the Arnold P. Gold Foundation. While we lost Arnold in 2018, Dr. Sandra Gold is still attending national meetings and encouraging and engaging with a sparkle in her eye. Without their belief in me so many years ago, if they had not said yes when I asked for the resources to support a sabbatical, this work would never have been done. Each year, I donate my book royalties back to the Gold Foundation to "pay this forward." Thank you.

In this second edition, I have revisited old relationships with contributing authors and forged new ones. To all, we did this together, it was hard, detailed work, and great fun.

I have been very well mentored (and remediated when need be) over the years. While the list is long, I will mention one. I am still reeling from the recent loss of Jo Anne Earp, ScD, in November 2022. JAE helped me find my voice, taught me to write, cheered me on at every step of the way, and adopted me into her enormous family of mentees. I am privileged to have been one of the "daughters" she has put on a path to make the world a better, more just place.

When you write something and send it out into the universe, you may never know where and how it lands. This book has been a "calling card" providing me many a grand adventure. Because of it, I have made many strong connections with changemakers around the globe. Thanks to Rachel Ellaway, PhD, now of the University of Calgary, for her wholehearted, deeply intellectual engagement in this work with us. Thanks also to Daniel Marom, PhD, who took me out to dinner in NYC "out of the blue" and introduced me to Dafna Meitar, MD, both from the Mandel School for Educational Leadership in Jerusalem. I cherish our annual "meetings" overlooking the Mediterranean. I have spoken on the topic of remediation in medical education to many schools and training programs in the United States, Canada, Israel, and Switzerland. These engagements have been invaluable to the work, forcing me to expand my perspective. Thank-you to the beautiful places—Brooklyn, NY; Lake Huntington, NY; and Milwaukee, WI, all fabulous places to live and write.

To my husband Mark, have I told you lately how your love and support make me brave? Thanks for taking the lead on keeping our home and family sacred while I have taken time to go on adventures. To my son Zachai and daughter Sara, remarkable adults who keep me humble and optimistic about the future. To my father Morton and my brother Michael and sister-in-law

Lorna, my in-laws Peter and Julie and Julie and Phil, and Lisa and Danny and Lisa and Leon, sisters and brothers of another mother. To my work spouse Sondra Zabar, sorry I moved away, and thank you for sticking with me. We have had some very painful losses these past years, and we have had much to celebrate.

Our world seems to be getting more worrisome. The pandemic has revealed many deep fissures in our society. Our planet is imperiled. But these challenges have also demonstrated how crucial our work is to society. When needed, the physicians, nurses, respiratory therapists, physician assistants, nurse practitioners, scientists, public health officials, and many other "essential" workers went to work so that we could be safe, so that lives could be saved. We should never forget the images of colleagues' faces bruised from wearing tight-fitting masks all day every day for months on end. This is not heroic; it is our work, it is what we prepare to do, and it is why we all train so seriously. When the time comes, everyone deserves to have caring and excellent health care. I am optimistic that we can make this a reality for most, but we are not there yet. It is with great honor that I have had a small role in the education of thousands of physicians. Thank you for the privilege.

Adina Kalet

2nd edition, July 2023

It is interesting (probably just to me) to read the acknowledgments from the last edition. Some things have stopped, e.g., my regular Oscar and Tony watching; some things have yet to happen, e.g., going to Dubrovnik; some things have receded, e.g., my hairline; and some things have not—my ongoing indebtedness to a burgeoning community of important supporters. In the same way that it takes many people to help a learner who struggles, so have I required a village of people to help me as I embarked on this volume.

Again, at the top of the list, Adina Kalet: it is an extraordinary privilege to work side by side with truly one of the titans of medical education. Even amidst the constellation of tasks needed to put together this book, I marvel at the powerhouse of your intellect, the broad knowledge of education theory and practice, the assiduousness of detailed and perspicacious editing, and the additional polymathy of your painting, guitar-playing, challah baking, and green thumb. I forever remain in your debt for taking me on over two decades ago as my first medical education mentor, through the Faculty-in-Training Program of the Academy of Communication in Healthcare (ACH). As we have grown as colleagues on this and other projects, our partnership and friendship remain deeply meaningful.

Anila Vijayan, Vishal Anand, and Miranda Finch at Springer—thank you for your ongoing support and forbearance.

I could not have focused on this book without the support of important people at my workplace at the VA in San Francisco, which I have experienced over the last 25+ years as a deeply nurturing and growth-oriented professional milieu. Rebecca Shunk, our indomitable Associate Chief of Staff for Education, and Jeff Kohlwes, our superbly visionary Chief of the Division of

General Medicine, relentlessly advocated for my educational leave so I could devote hours of blood, sweat, and tears (well, maybe not blood) to this book. I also fervently appreciate the leadership and support teams at the VA in San Francisco, starting with the Department of Medicine, including Ken McQuaid, Heather Nye, and Josue Zapata, for fording the labyrinthine logistics. The leadership teams at Medical Practice, including Maya Dulay, Krista Odden, and Sara Rumrill, and on the inpatient wards at the VA in San Francisco, particularly Nate Baskin (and Josue again), built critical coverage structures to reduce the ramifications of my educational leave. Kate Murphy and Lily Loew, you are intrepid and excellent clinicians who masterfully covered my complex panel of patients in my absence. I am also profoundly thankful to the many patients who asked after the progress of the book with curiosity and humor. Finally, but absolutely not least, deepest gratitude to my dear friend Jack Penner, for almost daily support and solidarity in the office and by phone, sometimes across time zones.

On the UCSF side, there are so many colleagues that have supported me and cheered me on: to name some important communities, the fantastic threesome of Anna Chang, Peter Chin-Hong, and Brian Schwartz, who continually impress me and keep me humble (and well fed), and our staunch LEAP leadership group, Carrie Chen, Gurpreet Dhaliwal, Ann Poncelet, and Lowell Tong, for breakfasts, tea, and cross-country Skypes and Zooms. In my Oscar moment, thanks to the Academy of Medical Educators at the UCSF, for the inaugural endowed chair that enabled me to embark on this work, and to the UCSF Center for Faculty Educators, for supporting innumerable feedback workshops over the past two decades that have sharply honed my feedback skills and teaching, and as I like to say, remediation is feedback on steroids.

In the intervening decade since the last edition, my community of collaborators and friends at the ACH (the other Academy) and associated programs at institutions around the country have grown astronomically. Your commitment, honesty, creativity, and expertise inspire me to be the best facilitator, communicator, and indeed person I can be. So many to name, and loath to exclude; yet I must mention my longest-term ACH work companions, Laura Cooley, Ellen Pearlman, Cathy Risdon, Denise Davis, Auguste Fortin, and Krista Hirschmann; some of the mentors who have guided our learning, including Amina Knowlan, Gerald Boyd, Charlie O'Leary (whom we lost and miss terribly), Ronke Tapp, and Ted DesMaisons; and some former mentees, who I pretended to have guided or supervised and who are now colleagues and friends, continually teaching me in every interaction with them: Lynn O'Neill, Jim Bell, Kara Myers, Ryan Laponis, Tim Gilligan, Laura Kirk, Barbette Weimer-Elder, and Sandi Moutsios. It is amazing to see the national and international reach of fundamental communication work, which of course is essential for effective remediation. I continue to have great pride that my half of proceeds from this book go to scholarships for underrepresented participants at the ACH's annual ENRICH faculty development course. We need to continue to build the pipeline to correct the representation gap, and then do much, much more.

To family: Craig Kliger, who put up with my being unbearable and frosty at times throughout the gestation of this book and who supports my hectic travel (and online) schedule with staunch equanimity; Beth Weise and Lisa Murphy: for raising our now college-age daughters—it is no accident that they have turned out so awesome; Eleanor and Margaret Murphy-Weise: you keep me accountable, entertained, and discovering depths of love and pride that I never thought possible; my siblings Homer and Carol, who teach me formally and informally how to be a better brother and who exhibit such patience for my shenanigans; our father Chris, whom we lost at 105 years old earlier this year, and who embodied perseverance and hardiness; and our mother Shufen, the epitome of patience and unconditional positive regard. In retrospect, those parental contributions set me up perfectly for this work.

As I reflect on these acknowledgments, one theme emerges. While learners (and children) start out needing structure, guidance, teaching, and feedback, as they develop into colleagues/adults, they themselves can pay forward to future learners and also pay back to their mentors, teachers, and parents in previously unimaginable ways. I hope that this volume provides some helpful direction to expedite progress in our complex systems of education and remediation. I also have high optimism for the field as the next generation of learners deploys their creativity, ingenuity, and commitment toward further growth and improvement.

Calvin L. Chou
2nd edition, July 2023

Contents

Part III Special Topics

Contributors

Eva Aagaard Washington University School of Medicine, St. Louis, MO, USA

Raghdah Al-Bualy Oman Medical Specialty Board, Muscat, Oman

Siham Al Sinani Oman Medical Specialty Board, Muscat, Oman

Muriel J. Bebeau School of Dentistry, University of Minnesota Twin Cities, Minneapolis, MN, USA

James Bell Institute for Healthcare Communication, Buffalo, NY, USA

Riley Brian Department of Surgery, University of California, San Francisco, CA, USA

Lynn Buckvar-Keltz Department of Medicine, New York University Grossman School of Medicine, New York, NY, USA

Justin Bullock Division of Nephrology, Department of Medicine, University of Washington, Seattle, WA, USA

Anna Chang Department of Medicine, University of California, San Francisco, CA, USA

Veterans Affairs Healthcare System, San Francisco, CA, USA

H. Carrie Chen Department of Pediatrics, Georgetown University School of Medicine, Washington, DC, USA

Calvin L. Chou Department of Medicine, University of California, San Francisco, CA, USA

Veterans Affairs Healthcare System, San Francisco, CA, USA

Carol M. Chou Department of Medicine, Perelman School of Medicine, University of Pennsylvania, Philadelphia, PA, USA

Irwin Clement Alphon Chung National Healthcare Group Polyclinics, Singapore, Singapore

Shaima Darwish Oman Medical Specialty Board, Muscat, Oman

Denise L. F. Davis Department of Medicine, University of California, San Francisco, CA, USA

Veterans Affairs Healthcare System, San Francisco, CA, USA

Marianne Mak-van der Vossen Department of General Practice, Amsterdam UMC, University of Amsterdam, Amsterdam, The Netherlands

Gurpreet Dhaliwal Department of Medicine, University of California, San Francisco, CA, USA

Veterans Affairs Healthcare System, San Francisco, CA, USA

Rachel H. Ellaway Community Health Sciences, Cumming School of Medicine, University of Calgary, Calgary, AB, Canada

Kathy Faber-Langendoen Center for Bioethics and Humanities, State University of New York Upstate Medical Center, Syracuse, NY, USA

Amber Fitzsimmons Department of Physical Therapy and Rehabilitation Science, University of California, San Francisco, CA, USA

Carol Flaten University of Minnesota School of Nursing, Minneapolis, MN, USA

Cha-Chi Fung Department of Clinical Medical Education, Keck School of Medicine, University of Southern California, Los Angeles, CA, USA

Rabih Geha Department of Medicine, University of California, San Francisco, CA, USA

Veterans Affairs Healthcare System, San Francisco, CA, USA

Eric Goren Department of Medicine, Perelman School of Medicine, University of Pennsylvania, Philadelphia, PA, USA

Suely Grosseman Department of Pediatrics, Federal University of Santa Catarina, Florianopolis, Santa Catarina, Brazil

Jeannette Guerrasio Medicine Within Reach, PLLC, Denver, CO, USA

David Hatem Department of Internal Medicine, University of Massachusetts TH Chan School of Medicine, Worcester, MA, USA

Neva Howard University of Colorado School of Medicine, Aurora, CO, USA

Jason Meng Huey Chan National Healthcare Group Polyclinics, Singapore, Singapore

Kimberly Illingworth Purdue University College of Pharmacy, West Lafayette, IN, USA

Jameze James Department of Pediatrics, Kaiser Permanente Medical Center, Oakland, CA, USA

Theresa Jaramillo Department of Physical Therapy and Rehabilitation Science, University of California, San Francisco, CA, USA

Lee Jones Georgetown University School of Medicine, Washington, DC, USA

Adina Kalet Kern Institute for the Transformation of Medical Education, Medical College of Wisconsin, Milwaukee, WI, USA

Kai Kennedy Department of Physical Therapy and Rehabilitation Science, University of California, San Francisco, CA, USA

Cedric Lefebvre Department of Emergency Medicine, Wake Forest University School of Medicine, Winston-Salem, NC, USA

Allison Ludwig Department of Medicine, Albert Einstein College of Medicine, Bronx, NY, USA

Andrew Lui Department of Physical Therapy and Rehabilitation Science, University of California, San Francisco, CA, USA

Kimberly Manning Department of Medicine, Emory University School of Medicine, Atlanta, GA, USA

Rebecca McAlister Department of Obstetrics and Gynecology, Washington University School of Medicine, St. Louis, MO, USA

Lynnea Mills Department of Medicine, University of California, San Francisco, CA, USA

Peter Moffett Department of Emergency Medicine, Virginia Commonwealth University, Richmond, VA, USA

Verna Monson Kern Institute for the Transformation of Medical Education, Medical College of Wisconsin, Milwaukee, WI, USA

Kendra Moore Department of Medicine, University of California, San Francisco, CA, USA

Ronald Olson Department of Family Medicine, Keck School of Medicine, University of Southern California, Los Angeles, CA, USA

Melissa Owen Nell Hodgson Woodruff School of Nursing, Emory University, Atlanta, GA, USA

Seattle University, College of Nursing, Seattle, WA, USA

Andrew S. Parsons Departments of Medicine and Public Health, University of Virginia School of Medicine, Charlottesville, VA, USA

John C. Penner Department of Medicine, University of California, Veterans Affairs Healthcare System, San Francisco, CA, USA

Abigail Phillips Department of Medicine, University of California, Veterans Affairs Healthcare System, San Francisco, CA, USA

Martin Pusic Harvard Medical School, Boston, MA, USA

Sanziana Roman Department of Surgery, University of California, San Francisco, CA, USA

Sara Rumrill Department of Medicine, University of California, Veterans Affairs Healthcare System, San Francisco, CA, USA

Antoinette Schoenthaler Department of Population Health, New York University Grossman School of Medicine, New York, NY, USA

Department of Medicine, New York University Grossman School of Medicine, New York, NY, USA

Darren Seah National Healthcare Group Polyclinics, Singapore, Singapore

Tahlia Spector Department of Emergency Medicine, David Geffen School of Medicine, University of California, Los Angeles, CA, USA

Archana Sridhar Department of Medicine, University of California, Veterans Affairs Healthcare System, San Francisco, CA, USA

Shareef Syed Department of Surgery, University of California, San Francisco, CA, USA

Sara Tariq University of Arkansas for Medical Sciences School of Medicine, Little Rock, AR, USA

Larissa Thomas Department of Medicine, University of California, San Francisco, CA, USA

Bau P. Tran Department of Physician Assistant Studies, University of Texas Southwestern, Dallas, TX, USA

Erica Traxel Division of Urology Surgery, Department of Surgery, Washington University School of Medicine, St. Louis, MO, USA

Sjoukje van den Broek Education Center, Department of Clinical Skills Training, University Medical Center, Utrecht, The Netherlands

Walther van Mook Department of Intensive Care Medicine, Academy for Postgraduate Training and School of Health Professions Education, Maastricht University and Maastricht University Medical Center, Maastricht, The Netherlands

Karen M. Warburton Department of Medicine, University of Virginia School of Medicine, Charlottesville, VA, USA

Andrew White Department of Pediatrics, Washington University School of Medicine, St. Louis, MO, USA

Department of Pediatrics, Saint Louis University School of Medicine, St. Louis, USA

Kelly Williamson Department of Emergency Medicine, Northwestern University, Chicago, IL, USA

Sarah Williams Department of Psychiatry, New York University Grossman School of Medicine, New York, NY, USA

Kalman Winston Cambridge University, Cambridge, UK

Paul Wise Department of Surgery, Washington University School of Medicine, St. Louis, MO, USA

Marian Wolters Center for Research and Development of Health Professions Education, University Medical Center, Utrecht, The Netherlands

Paul Yellin Department of Pediatrics, New York University Grossman School of Medicine, New York, NY, USA

Yellin Center for Mind, Brain, and Education, New York, NY, USA

Peter Yen Department of Medicine, Perelman School of Medicine, University of Pennsylvania, Philadelphia, PA, USA

Sondra Zabar Department of Medicine, New York University Grossman School of Medicine, New York, NY, USA

Part I
Overview and Framing

Remediation: The Measure of a Profession

Rachel H. Ellaway

I believe - I daily find it proved - that we can get nothing in this world worth keeping, not so much as a principle or a conviction, except out of purifying flame, or through strengthening peril. We err; we fall; we are humbled - then we walk more carefully. –Charlotte Brontë, *Shirley*

Introduction

It has been said that the measure of a civilization is how it treats its weakest members. As it is with civilization as a whole, so it is with health professions education. How we approach remediation, both of learners and of practicing health professionals, is a critical reflection of the professional values that we aspire to, that we espouse, and that we experience. Although a minority of learners, teachers, and practitioners will have firsthand experience of remediation during their careers, everyone is (or should be) aware of it, and everyone needs to be able to trust that it is effective, proportionate, and just. In this opening chapter, I consider some of the more intriguing and pressing issues in contemporary remediation practice in health professions education by taking a series of philosophical, ethical, systemic, and economic

R. H. Ellaway (✉)
Community Health Sciences, Cumming School of Medicine, University of Calgary, Calgary, AB, Canada
e-mail: rachel.ellaway@ucalgary.ca

perspectives on remediation. In doing so I seek to both situate and make strange existing practices and thinking in and around remediation in the health professions. I then draw these together to outline the challenges and agendas that a deep conceptual reading of remediation implies.

Unpacking Remediation

Let us begin by considering the original subtitle for this book: 'a mid-course correction'. This oft-used navigational metaphor for remediation suggests that there is a correct or optimal path to and through a health professional career, that some may lose their way, and that we should do what we can to help those individuals who do lose their way. As much as this seems benign on first reading, it does have deeper implications that should be unpacked and examined. Indeed, analyzing our metaphors can illuminate assumptions that may otherwise be inaccessible to us [1].

As we begin to deconstruct the pathway metaphor, we might ask whether there is one 'right' way of being or becoming a health professional, and whether a 'course correction' should be more concerned with proscribing and eradicating 'wrong' ways of being or becoming one. If so, then at what point does autonomy and individuality, or innovation and creativity in clinical learning and practice, turn into unacceptable deviation? And who decides these questions with

© The Author(s), under exclusive license to Springer Nature Switzerland AG 2023
A. Kalet, C. L. Chou (eds.), *Remediation in Medical Education*,
https://doi.org/10.1007/978-3-031-32404-8_1

what implications and accountabilities? It is easy to see, after all, how remediation (or the threat thereof) could become inappropriately coercive and controlling. *Whenever a judgment is made, both judge and judged must be prepared to come under scrutiny.*

While the use of remediation for coercive purposes is clearly problematic, the health professions cannot be so individualistic as to have no structure at all. We need to be able to guide learners and assess when they are failing or succeeding, while also allowing for their individual circumstances and trajectories. We therefore define broad corridors of acceptability in the form of outcomes and assessments, and more recently competencies, milestones, and Entrustable Professional Activities (EPAs). Learners and practitioners may wind their own way through these corridors, but they must still stay within their perimeters. We clearly need to be able to distinguish between individuals who are in trouble (and who need big 'R' remediation) and those who experience normal variations in performance. And that begs the question as to what role remediation has (if any) in defining the perimeters of these corridors. *Do remediators simply return strays to the fold, or should there be a dialogue between those who define the boundaries and those who police them?*

If there are many acceptable paths to independent practice, then perhaps our reading of the pathway metaphor should focus on how it is that some individuals lose their way, whatever path they are on. Or we might be more concerned with why it is that individuals stray or lose their way, than with when and how far they wandered. Reasons for failing are important both diagnostically (if we don't know what the problem is, then it's hard to do anything about it) and in determining their responsibility (more latitude is likely to be given to those who failed despite their best efforts than to those who failed because they just didn't try), and from those determinations arises our responsibilities for them. Indeed, it may turn out that we need to remediate the training or practice context, or the structures that define appropriate practice as well as, or instead of, the individual—see Fig. 1.1.

Failure or underperformance may be situated or contextual, only partially reflecting the abilities and failures of the individual. After all, when you are remediating an individual, are you truly remediating them or the circumstances they found themselves in? Lawyers, patient safety advocates, and human factors engineers will all point to institutional and other contextual factors that can compel or direct otherwise competent individuals to bad or incompetent behaviors. Remediating a person and returning them to a problematic context is unlikely to address the root problem. Remediation therefore also has a diagnostic component—one concerned with root causes and what is and can be changed in those causes, including but not limited to individual capabilities and dispositions. *Remediation is contextual; sometimes individuals need to be separated from their context to be remediated, and sometimes the context needs remediating more than the individual.*

Remediation is usually about individuals, and yet we are thinking more and more about contextual and social construction, team competence, workplace cultures, and macro and emergent (complex) outcomes and systems. This means we will need to think more about remediating other constructs than solitary individuals (see Chap. 2). How do we remediate groups and teams, organizations, cultures, and even societies? *Remediation involves more than a two-person dyadic relationship.*

Finally, our deconstruction of the pathway metaphor brings us to remedial actions (the focus of much of this book). Our first question might be whether we should act at all. When someone goes off the path, perhaps we should let natural selection ('sink or swim') be our model and expect individuals to recover (or not) according to their own abilities and opportunities. Or, if we have some sense of shared responsibility, perhaps we should be ready to send out search parties, or perhaps we should be on hand to help individuals when they stumble. Clearly, we do have some sense of shared responsibility, and both the individual and those around them have some responsibility to act. Again, this raises questions of autonomy and independence as well as being the key response to my opening comments on 'the

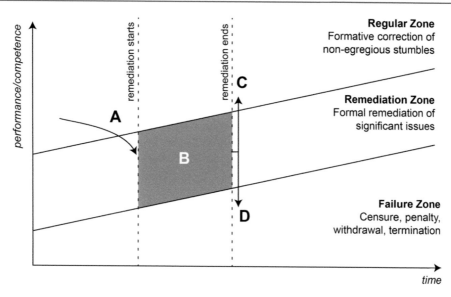

Fig. 1.1 Remediation takes place in a zone between regular practice and failure. Crossing the perimeter of regular acceptable practice (**a**) initiates a remediation episode (**b**), which can only end in three ways: return to the regular zone (**c**), move to the failure zone (**d**), or another episode of remediation (**b**). Eventually, remediation must end in either (**c**) or (**d**). Adapted from Ellaway et al. 2017 and Kalet et al. 2017

measure of a civilization'. *Remediation is not always the best response.*

We might also distinguish actions that are intended to keep people on their paths (maintenance) from those that are triggered when people deviate (as we perceive, which may involve assumptions and bias) from their paths (repair or restitution). Remediation as maintenance is perhaps more the concern of teachers and preceptors in that all learners will have small stumbles and wobbles. It is only when these stumbles cross the threshold between acceptable and unacceptable performance (however this is defined or justified) that remediation is triggered.

Boundary Practices, Liminal Spaces

Although departures from acceptable practice can trigger remediation, the remedial response is also outside 'normal' teaching practice. Remediation is higher stakes, involves greater scrutiny, and is personalized and temporary. Furthermore, the status of remediator and remediatee is not the same as between teacher and learner. Remediation is therefore a boundary practice [2]; it is not the same as regular practice. Remediation's thresholds are marked on one side by a return to normal practice (for those who successfully complete it) and on the other side by censure or termination of practice—see Fig. 1.1 [3, 4]. Within this Remediation Zone, remediator and remediatee share some responsibilities and have others that are unique to their roles.

Understanding remediation as a 'boundary practice' raises a number of important issues.

1. Remediation is triggered by crossing a boundary, typically defined in terms of one egregious event or an accumulation of problematic but not individually egregious events. We need to know that the boundary has been crossed, which in turn suggests monitoring and a triggering process that is tied to robust policies and procedures that define the boundaries for remediation and how these boundaries can be traversed.

2. Remediation is not an open-ended undertaking: it has a beginning, a set of activities that remediatee and remediator need to complete, some means by which the episode can be evaluated as having been completed, and,

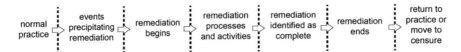

Fig. 1.2 Typical boundaries crossed during a remedial episode

once complete, it involves some kind of exit. Each episode of remediation involves crossing these boundaries (see also Fig. 1.2):

(a) Entering remediation means that the rules and expectations pertaining to the remediatee and remediator change. The remediatee loses a degree of agency and autonomy, they are given a different focus and set of objectives, their performances are under greater scrutiny, and the consequences of these performances have more significant consequences than before. The remediator is expected to monitor the remediatee more closely and critically, and they are required to make decisions or recommendations that have greater consequences.

(b) The point of remediation is to address or ensure the correction of the deficit(s) that precipitated the episode of remediation in the first place. Remediation is successful when the system's trust (invested in the remediator and their reporting to their oversight committee or other structure) is reestablished with respect to the deficit. If trust (or sufficient trust) is re-established, then another boundary is crossed by moving from the remediation back to the regular zone. What 'trust' entails, how it can be built, and how it can be lost are complex questions that have been attracting growing attention across much of health professions education in recent years [5, 6].

(c) Although one episode of remediation that is not fully resolved may lead to another, this cannot go on indefinitely—one of two boundaries must be crossed at its completion: a return to normal practice (regular zone) or censure or termination of practice (failure zone). The rules and expectations of remediation change and are replaced by those of the zone the remediatee now moves to.

3. While at any point in time, there may or may not be active remediations underway in a particular program, remediation is continuous as a potentialized space (in the form of policies and procedures, etc.). And yet, at an individual level, it is also intrinsically temporary. Nobody stays there indefinitely, save perhaps for full-time remediators who act like ferrymen: having helped one individual cross over, they cycle back to help the next. Like anything that requires boundary crossing, remediation is often seen as something additional and unusual rather than being intimately integrated into the ebb and flow of day-to-day practice.

For all its critical importance, both for those directly involved and as a reflection of the values of medicine and health professions education as a whole, remediation is a liminal undertaking consisting of a series of boundary practices and boundary crossings. It is distinctly 'other'; it has different rules, expectations, and outcomes from mainstream practice. And yet it is intimately bound up with the day-to-day nature of practice. Any one of us may stumble and fall, and any one of us may be called on to help those who do fall. *Not only is our approach to remediation a reflection of our values as a profession, but the way we engage with the boundaries and boundary practices of remediation is also a reflection of the values of remediation.*

In *Purgatorio*

Having raised the thorny issue of morality in remediation, we need to explore some of its consequences. Remediation is not unlike the Christian concept of purgatory, a state after death when sin must be cleansed to allow it to ascend; if it is not cleansed, the soul must fall into the abyss. Dante's vision of purgatory is of a mountain of seven terraces corresponding to the seven deadly sins: pride, envy, wrath, sloth, avarice, gluttony, and lust. These have all been linked to love—its absences, its excesses, its disorders, and its misdirection [7]. Substituting 'care' for 'love' provides an interesting template for remediation in health professions education, as it is so often about addressing absences, excesses, disorders, and misdirection in the enactment of care.

Purgatory also introduces concepts such as sin and remorse, penitence and atonement, and reconciliation and judgment. Not only can they be used, alongside concepts of love and compassion, to expand remediation's conceptual toolbox, it is also interesting to reflect on how perspectives such as these might shape our thinking about remediation. Indeed, we might consider other moral philosophies and existential worldviews in this light. For instance, we might ask how remediation might be reflected in 'tawba' in Islam, 'tshuva' in Judaism, or 'zhengming' in Confucianism (all meaning 'to return'). *While remediation in different cultures may well align with their distinct cultural philosophies, there are some absolute values and principles or remediation that transcend all cultures.*

A consideration of the moral dimension lets us consider the motives and responsibilities of the remediatee. As I noted earlier, we need to know why an individual stumbled, not least because this shapes what our collective responsibility for their fall is or should be. Usually, we seek to help those that get into trouble, but some acts are so egregious and some wanderings so problematic that we go (or should go) straight to censure. For example, acts that are criminal under the civil code (such as assault, theft, or criminal damage) may not be considered remediable, not least because the social contract requires higher standards of a profession than society sets for itself, not lower. The limits of what we are prepared to remediate can also depend on causes and underlying symptoms or indicators of failure (Table 1.1). *Remediation happens in a 'Goldilocks' zone: neither minor stumbles nor major failures usually attract remediation.*

Table 1.1 There is a continuum of severity of lapses, failures, or stumbles that ranges from minor problems that are to be expected of anyone in training to the deeply egregious ones that have major consequences whatever their causes. Remediation happens in this middle zone in the continuum, its upper and lower boundaries set by what is considered too little and too much to be remediated. Where these perimeters lie may vary from context to context, but the upper perimeter is defined by whether weaknesses or problems require additional scrutiny and assurance that they have been resolved, and the lower perimeter by acts that are too serious for remediation to be the means to resolve them

Zone	Lapse
Regular practice zone	Minor lapses, failures, stumbles in knowledge, skills, and/or attitudes
Remediation zone	Predictable significant yet remediable lapses, failures, or stumbles in knowledge, skills, and/or attitudes that need to be remediated to prevent future occurrences. Unpredicted significant lapses, failures, or stumbles whose causes may yield weaknesses that can be addressed through remediation
Failure zone	Egregious lapses, failures, or stumbles whose causes suggest fundamental irremediable causes and that attract automatic censure no matter their causes

Thinking about responsibility also allows us to reflect on the parallels between remediation and accommodations in health professions education and practice. Accommodations involve modifying practices to reduce the barriers for individuals with disabilities but who are otherwise competent to participate and thrive in what they do. Accommodations are often therefore unique to particular individuals and their circumstances, and they are another Goldilocks practice: neither minor barriers (such as having a bad hair day or having trouble parking) nor major barriers that make it impossible for someone to participate even with all the help we might provide, do not, by definition, require accommodating. Finally, and making the connection with remediation even more explicit, accommodations are in effect a remediation of the contexts and structures of everyday practice (see Chaps. 20, 26, 29). If these accommodations were not made, then the individuals they sought to accommodate would most likely need remediating in some other way or they may be excluded altogether. Not only does this reflect the relationships between individuals, contexts, and structures in remediation (see Fig. 1.3), it emphasizes the entanglement of performance with many parallel structures in health professions education and practice (including but not limited to remediation), and it reiterates the need for the perimeters of acceptable performance to be adjusted according to context and need. This also raises equity, diversity, and inclusivity issues in remediation (each of which also has boundary implications), topics that need much more attention than I can provide in this overview chapter (see Chap. 3). *For now, I will simply observe that remediation intersects with many other boundary practices in health professions education.*

A moral perspective on remediation also allows us to consider the motives, beliefs, and responsibilities of remediators and those that commission them and set the contexts for the work they do. First and foremost, remediation suggests hope; it is not a zero-tolerance policy. The health professions inherently encompass high stakes, so it is telling that we can accept and seek to fix individuals training for it rather than using a social Darwinist 'selection of the fittest' approach (unless the ability to subject oneself to

be remediated is itself a necessary if tacit competency). Not only can people be saved, but remediation also implies that they should be given the opportunity to atone and to improve. This reflects a sense of justice (everyone stumbles, a stumble may not be entirely your fault) and economy (a trained health professional is a big investment, so we repair them where we can). In this way, remediation could be seen as reflecting Japanese concepts of 'wabi sabi' (the beauty of imperfection) or ecological concepts of sufficiency and economy (we make the most of what we have by repairing and restoring things rather than replacing them). *Remediation implicitly embraces imperfection.*

Being identified as needing or requiring remediation can create strong feelings of anxiety and shame. Remediation marks an individual out as being flawed, and this can destabilize the remediatee's sense of identity and their standing with their peers. This loss may in turn trigger stages of grief (denial, anger, bargaining, and/or depression), before any sense of acceptance [8]. As I noted earlier, remediation necessarily changes the agency of the remediatee, which can be another source of shame and anxiety. Remediation is often perceived to be something individuals are obliged to submit to rather than, say, actively

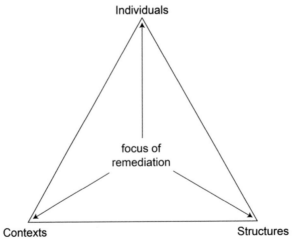

Fig. 1.3 While remediation traditionally tended to focus on underperforming or problematic individuals, considering the causes of underperformance or problematic behavior allows us to consider the entanglement of individuals with their contexts (places, teams, organizations) and the structures (rules, roles, cultures) that define expectations. For any given remediation, we might need to remediate more than just the individual

seeking out. The candidate for remediation is, of necessity, pulled out of their normal situation, they lose degrees of autonomy and trust, and they face increased doubt, scrutiny, and risk of failure. A remediatee may also experience negative emotions while being remediated, particularly if they cannot meet the standards required of them or experience other hardships (see Chap. 5). To some extent, it could be argued that this appropriately reflects the high-stakes nature of remediation and that some discomfort might be a positive contribution to remediatees resolving their shortcomings and an incentive for them to ensure they never need remediating again. There is also some sense that the shame of remediation can also serve as a disincentive to performance. Moreover, remediation can often be a distressing episode, and not just for the remediatee. Remediators can be distressed seeing their remediatees struggling or failing, particularly if this is accompanied by anger, frustration, or fear. *Whether or not it is intended, remediation can feel stressful and stigmatizing, but this is not always the case.*

Because of the high stakes of remediation outcomes, because of the emotional and physical effort remediation requires, and because of the necessity for fair and just practices, remediation is also subject to heightened scrutiny and accountability. Remediation practices, whatever they are, must work reliably and predictably, their outcomes must be proportionate to the effort required, and they must be fair (showing no bias toward or against anyone) and just (individuals get what they deserve within a shared moral code). The regulation of remediation, including setting policies and procedures and allocating resources, is often as much about meeting these requirements as it is about the actual processes of remediation. Indeed, accreditation standards for remediation often, I would suggest, appear to be more focused on fairness and justice than on efficacy or economy or on how these different drivers might be balanced. *Remediation need not be perfect but must be defensible; it must be effective, proportionate, just, and fair.*

The stigma attached to remediation, even if not intended, obscures some significant positive aspects of remedial episodes. For instance, reme-diation should involve higher levels of individual scrutiny, feedback, and guided improvement. That receiving expert one-to-one coaching is framed in such a negative way downplays the clear benefits of these focused and personalized learning experiences (for principles of coaching, see Chap. 6). *Given the opportunity for professional development that remediation affords, we might all seek to be remediated from time to time.*

An Expanding Discourse

Having explored some of the underlying challenges and issues in remediation, I turn now to the intersection of remediation with some of the key debates in health professions education and practice. A notable development since the first edition of this book has been the shift to competency-based education (CBE) in many countries around the world. There are many connections between CBE and remediation. For instance, continuous longitudinal assessment mapped to expected trajectories of development (defined by milestones) can be used to identify which learners are struggling and why they are struggling early enough to be able to address their shortcomings without formal remediation. If they need remediation, then can CBE more precisely identify what needs remediating and track whether the remediation goals are being met? There are also gaps. For instance, we (this volume's editors and your current interlocutor) critiqued the tendency of the CBE literature to focus on learner success at the expense of considering what should happen to failing learners and how remediation can address this deficit [3].

The International Competency-based Medical Education (ICBME) collaborators group identified five core components of CBE curricula: outcome competencies, sequenced progression, tailored learning experiences, competency-focused instruction, and programmatic assessment (PA) [9]. While the first four reflect good practices that are (or should be) well-layered into remediation practices, the links between PA and remediation bear further consideration. Introduced to and then developed within medical education by van der Vleuten and Schuwirth [10], PA itself has several key features, including the use of a variety of assessment methods, longitudinal aggregative data collection, separation between data and inferences, and attention to both summative and formative uses of assessment. Given that many programs are looking to implement PA in some way, not only does remediation within PA need attention, we might also consider what programmatic remediation might look like, and what the benefits and limitations of pursuing it as a kind of remediation practice might be. For instance, does remediation simply correct or can it also focus on learning more broadly? How might heterogeneous data sources map to an episode of remediation? The key issue of separating observation from judgment is well explored in this volume, but can we think more deeply about remediation evidence and the inferences we can make from such evidence as we have?

Another growing area of interest has developed around concepts of resilience and wellness (see Chap. 18). Clearly, as I discussed earlier, remediation can be a significant contributor to stress and to wellness; which strategies afford proportionate stress and wellness in remediation is an area that needs further consideration. We might also consider what role resilience to being remediated should play in admissions and policy; should we ever accept individuals into our programs and professions who cannot bear (for whatever reason) being remediated? If that is the case, then how do we identify those who are not susceptible to being remediated and what legal and ethical issues might this raise? Are resilience and receptivity to remediation intrinsic or developmental qualities?

I would argue that there is very little in the rich landscape of health professions education that does not have or could benefit from an exploration of its intersections and implications in and for remediation. For instance, we might consider the relationships between remediation and the social contract for medicine and health professions education. Arguably, remediation reflects a commitment to ensure those entering practice and already in practice are competent and safe.

However, by extending more and more opportunities to failing individuals to remediate, might we also be compromising that societal goal by contributing to the 'failure to fail' problem [11, 12]? On the other hand, it could also be argued that remediation actually reflects the social contract, through, for instance, protecting the substantial public investment in training healthcare providers.

That there are contrasting and at times conflicting drivers that shape remediation practice reflects the nature of health professions education governance in general. Programs and systems of health professions education are also defined by the ways that they balance their responses to the many requests made to them and the rules applied to them. Remediation is not and should not be thought immune from the political nature of policy and practice. *As much as it is a boundary practice, remediation is and must be understood as a part of larger systems of health professions education and practice.*

Scholarship and Remediation

In this chapter, I have considered many (although by no means all) of the conceptual and practical issues in remediation in contemporary health professions education and practice. Each and every topic and issue I have raised could (and should) be explored and tested further, and to that end, the italicized axioms I have woven throughout could serve as an outline agenda for scholarly inquiry in and through remediation's many spaces and dimensions—see Table 1.2.

Whatever its focus or starting point, ongoing scholarly inquiry is a necessary part of advancing both the practice and the theory of remediation. Much remediation research and the evidence it has generated has focused on what works at the sharp end of remediation, and as such, much of this work has been descriptive and evaluative in nature. While this is an appropriate reflection of the state of the art, as our thinking deepens, so should our approaches to inquiry.

Although Glassick et al.'s criteria for scholarly inquiry (clear goals, adequate preparation,

Table 1.2 A selection of the remediation axioms suggested in this chapter and their corresponding research questions. While equally valid axioms and questions may be posited, the issue in hand is that there is much more to remediation research than answering the question of 'what works?'

Suggested remediation axiom	Corresponding research question(s)
Remediation is contextual; sometimes individuals need to be separated from their context to be remediated, and sometimes the context needs remediating more than the individual	To what extent and in what ways do contextual factors contribute to individuals needing to be remediated? To what extent and in what ways do contexts need to be remediated rather than individuals?
The way we engage with the boundaries and boundary practices of remediation is a reflection of the values of remediation	What are the values of remediation and how well do they map to its practices?
While remediation in different cultures may well align with their distinct cultural philosophies, there are some absolute values and principles or remediation that transcend all cultures	Should remediation in different cultures be aligned with their distinct cultural philosophies? Are there absolute values and principles of remediation that unite or transcend all cultures?
Remediation happens in a 'Goldilocks' zone: minor stumbles and major failures do not usually attract remediation	How are the perimeters for what is considered remediable defined? Are these perimeters consistent and defensible?
Remediation intersects with many other boundary practices in health professions education	How is remediation shaped by and shaping of other practices in the health professions and health professions education?
Remediation implicitly embraces imperfection	What are the 'hidden curriculum' and other tacit messages that remediation sends to its different stakeholders?
Whether or not it is intended, remediation can feel stressful and stigmatizing, but this is not always the case	To what extent are affective aspects of remediation addressed or managed within current practices? What can a remediatee's affective response to remediation tell us about their suitability for their future practice?
Remediation need not be perfect but it must be defensible; it must be effective, proportionate, just, and fair	In what ways are remediation activities resisted or challenged and with what results?
Given the opportunity for professional development that remediation affords, we might all seek to be remediated from time to time	What impact does framing remediation as an optimal approach to professional development have on those involved?
Remediation is and must be understood as a part of larger systems of health professions education and practice	To what extent, in what ways, and with what consequences do remediation practices align with the systems within which they function?

appropriate methods, significant results, effective presentation, and reflective critique) set broad standards for scholarly inquiry [13], mapping a research landscape, particularly for a multidimensional undertaking such as remediation, can be challenging. These challenges are, I would argue, to some extent exacerbated in health professions and academic cultures that value epidemiological and post-positivist approaches to science above all others. Given the relatively small numbers of individuals involved, the unpredictable timing, and the idiosyncratic nature of remediation practices, randomized controlled trials, and cohort studies are neither feasible nor a particularly logical study design in remediation

research. Smaller, qualitative studies based on participant experiences (phenomenology) and practices (ethnography) are better aligned with the dynamics of remediation but can be hard to generalize to other settings. Middle-range approaches such as realist inquiry [14] that focus on explaining how systems and innovations 'work' by exploring "what works for whom in what circumstances and in what respects, and how?" [15] may be a better fit in remediation research, particularly in explaining why different approaches to remediation are more or less effective in different contexts.

Boyer described scholarship in terms of four areas of activity: the scholarships of discovery (research, innovation), of integration (synthesis, crossing domains), of application (effectiveness), and of teaching and learning (systematic evaluation and exploration) [16]. Unpacking this further to identify discrete kinds of scholarly inquiry, our METRICS framework can be used to outline the landscape for remediation scholarship [17]. METRICS reflects seven kinds of scholarly inquiry found in health professions education:

- Meta-scholarship inquiry explores the nature of scholarly activity. This includes appraising approaches to scholarship, patterns in scholarly inquiry, and professional development. Applied to remediation, meta-scholarship can be used to consider where the evidence for remediation is coming from (wealthier research-focused institutions in higher-income countries most likely, which in turn raises issues of epistemic (in)justice and equity [18]), how it is articulated (evaluative and practical guides), and where more attention is needed (for instance into equity and diversity concerns).
- Evaluation inquiry explores the value of things. This includes studies that compare alternatives to rank them according to their qualities, and those that seek to appraise the value of things relative to some ideal. Applied to remediation, evaluation is reflected throughout this book, whenever better (rather than 'best') practices are advanced. Indeed that evaluative approaches are the most common in and around remediation. However, asking why something is better or worse and what role context plays in shaping this value is perhaps less well developed, and to that end realist evaluation [19] offers great potential to contribute to this dimension of scholarly inquiry.
- Translation inquiry explores how practices or knowledge can be moved from one domain to another. This includes translating research findings into practice, translating concepts or perspectives between disciplines, and translating practices between contexts. Applied to remediation, translation can be used to explore how evidence can and does inform practice

(the main focus of implementation science [20]), what might be learned from other disciplines and discourses (such as from cognitive psychology or human factors research), and how knowledge and practice changes across contexts and cultures (for instance reflecting my earlier questioning whether different cultural contexts might consider remediation in quite different ways).

- Research inquiry focuses on inductive theory generation and testing. This includes any acts that are experimental, descriptive, or explanatory that involve an interplay between empiricism and theory. Applied to remediation, robust research is definitely needed in order to develop a better theoretical understanding of its nature and practice. While large-scale systematic inquiry is (as I argued earlier) challenging in remediation, much current remediation practice is heuristic (lean but imprecise approaches to practical problem solving). A rigorous and systematic testing of practices and their outcomes should support greater precision and help to emphasize some aspects while deprecating others. More importantly, research (defined more narrowly in this way) can challenge faulty or biased assumptions and beliefs.
- Innovation inquiry focuses on the scholarly creation of things such as instruments, techniques, practices, or organizations (of things, people, and ideas). Applied to remediation, innovation (exploring novel approaches) is important and there are many innovations or ideas developed from innovations described in this volume. However, scholarly innovation involves more than trial and error and divine inspiration. Structured approaches such as design-based research, can help here, as can the use of experimental techniques to identify likely candidates for innovative exploration. Holding to the principles of scholarly inquiry is critical in whatever aspect of remediation it is pursued.
- Conceptual inquiry explores and develops the conceptual and philosophical basis of a field. This includes the deductive development of new models, concepts, theories, and para-

digms. Applied to remediation, conceptual inquiry is also needed, both to guide thought and to render complex ideas in easier-to-understand (and therefore use) ways. As an example, I have focused much of this chapter on forms of conceptual inquiry, critical analysis, deconstruction, and model generation.

- Synthesis inquiry focuses on appraising and mobilizing existing knowledge. This can include literature reviews, scoping reviews, systematic reviews, and meta-analyses. Applied to remediation, synthesis can be used to appraise what has been published on and around remediation (strengths and limitations of the research effort, future directions), to extract the key messages (systematic review and meta-analysis), and to more clearly articulate the knowledge gaps that need to be addressed. Again, much of this book reflects syntheses of the existing research effort in its many literature reviews and appraisals.

A third approach to mapping the remediation research landscape is to use Lingard's 'problem-gap-hook' framing of scholarly inquiry [21]. For instance, I have spent much of this chapter considering the problem areas of remediation, as others in this volume have also done. Individual practitioner and program problems and needs associated with remediation may be easier to articulate. Indeed, from a practitioner's perspective, the problem-gap-hook heuristic for framing scholarly inquiry may be the most accessible and immediately valuable approach.

In summary, rather than simply repeating the tired assertion that 'more research is needed', I would argue that broader, deeper, and more scholarly approaches to inquiry are needed to respond to the needs, challenges, and opportunities in the changing remediation landscape in the health professions.

The Better Angels of Our Nature?

In this chapter, I have explored a range of conceptual, theoretical, and philosophical lenses through which we can ask fundamental questions about remediation, and from which we can deepen and expand our thinking and practice. I have argued that scholarly inquiry is necessary for the advancement of remediation thinking and practice. However, I would expand on this to suggest that there is a bigger opportunity (and responsibility) here to consider remediation as representing the system as a whole and that we should consider what remediation-related inquiry may tell us about health professions education and practice in general. This reflects my opening assertion that remediation is a measure of the educational and practice-based aspects of the professions, as it is here that things get the thinnest, riskiest, and the most telling as to what we really believe and are prepared to do to and with our weakest members. We are all flawed and sometimes we stumble. What happens next says everything about who we are and who we aspire to be.

References

1. Lakoff G, Johnson M. Metaphors we live by. Chicago, IL: University of Chicago Press; 2008.
2. Wenger E. Communities of practice: learning, meaning and identity. Cambridge, UK: Cambridge University Press; 1999.
3. Ellaway RH, Chou CL, Kalet AL. Situating remediation: accommodating success and failure in medical education systems. Acad Med. 2017;93:391–8.
4. Kalet A, Chou CL, Ellaway RH. To fail is human: remediating remediation in medical education. Perspect Med Educ. 2017;6:418–24.
5. ten Cate O. Trust, competence, and the supervisor's role in postgraduate training. BMJ. 2006;333:748–51.
6. Damodaran A, Shulruf B, Jones P. Trust and risk: a model for medical education. Med Educ. 2017;51:892–902.
7. Reynolds B. The passionate intellect: Dorothy L. Sayers's encounter with Dante. Kent, OH: Kent State University Press; 1989.
8. Kübler-Ross E. On death and dying. New York: The MacMillan Company; 1969.
9. Van Melle E, Frank JR, Holmboe ES, Dagnone D, Stockley D, Sherbino J, International Competency-based Medical Education Collaborators. A core components framework for evaluating implementation of competency-based medical education programs. Acad Med. 2019;94:1002–9.
10. Van der Vleuten CP, Schuwirth LW. Assessing professional competence: from methods to programmes. Med Educ. 2005;39:309–17.

11. Dudek NL, Marks MB, Regehr G. Failure to fail: the perspectives of clinical supervisors. Acad Med. 2005;80:S84–7.

12. Yepes-Rios M, Dudek N, Duboyce R, Curtis J, Allard RJ, Varpio L. The failure to fail underperforming trainees in health professions education: a BEME systematic review; BEME Guide No. 42. Med Teach. 2016;38:1092–9.

13. Glassick CE, Huber MR, Maeroff GI. Scholarship assessed: evaluation of the professoriate. San Francisco, CA: Jossey-Bass; 1997.

14. Ellaway RH, Kehoe A, Illing J. Critical realism and realist inquiry in medical education. Acad Med. 2020;95:984–8.

15. Pawson R, Tilley N. Realistic evaluation. Thousand Oaks, CA: SAGE; 1997.

16. Boyer EL. Scholarship reconsidered: priorities of the professoriate. Princeton, NJ: Carnegie Foundation for the Advancement of Teaching; 1990.

17. Ellaway RH, Topps D. METRICS: a pattern language of scholarship in medical education. MedEdPublish; 2018. p. 1305. https://www.mededpublish.org/manuscripts/1305.

18. Fricker M. Epistemic injustice: power and the ethics of knowing. Oxford, UK: Oxford University Press; 2007.

19. Pawson R. The science of evaluation: a realist manifesto. Thousand Oaks, CA: SAGE; 2013.

20. Bauer MS, Damschroder L, Hagedorn H, Smith J, Kilbourne AM. An introduction to implementation science for the non-specialist. BMC Psychol. 2015;3:32.

21. Lingard L. Joining a conversation: the problem/gap/hook heuristic. Perspect Med Educ. 2015;4:252–3.

Toward a Programmatic Approach for Remediation: Evidence-Based Goals for Institutions

Bau P. Tran and Calvin L. Chou

Introduction

The advent of competency-based education has provided health professions education programs with more objective criteria to detect trainees with academic difficulties. Typically, accrediting bodies determine standards that each program must monitor to longitudinally document learners' progress, promptly identify deficiencies in fundamental knowledge or gaps in skills, and provide a threshold for remediation. However, these standards do not offer specific methodologies for constructing remediation paths or processes. The overall benefits of remediation for individual learners remain clear, but optimal methods on the institutional level presently are currently largely undefined.

Ideally, a programmatic remediation strategy would strengthen learners both effectively and compassionately. Of course, this balance is difficult to strike. As programs bear responsibility for training graduates who will ably serve society, they must uphold rigorous standards, identify trainees needing support early, and guide them toward competence, while simultaneously addressing the emotional effects of the stigma that learners frequently perceive [1]. To remediate compassionately, as befits the healing professions, entails assembling resources that may require trainees to undergo alternative training tracks, which in turn necessitate extra and often unfunded support from faculty and sometimes other trainees. Furthermore, compassionate programs may wish to attend to the collateral negative long-term effects that may arise, including the loss of peer relationships, suspension of professional identity formation, and personal mental health sequelae, not to mention increased tuition costs [2].

In this chapter, we offer a series of overarching goals to institutions and programs to guide the development of a programmatic remediation process that aspires to both effectiveness and compassion. Understanding the complexity of remediation processes, we roughly divide these goals into three temporally sequenced phases: setting up the institution's remediation system, constructing remediation programs, and follow-through. We recognize that many institutions may not have the resources available to achieve all these goals; however, by describing the goals explicitly, we expect that remediation processes and structures will become more accepted, integrated throughout educational programs with adequate longitudinal oversight, and potentially standardized across institutions.

B. P. Tran
Department of Physician Assistant Studies,
University of Texas Southwestern, Dallas, TX, USA
e-mail: bau.tran@utsouthwestern.edu

C. L. Chou (✉)
Department of Medicine, University of California,
San Francisco, CA, USA

Veterans Affairs Healthcare System,
San Francisco, CA, USA
e-mail: calvin.chou@ucsf.edu

Phase 1: Setting Up the Institution's Remediation Process

Goal 1A: Ensure Due Process to Uphold the Professional Compact with Society, While Maintaining Empathy for Individual Learners' Struggles

In the United States, even prior to trainee matriculation, institutions are obligated by the Family Educational Rights and Privacy Act (FERPA) to uphold each learner's privacy. Institutions must delineate and clarify principles of transparency, equity, confidentiality, and informed consent throughout the remediation process. All learners must understand and be able to refer to objectives, expectations, evaluation practices, and methods for all courses or rotations; supervisors must provide regular feedback on learner performance with frequent documentation thereof; and institutions must provide and follow evaluation and grievance policies. This essential groundwork becomes critical when institutions must consider the dismissal of a trainee (see Chap. 29).

We further enumerate components of effective and ethical institution-based remediation processes: (1) documentation of open discussions with program leadership and stakeholders that delineate decisions and reasons for remediation; (2) a written individualized remediation plan, including goals for remediation, instructional strategies, assessments, lists of responsible parties for each remediation area, and learner attestations to their plans; and (3) clear descriptions of observed outcomes, ongoing summaries of discussion with learners, and assessments to determine whether learners are meeting goals, time frame, and decision making [3, 4]. Institutions must also construct ongoing quality improvement processes to assess the overall success of remediation programs.

Moreover, institutions must ensure that successfully remediated learners achieve at least minimum competency, based on measurable performance benchmarks, as well as proof of continuous ongoing improvement. Conversely, failure to meet these standards would signal the need to transition to consequential administrative review; remediation teams cannot support learners who struggle indefinitely. Though these claims may seem obvious, institutions commonly graduate learners who are not ready [5]. Ultimately, in our compact with society, our educational processes must ensure the competence of the professionals we train [3, 4]. Legal precedent in the US and several other countries emphasizes due process and ensures nondiscrimination in supporting final academic decisions. Yet, as all programs and institutions are aware, these legal protections do not necessarily decrease the emotional, financial, and time commitments necessary to arrive at these determinations. In the pursuit of these goals, institutions likely underestimate the emotional effects of remediation on learners [1]. In addition, given the significant investment of time, money, and other resources in health professions training, "compassionate off ramps" have recently been suggested but incompletely implemented ([6, 7]; see Goal 3A below).

Goal 1B: Ensure That Admissions and Selection Processes Correspond with Desired Outcomes, Including Diversifying the Workforce—And Don't Stop There

Challenges abound in developing a fair, equitable, and accurate selection process for admission to health professions schools [8, 9]. Due to the range of admission processes between educational institutions, research to identify generalizable selection criteria is lacking, and possibly undesirable [10]. Instead, institutions should focus on defining the desired health professional graduate competencies and using these as the basis of an outcome-based selection procedure [11–13].

Evidence of the capacity to be academically successful is important in selecting candidates for health professions training but is complex. For medical school applicants, a review of qualifications has traditionally included standardized exam performance (e.g., Medical College

Admission Test [MCAT]) and undergraduate grade-point average (GPA). A recent large-sample longitudinal study correlated frequently-used admission measures with disenrollment, probation, or termination in undergraduate and graduate medical education settings [14]. Although not statistically significant, learners who appeared before promotion committees during probation or termination proceedings tended to have lower MCAT scores when compared to classmates. Similarly, nurse practitioner training programs show that standardized exams, specifically total and verbal Graduate Record Examination (GRE) scores, may predict both success in program completion and difficulty in program completion, such as prolonged time to graduation [15]. However, other health professions programs, like physician assistant schools, have generally found little correlation between admissions predictors (e.g., GRE, GPA, multiple mini-interview) and successful student matriculation. A new entrance exam, the Physician Assistant College Admission Test (PA-CAT), is currently being piloted to strengthen the admissions process and select candidates with the highest likelihood of successful program completion. Before anchoring on the viability of these criteria, however, programs must understand that standardized exams often reflect specific demographic or socioeconomic characteristics of examination-takers unrelated to their diligence, willingness, and grit [16, 17]. It is important to note that most matriculants with relatively low standardized test scores successfully complete health professions education, and there is little evidence that these metrics, in and of themselves, predict-long term clinical competence or practice outcomes.

Importantly, admissions committees across the health professions have widely increased and embraced the use of holistic approaches that consider a wide range of eligibility criteria [18–20]. These processes aim to reduce the known biases in standardized testing and other traditional metrics which are associated with low representation among ethnic and racial minority applications [21, 22]. By balancing standardized exams with other cognitive and noncognitive criteria impor-

tant to health professions practice in the admissions process, we address the societal imperative to develop a more diverse and representative professional workforce, a goal which far outweighs the theoretical risk of low academic performance.

Achieving representation in programs and institutions, though necessary and an uphill climb by itself, is insufficient. Despite recent attention due to national events in and out of healthcare, implicit and explicit bias persist throughout health professions education, on the part of patients, learners, colleagues, and supervisors. Indeed, it is likely impossible to achieve a bias-free state [23]. Yet we emphasize that programs and institutions must strive continuously to address systemic factors that minimize prejudice in favor of diversity, equity, and inclusion. Sobering data show that when otherwise demographically adjusted, students underrepresented in medicine receive fewer honors grades and fewer selections for honor society membership than those not underrepresented [24, 25]. Systems that can mitigate the effect of bias on perceptions of learners' performance include an explicit institutional mission of confronting bias, policies that address violations of behavioral expectations, emphasis on growth mindset, diverse role models, sound assessments that use narratives and incorporate frequent direct observations with feedback, longitudinal clinical supervision, avoidance of comparisons with peers, and cultural expectations that support diversity, accountability, inquiry rather than judgment, and restorative justice ([23, 26, 27]; also see Chap. 3).

Goal 1C: Transparently Align Instructional Paradigms with Defined Outcomes

A program's success stems from the active engagement of learners in their development as health care providers. If concerns about competence are significant, learners should be required to participate in remediation and be held accountable to engage actively with the remediation team to create an individualized remediation plan, initiate and complete remediation activities, and successfully undertake appropriate performance assessments. Rather than viewing this as punitive, the coach–learner team should embrace this approach as a structure that facilitates the attainment of the life-long learning strategies that ensure the mainte-nance of competence throughout a practice career (see Goal 2A). These processes often require robust and ongoing faculty development (see Goal 1F and Chap. 19) so that coaches can offer structured, compassionate, and rigorous support to learners.

Ideally, in the competency-based approach that health professions education has increasingly adopted, learners undergo continual and more individualized assessment, de-emphasizing time-based training [28–32]. There are stark differ-ences between programs, with different approaches and philosophies toward measuring competencies. Such differences can lead to confu-sion for learners [33]. For example, a recent study examined the paradox that arises in simulation-based education, where stated ground rules of the benefits of making errors in the pursuit of deeper learning may conflict with larger values of medi-cal culture that emphasize performance, certainty, and confidence [34]. These factors risk becoming even more amplified in remediation contexts. Educators and education administrators involved in assessment and, by extension, remediation, will strongly benefit from knowledge of, and discern-ment between, the many different approaches to teaching and learning, all based in educational theories that have been advanced over the past century: behavioral, cognitive, cognitive con-structivist, sociocultural, humanist, and transfor-mative [35]. To avoid educational incongruities that confuse all learners, and particularly those in remediation, instructional processes must align with desired outcomes.

It follows that how we measure these out-comes depends strongly on best practices in cur-ricular and instructional design, delivery, and assessment. Rarely is a learner solely to blame for their inability to achieve competencies, espe-cially after surviving the rigorous admissions selection processes of many health professions education programs. An institutional commit-ment to ongoing quality improvement of all edu-cational processes comprises one of the most important pillars of successful student perfor-mance and remediation.

Goal 1D: Cultivate Effective Support Systems to Avert the Need for Remediation, Including Mentoring and Developing a Culture of Feedback

Realistically, the need for remediation is ever-present [36]. Accordingly, it is necessary for pro-grams to cultivate a learning environment that proactively provides support for any learner who requires course correction. Anticipatory support mechanisms include encouraging specific learn-ing strategies that enable long-term learning (see Chap. 4), effective mentoring, and an overarching institutional approach to constructive feedback.

Mentoring

As trainees navigate clinical training and develop their professional identity, many stressors, particu-larly those fostered by the implicit curriculum, can influence the need for future remediation. Trainees report feeling that they constantly undergo evalua-tion, particularly in the setting of clerkships, where the criteria and expectations for grades are subjec-tive and can appear arbitrary and whimsical [37–39]. To alleviate some of the stress, a program-facilitated support group with sessions aimed at increasing self-awareness, self-care, and mindfulness training benefits learners [40–42].

Providing high-quality mentorship to learners arguably has many benefits, including better alignment of career goals with a suitable spe-cialty, improved professional development, and attainment of successful clinical outcomes [43]. As health care becomes increasingly complex, McBride et al. suggest that healthcare providers need new options for competency and capacity development fostered by strong mentoring rela-tionships [44]. This long-term professional mentee-mentor relationship will continue to engage and focus on the mentee's competency development, which will aid in identifying areas of struggles or adversity.

Culture of Feedback

As part of academic development, feedback is expected, essential, and intended to be formative, developmental, and growth-oriented regardless of the context. However, giving and receiving feedback are often accompanied by angst, misperception, dread, and denial [45, 46]. Though 'feedback is an emotional business' [47], it is an essential component in medical education: the importance of a robust feedback culture is one of the best-documented aspects of effective education [48–50]. Merely instituting unstructured forms of feedback without changing the culture vastly limits the potential for improving learner performance. All learners, whether they struggle or not, benefit from close observation, effective feedback, and ongoing formative assessment [51]. Immersing learners fully and actively in ongoing feedback processes increases their motivation and engagement in the lifelong learning that characterizes ideal clinical practice [52, 53]. Sadly, trainees regularly discount feedback they receive [54–56]. In addition, faculty often feel uncomfortable holding feedback conversations that honestly and compassionately address trainees' areas of struggles (see Goal 1F). Though feedback has been a research focus for many years, investigation continues about how best to support clinical teachers in optimizing feedback to learners.

Feedback from multiple sources across the health professions can deepen the impact of recommendations for improvement. For example, compared with controls, pediatric residents who received multisource feedback on their professionalism and communication skills received higher ratings from nurses on their professionalism [57]. A similar approach to the establishment of a feedback culture can particularly help learners who struggle. A learner-centered, explicit, and relationship-based feedback culture [58, 59], where everyone (faculty and learners) in health professions education programs can regularly engage in respectful, bidirectional, and growth-oriented feedback conversations, will ultimately guide learners in remediation toward success ([60]; see Chap. 6).

Goal 1E: Promote the Availability of Remediation Resources to All Learners and Health Professions Education Community Members

As previously noted, most learners will need support at one time or another during training (Goal 1D), and early discussions with learners should communicate that remediation is a component of professionalism. We advocate explicitly reframing, and thereby destigmatizing, remediation as a special zone of learning (Chap. 1), with support for personal development, resilience building, and opportunities to practice with feedback, all to develop the adaptive capacity needed by all medical professionals [61, 62].

A culture where faculty and learners form educational partnerships can fortify a growth mindset that underpins lifelong learning [63]. A deficit-based approach, on the other hand, can reinforce maladaptive behaviors that continue the spiral of a learner's struggles. Therefore, we strongly recommend that institutions transparently recognize that the need for remediation occurs regularly and adequately supports the remediation process, thereby minimizing the association of shame or disgrace [1, 64]. For example, after creating an academic policy with clearly communicated benchmarks and early support for learners who struggled, one school significantly increased the number of learners attending voluntary remediation sessions [65]. We assert that this transparency coupled with accessible resources will maximize success.

Goal 1F: Support Faculty Development Initiatives for All Steps of the Remediation Process, Including Early Identification, Intervention, and Referral

A key component in the remediation process is faculty development (see Chap. 19). Many faculty remediators, including program directors, feel ill-prepared [66] or have little self-confidence in their abilities to identify a need for, or to conduct, remediation [3, 67], particularly in professionalism

[68]. Faculty with more experience as educators likely remediate more effectively than their less experienced colleagues [69, 70]. Moreover, many programs and faculty members underestimate the time commitment, not to mention the expertise and resources, needed to coach a learner through the remediation process [71, 72]; therefore, programs must select and develop appropriate faculty for remediation programs. We believe that institutions must commit adequate resources for remediation and not rely on volunteers.

The selection of personnel to develop into remediation coaches is also critical. Though programs may instinctively gravitate toward the selection of master clinicians as remediators, clinical experts display unconscious competence in fundamental skills and are unlikely to have experience or expertise in remediation. Therefore, this choice may not achieve optimal results. Contrastingly, experts in remediation have high clinical virtuosity, the ability to both recognize and motivate learners where they struggle, and a wealth of patience and support. One institution has developed an initiative in which advanced medical students act as remediation coaches, with faculty guidance, for near-peers with struggles [73]. This approach takes advantage of cognitive and social congruence, hallmarks of other successful near-peer programs [74]. While promising, it requires further evaluation of its outcomes.

Given the inherent complexity of remediation, the overall goal of faculty development programs should produce effective remediation coaches who can enhance the competency-based performance of learners longitudinally, rather than "teaching toward the test." Components of effective faculty development would ideally include cultivating deep expertise in not only the specific competency or competencies in which the faculty member desires concentrated effort, but also fundamental learning theories, relationship-centered mentoring, facilitation, antibias practices, and observation and feedback [26, 75–77]. Ultimately, these programs should foster development of a community of practice among committed remediation experts who collectively are equipped to address a broad range of common learner struggles [78].

Phase 2: Structural Elements of the Remediation Process

Goal 2A: Tailor Remediation Plans to Individual Learners' Needs

Learners who struggle comprise a very heterogeneous group ranging from students with academic difficulties to learners in clinical training grappling with clinical reasoning, to colleagues displaying unprofessional behaviors. As remediation for any given learner typically depends on the specific blend of observed struggles that stem from the learner's distinctive background or concurrent life experiences, many remediation efforts are more successfully addressed individually. Common institutional resources to address these overarching needs can be assembled for a given learner, including faculty with deep expertise in particular areas (e.g., communication skills, clinical reasoning), learning specialists, standardized patient trainers, mental health professionals, public speaking coaches, drama therapists, yoga instructors, among many others [75]. This team-based approach allows for the highly customized, multipronged remediation that learners who struggle need to succeed. In addition, encouraging learners to develop their own remediation plans can help develop autonomy and competence, two elements necessary for self-regulation and that enhance continuous professional development ([79–81]; also see Chap. 4).

In some circumstances, remediation in groups can parlay the benefits of social cognitive theory to develop critical thinking, group identity, and social regulation, which then can further influence self-regulation [82–86]. For example, professional identity formation curricula can identify broader motivations for staying in training (see Chap. 13); with expert faculty facilitation, classroom-based and clinical skills remediation can also succeed [87–91].

Both individualized and group remediation experiences should inform ongoing curricular and systems improvements for all trainees.

Goal 2B: Construct Effective and Nonjudgmental Processes to Share Evolving Information About Learners Who Struggle

As previously noted (Goal 1D), effective feedback to learners is crucial to the remediation process. Effective feeding forward (sometimes called "learner handover"), a process where educational supervisors communicate details about learners who struggle to upcoming supervisors, can also provide benefits (see Chaps. 20, 26 and 29). Certainly, concerns of bias can unduly influence these conversations [92]. In a recent scoping review, mostly in settings outside healthcare, feeding forward can lead to more negative than positive bias in subsequent performance evaluations [93]. Therefore, such practices would require close attention to potential bias. Further apprehensions with this practice would be privacy concerns, as university officials with legitimate educational interests may legally engage in such activities without explicit student consent [94–96]. Finally, institutional and individual approaches to feeding forward appear to be highly variable and inconsistent [97].

Equally, others may view that a lack of continuity in communication of valuable information may hinder the early identification of trainees who need it, thereby preventing early and effective interventions [98–102]. While the use of feeding forward is controversial and highly debated in the United States, it is a common practice in other countries, including the United Kingdom. Sharing educational information about at-risk learners (e.g., from minoritized backgrounds) gave rise to enhanced resources and improved grades for learners who struggled [92]. At one school, feeding forward in preclerkship curricular contexts increased early identification, contextualized concerns, and uncovered professionalism issues [103]; four additional schools have described their feed forward process and the benefits that have accrued [104]. In addition, FERPA includes specific exclusions from privacy at educational institutions to allow for research.

In either case, making the judgment about whether to feed forward is complex, and we understand that it may have implications, both beneficial and harmful, to the remediation of a learner. However, we recommend it because of health professions' contract with society, with important stipulations: (1) transparency to the learners, considering privacy concerns; (2) communication of specific, low-inference information that will effectively contribute to remediation success; (3) incorporation of appreciative approaches, when possible, to reduce negative judgments; and (4) limitation of information-sharing only with members of the remediation and decision-making teams. As the story in Dr. Manning's foreword illustrates, feeding forward, if done with the intention of supporting the student's growing competence, enables effective remediation.

Goal 2C: Avoid Conflicts of Interest When Distributing Remediation Roles

A robust relationship with a learner in remediation must optimally incorporate trust and confidentiality, as well as clear boundaries [4, 62]. Because learner difficulties have a multitude of causes and manifestations, a single course/program director, while essential to guide and coordinate remediation, cannot adequately synthesize all the skills necessary to conduct impactful remediation. In addition, when the responsibility lies solely with one individual, such as their mentor or remediation coach, to decide whether to promote or dismiss a learner, the perceived conflict of interest may strain the working relationship with the learner [105]. To facilitate defensible judgments, we strongly recommend that those conducting the remediation with the trainee (the remediation team of interdisciplinary experts listed in Goal 2A) should differ from the individual making the ultimate adjudication decisions [4]. This structure could decrease the perceptions by learners that institutions act as both 'judge and jury' [106]. We recognize that in smaller programs, it may not be feasible to separate these roles; in those cases, it can be worthwhile to form a community of remediation resources independent of departmental divisions, so that remediation experts in parallel programs may provide support. For example, a need to remediate a learner in otolaryngology with gaps in procedural skill could be referred to a colleague with that expertise in plastic surgery, with a reciprocal agreement as needed.

Phase 3: Supporting the Ultimate Decision

Goal 3A: Develop Compassionate "Off-Ramps" for Learners Who Must Discontinue Training

Learners early in their journeys of health professions education must undergo a significant acculturation process. Many, if not most, learners cannot foresee their future development, and others experience external pressure to enter health professions training. It is notable that many other professions, including business and the law, have higher levels of learner attrition over time than do the health professions. Health professions programs should expect that some learners will not complete their training (see Chap. 29), but professional and regional variation in remediation practices limits standardization and ultimately may undermine the trust that society places on us to graduate competent professionals.

For health professions training, with its heavy time and financial commitments, various structures have been proposed to mitigate the portentous burden of withdrawal or dismissal. Already mentioned above is the implementation of competency-based education and training to identify learners needing support and to specify the areas of improvement. Systems that all programs can implement for all trainees include the assessment of learners' motivations to continue in a health professions program by ongoing career counseling, curricula emphasizing profes-

sional identity formation, and financial counseling to manage debt. For learners contemplating or needing to leave training, a means of officially recognizing and credentialing work already undertaken in training does not yet exist except as a blight on one's resumé. Additionally, institutions can provide advising for alternative pathways in education, research, or industry. Studies of alternate pathways taken in countries where many who enter health professions training do not complete would inform the development of such policies elsewhere [6, 7].

Conclusion

Remediation is a complex process that is multifactorial and often requires interdisciplinary support. Balancing the many tasks involved in the remediation process is complicated and time-consuming; striving to achieve some balance between structure and compassion also takes effort and nuance. Therefore, it is essential to implement a system that reduces the need for remediation and maximizes educational outcomes for all learners, including those who struggle. These goals highlight important components of a holistic remediation process that fosters transparency in the academic policies and structures, allows for an environment conducive to learning for both the trainee and faculty, and compassionately reinforces our commitment to both learner and profession. We acknowledge a continual need for research in this area of concern and hope that future studies will facilitate further consistency and standardization across institutions. In the interim, we hope that providing these goals will allow institutions and programs a framework to develop or revise their current remediation strategies to enhance our support for learners while upholding our obligation to institution, profession, and society.

Acknowledgments We are indebted to Rob Foshay for reading a prior draft of this manuscript. This chapter is a revised and updated version of a previously published paper [107].

References

1. Mills LM, Boscardin C, Joyce EA, ten Cate O, O'Sullivan PS. Emotion in remediation: a scoping review of the medical education literature. Med Educ. 2021;55:1–13.
2. Hardinger K, Garavalia L, Graham MR, et al. Enrollment management strategies in the professional pharmacy program: a focus on progression and retention. Curr Pharm Teach Learn. 2015;7:199–206.
3. Cleland JA, Knight L, Rees C, Tracey S, Bond CB. 'Is it me or is it them?' Factors influencing assessors' failure to report underperformance in medical students. Med Educ. 2008;42:800–9.
4. Kalet A, Chou CL, Ellaway RH. To fail is human: remediating remediation in medical education. Perspect Med Educ. 2017;6:418–24.
5. Yepes-Rios M, Dudek N, Duboyce R, Curtis J, Allard RJ, Varpio L. The failure to fail underperforming trainees in health professions education: a BEME systematic review; BEME guide no. 42. Med Teach. 2016;38:1092–9.
6. Bellini LM, Kalet A, Englander R. Providing compassionate off-ramps for medical students is a moral imperative. Acad Med. 2019;94:656–8.
7. Aagaard E, Moscoso L. Practical implications off compassionate off-ramps for medical students. Acad Med. 2019;94:619–22.
8. MacKenzie RK, Dowell J, Ayansina D, Cleland JA. Do personality traits assessed on medical school admission predict exit performance? A UK-wide longitudinal cohort study. Adv Health Sci Educ. 2017;22:365–85.
9. Hecker K, Norman G. Have admissions committees considered all the evidence? Adv Health Sci Educ. 2017;22:573–6.
10. Brown G, Imel B, Nelson A, Hale LS, Jansen N. Correlations between PANCE performance, physician assistant program grade point average, and selection criteria. J Physician Assist Educ. 2013;24:42–4.
11. Wilkinson TJ, McKenzie JM, Ali AN, Rudland J, Carter FA, Bell CJ. Identifying medical students at risk of underperformance from significant stressors. BMC Med Educ. 2016;16:43.
12. Frank JR, Snell L, Englander R, Holmboe ES. Implementing competency-based medical education: moving forward. Med Teach. 2017;39:568–73.
13. Gruppen LD, Burkhardt JC, Fitzgerald JT, et al. Competency based education: programme design and challenges to implementation. Med Educ. 2016;50:532–9.
14. Dong T, Gilliland WR, Cruess D, Hutchinson J, Morres L, Curtis J, Hewitt-Clarke GS, Durning SJ. A longitudinal study of commonly used admissions measures and disenrollment from medical school and graduate medical education probation or termination from training. Mil Med. 2018;183:e680–4.
15. Richard-Eaglin A. Predicting student success in nurse practitioner programs. J Am Assoc Nurse Pract. 2017;29:600–5.
16. Davis D, Dorsey JK, Franks RD, Sackett PR, Searcy CA, Zhao X. Do racial and ethnic group differences in performance on the MCAT exam reflect test bias? Acad Med. 2013;88:593–602.
17. Miller C, Stassun K. A test that fails. Nature. 2014;510:303–4.
18. Aibana O, Swails J, Flores J, Love L. Bridging the gap: holistic review to increase diversity in graduate medical education. Acad Med. 2019;94:1137–41.
19. Robinett K, Kareem R, Reavis K, Quezada S. A multi-pronged, antiracist approach to optimize equity in medical school admissions. Med Educ. 2021;55:1376–82.
20. Glazer G, Bankston K, Stacy K. The University of Cincinnati College of nursing case study: bias and discriminatioin in the nursing learning environment. Acad Med. 2020;95:S23–7.
21. Lucey CR, Saguil A. The consequences of structural racism on MCAT scores and medical school admissions: the past is prologue. Acad Med. 2020;95:351–6.
22. Rubright JD, Jodoin M, Barone MA. Examining demographics, prior academic performance, and United States Mediical licensing examination scores. Acad Med. 2019;94:364–70.
23. Plews-Ogan ML, Bell TD, Townsend G, Canterbury RJ, Wilkes DS. Acting wisely: eliminating negative bias in medical education—part 2: how can we do better? Acad Med. 2020;95:S16–22.
24. Teherani A, Hauer KE, Fernandez A, King TE Jr, Lucey C. How small differences in assessed clinical performance amplify to large differences in grades and awards: a cascade with serious consequences for students underrepresented in medicine. Acad Med. 2018;93:1286–92.
25. Low D, Pollack SW, Liao ZC, Maestas R, Kirven LE, Eacker AM, Morales LS. Racial/ethnic disparities in clinical grading in medical school. Teach Learn Med. 2019;31:487–96.
26. Teherani A, Perez S, Muller-Juge V, Lupton K, Hauer KE. A narrative study of equity in clinical assessment through the antideficit lens. Acad Med. 2020;95:S121–30.
27. Elks ML, Johnson K, Anachebe NF. Morehouse School of Medicine case study: teacher-learner relationships free of bias and discrimination. Acad Med. 2020;95:S88–92.
28. Ten Cate O. Competency-based postgraduate medical education: past, present and future. GMS J Med Educ. 2017;34:Doc69.
29. Whittaker JL, Ellis R, Hodges PW, et al. Imaging with ultrasound in physical therapy: what is the PT's scope of practice? A competency-based educational model and training recommendations. Br J Sports Med. 2019;53(23):1447–53.
30. Croft H, Gilligan C, Rasiah R, Levett-Jones T, Schneider J. Current trends and opportunities for

competency assessment in pharmacy education: a literature review. Pharmacy. 2019;7:67.

31. Chimea T, Kanji Z, Schmitz S. Assessment of clinical competence in competency-based education. Can J Dent Hyg. 2020;54(2):83–91.

32. Knebel E, Puttkammer N, Demes A, Devirois R, Prismy M. Developing a competency-based curriculum in HIV for nursing schools in Haiti. Hum Resour Health. 2008;6:17.

33. Baker LR, Phelan S, Woods NN, Boyd VA, Rowland P, Ng SL. Re-envisioning paradigms of education: towards awareness, alignment, and pluralism. Adv Health Sci Educ Theory Pract. 2021;26:1045–58.

34. Ng SL, Kangasjarvi E, Lorello GR, Nemoy L, Brydges R. There shouldn't be anything wrong with not knowing: epistemologies in simulation. Med Educ. 2019;53:1049–59.

35. Baker L, Shing LK, Wright S, Mylopoulos M, Kulasegaram K, Ng S. Aligning and applying the paradigms and practices of education. Acad Med. 2019;94(7):1060.

36. Ellaway RH, Chou CL, Kalet AL. Situating remediation: accommodating success and failure in medical education systems. Acad Med. 2018;93:391–8.

37. Bullock JL, Lai CJ, Lockspeiser T, et al. In pursuit of honors: a multi-institutional study of students' perceptions of clerkship evaluation and grading. Acad Med. 2019;94:S48–56.

38. Hays RB, Lawson M, Gray C. Problems presented by medical students seeking support: a possible intervention framework. Med Teach. 2011;33:161–4.

39. Hauer KE, Lucey CR. Core clerkship grading: the illusion of objectivity. Acad Med. 2019;94:469–72.

40. Krasner MS, Epstein RM, Beckman H, et al. Association of an educational program in mindful communication with burnout, empathy, and attitudes among primary care physicians. JAMA. 2009;302:1284–93.

41. Dyrbye LN, Shanafelt TD, Werner L, Sood A, Satele D, Wolanskyj AP. The impact of a required longitudinal stress management and resilience training course for first-year medical students. J Gen Intern Med. 2017;32:1309–14.

42. Chou CL, Johnston CB, Singh B, et al. A 'safe space' for learning and reflection: one school's design for continuity with a peer group across clinical clerkships. Acad Med. 2011;86:1560–5.

43. Disch J. Rethinking mentoring. Crit Care Med. 2018;46:437–41.

44. McBride AB, Campbell J, Woods NF, Manson SM. Building a mentoring network. Nurs Outlook. 2017;65:305–14.

45. Moore S, Kuol N. Students evaluating teachers: exploring the importance of faculty reaction to feedback on teaching. Teach High Educ. 2005;2005(10):57–73.

46. Stone D, Heen S. Thanks for the feedback: the science and art of receiving feedback well. New York: Penguin Books; 2014.

47. Forsythe A, Johnson S. Thanks, but no-thanks for the feedback. Assess Eval High Educ. 2017;42:850–9.

48. Lefroy J, Watling C, Teunissen PW, Brand P. Guidelines: the do's, don'ts and don't knows of feedback for clinical education. Perspect Med Educ. 2015;4(284):99.

49. Hattie J, Timperley H. The power of feedback. Rev Educ Res. 2007;77:81–112.

50. Watling CJ, Ginsburg S. Assessment, feedback and the alchemy of learning. Med Educ. 2019;53:76–85.

51. Rougas S, Clyne B, Cianciolo AT, Chan TM, Sherbino J, Yarris LM. An extended validity argument for assessing feedback culture. Teach Learn Med. 2015;27:355–8.

52. Cleland JA, Cilliers F, van Schalkwyk S. The learning environment in remediation: a review. Clin Teach. 2018;15:13–8.

53. Boud D, Molloy E, editors. Feedback in higher and professional education. London: Routledge; 2013.

54. Higgins R, Hartley P, Skelton A. Getting the message across: the problem of communicating assessment feedback. Teach High Educ. 2001;6:269–74.

55. Gibbs G. How assessment frames student learning. In: Bryan C, Clegg K, editors. Innovative assessment in higher education. London: Routledge; 2006.

56. Poulos A, Mahony MJ. Effectiveness of feedback: the students' perspective. Assess Eval High Educ. 2008;33:143–54.

57. Brinkman WB, Geraghty SR, Lanphear BP, et al. Effect of multisource feedback on resident communication skills and professionalism: a randomized controlled trial. Arch Pediatr Adolesc Med. 2007;161:44–9.

58. Winstone NE, Nash RA, Parker M, Rowntree J. Supporting learners' agentic engagement with feedback: a systematic review and a taxonomy of recipience processes. Educ Psychol. 2017;52:17–37.

59. Carless D, Salter D, Yang M, Lam J. Developing sustainable feedback practices. Stud High Educ. 2011;36:395–407.

60. Telio S, Ajjawi R, Regehr G. The 'educational alliance' as a framework for reconceptualizing feedback in medical education. Acad Med. 2015;90:609–14.

61. Cutrer WB, Miller B, Pusic MV, et al. Fostering the development of master adaptive learners: a conceptual model to guide skill acquisition in medical education. Acad Med. 2017;92:70–5.

62. Bennion LD, Durning SJ, LaRochelle J, et al. Untying the Gordian knot: remediation problems in medical schools that need remediation. BMC Med Educ. 2018;18:120.

63. Dweck CS. Mindset: the new psychology of success. New York: Ballantine Books; 2016.

64. Bynum WE IV, Varpio L, Lagoo J, Teunissen PW. "I'm unworthy of being in this space": the origins of shame in medical students. Med Educ. 2021;55:185–97.

65. Stegers-Jager KM, Cohen-Schotanus J, Splinter TA, Themmen AP. Academic dismissal policy for

medical students: effect on study progress and help-seeking behaviour. Med Educ. 2011;45:987–94.

66. Caligor E, Levin ZE, Deringer E. Preparing program directors to address unprofessional behavior. In: Kalet A, Chou C, editors. Remediation in medical education: a mid-course correction. New York (NY): Springer; 2014. p. 285–96.

67. Dudek NL, Marks MB, Regehr G. Failure to fail: the perspectives of clinical supervisors. Acad Med. 2005;80:S84–7.

68. Mak-van der Vossen MC, de la Croix A, Teherani A, van Mook WN, Croiset G, Kusurkar RA. A road map for attending to medical students' professionalism lapses. Acad Med. 2019;94:570–8.

69. Saxena V, O'Sullivan PS, Teherani A, Irby DM, Hauer KE. Remediation techniques for student performance problems after a comprehensive clinical skills assessment. Acad Med. 2009;4:669–76.

70. Winston KA, Van Der Vleuten CPM, Scherpbier AJJA. The role of the teacher in remediating at-risk medical students. Med Teach. 2012;34:e732–42.

71. O'Neill LD, Norberg K, Thomsen M, et al. Residents in difficulty—just slower learners? A case-control study. BMC Med Educ. 2014;14:1047.

72. Klamen DL, Williams RG. The efficacy of a targeted remediation process for students who fail standardized patient examinations. Teach Learn Med. 2011;23:3–11.

73. Chang CC, Phillips A, Rumrill SM. Developing a tutor curriculum for the Clinical Skills Tutoring Program (CSTP) at UCSF. Oral presentation. Society of General Internal Medicine, California-Hawaii regional conference; 2021.

74. Lockspeiser TM, O'Sullivan P, Teherani A, Muller J. Understanding the experience of being taught by peers: the value of social and cognitive congruence. Adv Health Sci Educ Theory. 2008;13:361–72.

75. Kalet A, Zabar S. Preparing to conduct remediation. In: Kalet A, Chou CL, editors. Remediation in medical education: a mid-course correction. New York: Springer; 2014.

76. Shearer C, Bosma M, Bergin F, Sargeant J, Warren A. Remediation in Canadian medical residency programs: established and emerging best practices. Med Teach. 2019;41:28–35.

77. Bearman M, Tai J, Kent F, Edouard V, Nestel D, Molloy E. What should we teach the teachers? Identifying the learning priorities of clinical supervisors. Adv Health Sci Educ. 2018;23:29–41.

78. Irby DM, O'Sullivan PS. Developing and rewarding teachers as educators and scholars: remarkable progress and daunting challenges. Med Educ. 2018;52:58–67.

79. Neville S, French S. Clinical education: students' and clinical tutors' views. Physiotherapy. 1991;77:351–4.

80. Bearman M, Molloy E, Ajjawi R, Keating J. 'Is there a plan B?': clinical educators supporting under performing students in practice settings. Teach High Educ. 2013;18:531–44.

81. Yellin PB. Learning differences and medical education. In: Kalet A, Chou CL, editors. Remediation in medical education: a mid-course correction. New York: Springer; 2014.

82. Bierer SB, Dannefer EF, Tetzlaff JE. Time to loosen the apron strings: cohort-based evaluation of a kearner-driven remediation model at one medical school. J Gen Intern Med. 2015;30:1339–43.

83. Ryan RM, Deci EL. Self-determination theory: basic psychological needs in motivation, development, and wellness. New York: The Guilford Press; 2018.

84. Dewey J. How we think. Lexington MA: D C Heath and Co; 1910.

85. Mercer N. Words & minds: how we use language to think together. London: Routledge; 2000.

86. Volet S, Vauras M, Salonen P. Self- and social regulation in learning contexts: an integrative perspective. Educ Psychol. 2009;44:215–26.

87. Winston KA, Van Der Vleuten CPM, Scherpbier AJJA. Remediation of at-risk medical students: theory in action. BMC Med Educ. 2013;13:132.

88. Hmelo-Silver CE, Barrows HS. Facilitating collaborative knowledge building. Cogn Instr. 2008;26:48–94.

89. Winston KA. Core concepts in remediation: lessons learned from a six year case study. Med Sci Educ. 2015;25:307–15.

90. Zbieranowski I, Takahashi SG, Verma S, Spadafora SM. Remediation of residents in difficulty: a retrospective 10-year review of the experience of a postgraduate board of examiners. Acad Med. 2013;88:111–6.

91. Stegers-Jager KM, Cohen-Schotanus J, Themmen AP. Motivation, learning strategies, participation and medical school performance. Med Educ. 2012;46:678–88.

92. Cox SM. 'Forward feeding' about students' progress: information on struggling medical students should not be shared among clerkship directors or with students' current teachers. Acad Med. 2008;83:801.

93. Humphrey-Murto S, LeBlanc A, Touchie C, et al. The influence of prior performance information on ratings of current performance and implications for learner handover: a scoping review. Acad Med. 2019;94:1050–7.

94. Rinehart-Thompson LA. Amendments to FERPA regulations. JAHIMA. 2009;80:56.

95. Graham R, Hall R, Gilmer WG. Connecting the dots: information sharing by post-secondary educational institutions under the Family Education Rights And Privacy Act (FERPA). Educ Law. 2008;20:301–16.

96. Schulze LN Jr. Balancing law student privacy interests and progressive pedagogy: dispelling the myth that FERPA prohibits cutting-edge academic support methodologies. Widener Law J. 2009;19:215.

97. Gold WL, McArdle P, Federman DD. Should medical school faculty see assessments of students made by previous teachers? Acad Med. 2002;77:1096–100.

98. Frellsen SL, Baker EA, Papp KK, Durning SJ. Medical school policies regarding struggling medical students during the internal medicine clerkships: results of a national survey. Acad Med. 2008;83:876–81.

99. Cleary L. 'Forward feeding' about students' progress: the case for longitudinal, progressive, and shared assessment of medical students. Acad Med. 2008;83:800.

100. Cohen GS, Blumberg P. Investigating whether teachers should be given assessments of students made by previous teachers. Acad Med. 1991;66:288–9.

101. Pangaro L. 'Forward feeding' about students' progress: more information will enable better policy. Acad Med. 2008;83:802–3.

102. Warm EJ, Englander R, Pereira A, Barach P. Improving learner handovers in medical education. Acad Med. 2017;92:927–31.

103. Price JA. Sharing student background information with faculty: does it make a difference? Dissertation. Harvard University; 2012.

104. Masangkay N, Adams J, Dwinnell B, Hanson JT, Jain S, Tariq S. Revisiting feed forward: promoting a student-centered approach to education handoffs, remediation, and clerkship success. Teaching Learn Med. 2022. https://doi.org/10.1080/10401334.2022.2082433.

105. Wilkinson TJ, Tweed MJ, Egan TG, et al. Joining the dots: conditional pass and programmatic assessment enhances recognition of problems with professionalism and factors hampering student progress. BMC Med Educ. 2011;11:29.

106. Patel RS, Tarrant C, Bonas S, Shaw RL. Medical students' personal experience of high-stakes failure: case studies using interpretative phenomenological analysis. BMC Med Educ. 2015;15:86.

107. Chou CL, Kalet A, Joao Costa M, Cleland J, Winston K. Guidelines: the do's, don'ts and don't knows of remediation in medical education. Perspect Med Educ. 2019;8:322–38.

Diversity, Inclusion, and Remediation: Excellence Requires Equity

3

Denise L. F. Davis, Justin Bullock, John C. Penner, and Calvin L. Chou

Introduction

You have some anxiety as you prepare to meet with Mary (she/her), a student who excelled in her undergraduate work and during a gap year in which she did research at a large academic medical center. The Associate Dean for Students in your institution recommends she work with you, as she has struggled; She barely passed her clerkships. She plans to apply to a very competitive specialty.

Mary identifies as Black. She reports that she has received scant mentoring and that there are few Black role models and mentors in your institution. She entered health professions school as one of three people of color in a class of 100. There was one person of color on faculty, the dean of diversity, who seemed well-meaning and also very busy. Paintings and photographs on the walls of the entry to the school all depict white men. Case materials to illustrate clinical concepts mostly described white patients, and the few patients of color featured in the cases were characterized as poor and/or "substance-abusing." Mary didn't feel she belonged, and that her own experiences were less meaningful than the talk of valuing diversity that she heard during interviews and in orientation sessions upon matriculation.

How should you prepare to earn Mary's trust and help her improve her clinical performance?

D. L. F. Davis (✉) · C. L. Chou
Department of Medicine, University of California, San Francisco, CA, USA

Veterans Affairs Healthcare System, San Francisco, CA, USA
e-mail: denise.davis@ucsf.edu; calvin.chou@ucsf.edu

J. Bullock
Division of Nephrology, Department of Medicine, University of Washington, Seattle, WA, USA
e-mail: justinbu@uw.edu

J. C. Penner
Department of Medicine, University of California, Veterans Affairs Healthcare System, San Francisco, CA, USA
e-mail: john.penner@ucsf.edu

Increasing the proportion of trainees who are from racial and ethnic backgrounds underrepresented in the health professions (URHP) is crucial in addressing the well-documented racial disparities in the health professions workforce and in health outcomes [1]. Patients in race-concordant relationships with their physicians perceive their care to be of higher quality than those in race-discordant relationships [2, 3]. A systematic literature review found that racial discordance predicts poorer communication in several domains including information-giving, partnership-building, and participatory decision-making [4]. Similar dynamics may affect the well-being and success of learners in race-discordant relationships with supervisors [5]. Unfortunately, URHP trainees encounter additional pressures beyond those of their represented peers, including bias from supervisors, stereotype threat, and inequities in housing, education, and social opportunities [6–12]. Differences in academic outcomes ensue, including lower results on high-stakes standardized exams, clerkship grades, and performance ratings, leading to a higher risk for remediation and differences in ultimate career choice [13–15]. Schools have begun to identify and implement systemic countermeasures to address this "amplification cascade" [13].

To help URHP learners identified as struggling to reach their full potential, we must recognize, examine, and address complex and reciprocal interpersonal, institutional, and structural processes. Learners' struggles are rarely simple or solely attributable to learner characteristics. After a brief section on theoretical framing, we will adapt Jones' allegory about bias [16] as a conceptual framework to address *intrapersonal* work that faculty must confront; *interpersonal* interactions with individual learners; and *systems-level* interventions, all of which must work together for ultimate success in remediating learners across differences. Specifically, we will describe the effects of implicit bias, stereotype threat, and microaggressions (see Box for definitions) on learners who struggle and outline some actionable recommendations to address them.

Definitions of Major Concepts in Diversity, Equity, and Inclusion in Remediation

Implicit bias: an automatic, unconscious set of negative beliefs or attitudes about people from a particular social group, leading to perceptions based on social stereotypes [17].

Stereotype threat: an anxiety state in which one perceives that one's identity is threatened by a negative stereotype [18].

Microaggressions: common everyday slights, verbal or non-verbal, intentional or unintentional, that target people with marginalized identities and reinforce privilege and power [19].

Minority taxes: burdens of extra responsibilities placed on minoritized learners and faculty in the name of diversity [20].

As an important aside, writing a chapter on diversity brings significant challenges and much humility. No guidelines can eliminate the effects of oppression on individuals or groups; we can merely enumerate aspirational attitudes and wise actions that reflect our current and limited perspectives, informed and restricted by our identities that exist in a matrix of marginalized and privileged social locations. We acknowledge our limitations and commit to lifelong learning. We hope that you will, too.

The Social Identity Approach

The social identity approach, a collection of theories including social identity theory and social categorization theory, can help explain how dynamics that underlie our relationship with difference may develop [21]. As individuals, we maintain a sense of self that is influenced by our social groups. We assimilate into our own "ingroups" with people with whom we share common characteristics and view favorably. We also differentiate from people in "out-groups," which helps maintain the positive self-image of the in-group. Our perception of our own social identities is a combination of how we view ourselves and how we perceive others view us. Comparisons between groups may result in expressions of power, privilege, and depersonalization, where individuals are viewed as prototypical of a particular group rather than as unique [22]. These dynamics form the basis for xenophobia and racism. The health professions are subject to these insidious effects, as evidenced by a longstanding and ongoing inability to include learners and health professions educators from historically URHP backgrounds that is commensurate with their proportion of the population.

Intrapersonal Work: An Inside Job

We must reject not only the stereotypes that others hold of us, but also the stereotypes that we hold of ourselves.—Shirley Chisholm

> *DD: As a Black woman in medicine, with both humility and urgency for my colleagues who coach learners in the health professions, my message is to be better prepared. Remediate yourself as a first step in working with struggling learners.*

Implicit Bias

Committing to support learners who struggle requires that we become aware of the biases that we hold. Our implicit bias is the intrapersonal broad brush we use as a shortcut when judging another person or situation. It is not a moral failing but a habit of mind, leading to perceptions based on social stereotypes [17]. Kahneman described this process as System 1 thinking: instinctual, intuitive, automatic, "thinking fast"

[23], arising out of the need for efficiency, and reinforced in fast-paced clinical settings. Similarly, our System 1 thinking figures prominently in our work with learners, potentially leading to bias when encountering a mentee with historically marginalized identities. Implicit bias based on learner race/ethnicity is associated with poorer learner outcomes for Black and Latinx students [24, 25]. Furthermore, clinical evaluations of women and URHP students tend to emphasize descriptions of personal attributes rather than competency, which can lead to discriminatory academic assessment [9, 26]; minoritized medical students are judged more harshly than white students by faculty from both majority and minority groups [19, 27]. Awareness of these implicit biases can be highlighted by taking implicit association tests [28–30].

Everyday societal messaging reinforces implicit biases, which are insidiously integrated into our everyday lives, and notoriously challenging to recognize and correct [31–34]. As a woman of color, Mary may be subject to implicit bias from faculty who typically represent majority identities, and subject to her own stereotype threat (see section below). Additionally, as someone referred for remediation, she holds a new identity in a marginalized social group. The intersection of these identities is greater than any individual element.

Mitigating implicit bias is not straightforward. "Cultural competence" training may help raise awareness but is insufficient for abiding change. If consciously activated, System 2 thinking, a rational, deliberate, and energy-intensive process of "thinking slow" [23], theoretically can disrupt automatic implicit bias. Unfortunately, urgency, stress, and fatigue, elements endemic throughout health professions practice and training, likely detract from System 2 thinking. In addition, attempting to change one's thinking inherently increases cognitive load and can exacerbate biased behaviors. For example, a remediation coach who is self-conscious about their own potentially biased language may stammer, make less eye contact, fail to detect subtle emotional cues, and appear emotionally restricted and therefore less empathic than they actually feel with a learner who struggles [35–38].

Recommendations: Several learner-based interventions to mitigate implicit bias may apply to remediation faculty [39]. Merely understanding that implicit bias has neurobiological roots is an ineffective approach [40]. Deliberately practicing mindfulness and self-regulation strategies (Table 3.1) can bring about changes in automatic processes that control stereotype activation, and they lessen cognitive load [41–43].

These recommendations are not that easily described, and are even more difficult to operationalize and sustain [44]. Perhaps more than any other paradigm of lifelong learning, the process of recognizing, examining, and addressing implicit bias forces us to uncomfortably confront entrenched assumptions. Acting with honesty, courage, and commitment in the face of the discomfort and associated negative emotions, such as disdain, contempt, and defensiveness, that arise when addressing implicit bias can facilitate transformative learning [45]. We need self-compassion and grace to work on this incrementally and relentlessly, "striving while accepting"

Table 3.1 Strategies to mitigate implicit bias [39, 41, 42]

Strategy	Examples
Counter-stereotypic imaging	Visualizing positive exemplars of minoritized groups: abstract (e.g., photos or symbols), well-known, or direct (from people you know)
Individuation	Spending one-on-one time meeting with individuals about whose identities you have biases or who have different life experiences, rather than making generalized assumptions about them as part of their minoritized group
Perspective-taking	Finding respectful ways to inhabit viewpoints of people in marginalized groups (e.g., watching a documentary or reading a thought piece)
Values affirmation	Reinforcing values of equity, both as a mental subroutine and explicitly to learners
Framing every encounter with a URHP learner as a commitment to equity and fairness reinforces those values

[46]. URHP learners do not have the privilege of respite from the implicit bias and assumptions of others that impede their progress.

Interpersonal Work: Interacting with Learners

We now move to interactions with learners who struggle, integrating some awareness of our identities and biases with the humility that we will never fully know everything, and with the commitment to learn more about ourselves and the social contexts that influence our perspectives. With this admittedly incomplete toolbox of potential resources and perspectives, we can increase our awareness of the cultural forces that impact mentoring and remediation relationships across power and privilege.

Start with "Location of Self"

To optimize the remediation, educators must, from the very first interaction, create a sense of safety for learners who are often dealing with fear of the required remediation and concerns about bias, both of which negatively influence performance and well-being [47]. How is this accomplished? Educators can openly welcome the URHP learner's identities as a strength (for instance, because it often serves as an advantage when interacting with patients of similar backgrounds) and acknowledge that assessments may be biased and inequitable [48].

Therefore, in any new mentoring relationship, we start with a "location of self" introduction, where we briefly explain our own key identities (Table 3.2) and how they may potentially influence the remediation work to ensue [49]. Though this suggestion may seem contrary to the caution against self-disclosure in patient interactions [50], by modeling vulnerability, the remediation coach can help flatten the inherent hierarchy in this high-stakes learning relationship. The ensuing psychological safety can augment a learner's comfort to speak their thoughts, lead with their differences, admit their mistakes, and ask for

Table 3.2 Sample location of self-introductions, as if spoken directly to Mary

DD: Mary, may I tell you a bit more about my journey? As the first physician in my family, I am grateful that my mother, a Registered Nurse, shared her textbooks with me, and my father, quizzed me and my brother at the dinner table about world history, focusing intentionally on the African diaspora as well current events. They wanted me to be proud of who I am, and they succeeded. But, there have been rough spots in between, as when I was the only African American trainee in a large academic hospital, and I was struggling and left the program after a year. I look back and see that the learning environment affected me and that I needed time and guidance to regain my sense of confidence and joy. I am dedicated to supporting you and your success.

JB: During medical school, I failed my clinical skills final examination. To that point, I had never failed anything. I remember my feelings of embarrassment. In addition to the disappointment in myself, a lot of my shame came from the fact that as a Black man, I felt that I was fulfilling the stereotypes that others had about medical trainees who shared my racial background. As I went to the group remediation session, I felt there were a disproportionate number of students from underrepresented backgrounds who apparently had failed the test. After the group remediation session, I was paired with a chief resident who would help me to work on my clinical skills. Notably, he was a white man, whom I did not expect to relate very much to aside from a mutual interest in medicine (yes, I was stereotyping him). I found myself pleasantly surprised when on our first session, he opened with the fact that he too had failed something in medical school and was very excited at the opportunity to work with me and hopefully help me. By sharing an inconspicuous part of his identity (as one who had failed), he created a safe space which helped to lower my veil of shame and to focus on learning from him. That's my goal for you.

JCP: As a cisgendered, straight, white man, I carry many privileged identities in my personal and professional lives. I also carry one of someone who struggled throughout medical school, especially on standardized tests and high-stakes exams throughout the preclerkship curriculum. Even with the unearned privilege of my identities, I've felt the toll of how lonely and isolating that experience of struggling to keep up can be, the ways it can ripple out into one's sense of self, and the impact it can have on one's mental health. While I will never know exactly what your experience is as a Black woman in medicine, I sincerely hope to earn your trust so that I can come to better know and understand it through whatever you may choose to share so that I can leverage the privilege I carry to help you thrive in whatever ways that looks like to you. That is my commitment to you in our time working together and beyond.

CLC: As a gay Chinese doctor, son of immigrants, there were—and still are—many times when I am reminded that I am an outsider. I felt society was telling me that it wasn't ok to be Chinese, and when I was younger, I internalized a lot of that. Then as my sexuality was dawning on me, in the very beginning of the AIDS epidemic, it was clear that society was telling me several ways that it wasn't ok to be gay, either. It has taken a lot of hard knocks, some of them physical, all of them emotional, and a lot of processing and therapy to get to this place of being not just ok with but actually proud of myself. And so I resolve to pay that belonging and pride forward to you. I am sure I don't know what it is like to be a Black woman at this stage of your development. I am working on understanding the experiences of women, Black people, and the intersections between those and other identities you might eventually be willing to share with me. Please know that our work together is fully in support of you, to be the best you that you can be.

help [51]. Contrastingly, a lack of psychological safety may lead to negative effects on career, status, or self-image [52]. Explicitly stating one's location of self also brings intellectual and moral integrity to a coaching or learning relationship: we invoke the social identity approach by demonstrating awareness of not only the in-groups we belong (or appear to belong) to, but also the possible bias we bring to out-group members and our willingness to mitigate it [22].

Openly discussing our identities and the relationship of those identities to power, privilege, and marginalization takes courage. Faculty remediators, especially those from majority identities, may state *"there's nothing interesting about my*

background; I'm average." Many people of color, as well as queer and transgender people, must frequently and involuntarily address their identities [18, 53–55]. Similarly, URHP learners see an educator not as Italian, for example, but as White; avoiding an overt self-description as "White" may thereby interfere with developing trust in that learning relationship. Vulnerably introducing our identities, strengths, and limitations helps build an alliance across differences, which is necessary for the success of crucial feedback conversations in remediation [56].

Recommendation: We support overt acknowledgment of our positions of power, privilege, and hierarchy, coupled with a commitment to use those positions to help the learner, an expectation that we will commit errors in the mentoring process, and ongoing humble commitment toward continuous improvement. Starting mentoring relationships with honesty about who we are invites co-construction of the trust that is so influential in maximizing the success of the remediation process.

An Exercise

For faculty remediators, talking through these issues with trusted peers and practicing addressing identity (with feedback) is a very effective way to build skills in working across differences.

Think now about a striving and struggling learner you know who identifies with a marginalized group. Please take 30 seconds right now to imagine how that person might feel in their academic and clinical life.

Now think about your own identities—race/ethnicity, gender, social class, body size, sexual orientation, ability, language preferences, and others. How would you describe yourself to learners? How comfortable do you feel in talking about your own identities? How might Black, Indigenous, and People of Color (BIPOC) see you? How might queer, transgender, and non-binary learners see you? Their identities matter and how they see you matters, and in your role as a coach and remediator, your identities, when addressed early in the relationship, matter just as much because they have the potential to earn the trust of the learner.

Recognize and Diminish Stereotype Threat and Microaggressions

Though failure to meet educational standards is often attributed solely to the learner's cognitive capabilities, lack of preparation, or low motivation, strong evidence indicates that perceptions that one's identity is threatened by a negative stereotype measurably undermines performance [18]. This anxiety state, or "stereotype threat," is common in minoritized learners, who may feel alienated by constant reminders that they don't belong in the face of verbal and nonverbal cues throughout the healthcare environment [57, 58]. These implicit messages reinforce a dynamic of "internalized oppression," the belief that there is truth underlying these reminders. For example, even in the absence of overt sexism and racism, when negative stereotypes were merely present in the environment, women and African Americans underperformed compared to men and white people [18].

Minoritized medical students undergo three stages of stereotype threat: *triggering*, where an experience activates stereotype threat; *internal dialogue*, in which the learner expends significant energy questioning and processing their experiences; and *response*, which takes numerous potential forms including avoidance, denial, prevention, deferral, and confrontation [59]. Learners in remediation settings experience additional stereotype threat when seen as struggling and often adopt maladaptive behaviors that further impede progress [60, 61].

Stereotype threat is perpetuated with ongoing microaggressions, defined as common everyday slights, verbal or non-verbal, intentional or unintentional, that target people with marginalized identities and reinforce privilege and power [19]. Microaggressions can seem innocuous to the uninformed, while the ambiguity can create stress for the target of the offense. A common microaggression, "Mary, your hair is so unique," targets Black people, especially Black women's hairstyles, even though it may be intended as a compliment. Microaggressions that trigger identity threat can also be environmental (e.g., paintings depicting only white male progenitors). The effects of microaggressions range broadly. First, they increase cognitive load (see Chap. 10): having to hear, process, and decide how to respond to interpersonal microaggressions interfering with academic performance [58]. Second, since microaggressions often occur without response from supervisors or team members, trainees can feel alone in that silence [62, 63]. Finally, there is a dose-response relationship between the number of reported microaggressions experienced by medical students and depression and anxiety, which lead to further deleterious mental and physical outcomes, and an increased incidence of thoughts of withdrawing from school [64, 65]. Microaggressions poison the learning climate and require learner and mentor preparation, debriefing, and allyship [18, 54, 55].

Stereotype threat and microaggressions are two interconnected forms of identity threat which detract from trainees' ability to learn and demonstrate learning. Fostering a sense of *identity safety* may promote successful remediation across differences. Identity safety is an evolving construct, defined by some as absence of identity threat and by others as respect and appreciation. The most extensive characterization of identity safety is in elementary school students, defined by four pillars: learner-centered teaching, cultivating diversity as a resource, classroom relationships, and caring environments [66]. Preliminary research on identity safety in health professions trainees highlights the importance of adopting an anti-deficit mindset to create safe environments in which identity is viewed from a positive lens (e.g., the assets one brings because of their diverse identities) as opposed to the deficit framework (e.g., predominantly thinking about the negative associations with minoritized identities). This results in cultivating diversity as a resource [67]. For JB (Table 3.2), his mentor successfully leveraged his identity by disclosing that he was a former trainee who failed and now was a successful chief resident using his experience to give back to other learners who had failed.

Recommendations: Clinical supervisors and remediation coaches can use several helpful strategies to decrease stereotype threat and demonstrate allyship. In most ways, URHP struggling learners' needs are similar to other learners who need coaching for success. Though using an anti-deficit mindset seems paradoxical and perhaps even antithetical in the realm of remediation, all learners deserve the relationship-centered processes of respect, beneficial and brave feedback, and mentoring. Because URHP learners learn in the universe of health professions education that treats some differently than others due to long-standing systems of privilege, power, marginalization, and oppression, we describe additional approaches that have salience for URHP learners (Table 3.3).

Table 3.3 Strategies to mitigate stereotype threat, microaggressions, and identity threat

1. **Self-affirmation and values affirmation** [68]
   (a) *"Mary, I would love to know things that you value about clinical learning environments."*
   (b) *"I'd like to hear whatever you feel comfortable telling me about a recent success."*
   (c) Deferring extensive modifying feedback at the outset of a coaching relationship and emphasizing validating feedback: *"I noticed how you quickly developed rapport with your patient by introducing yourself with a warm greeting and apologizing for interrupting the patient's day. Please keep doing that."*

2. **Defined structure to remediation programs**, making very explicit the specific details of the road map that will lead to learner success [56, 69]. Even with delineation of precisely defined objectives, the clinical training pathway is fraught with implicit curricular expectations, some of which are further accompanied by implicit bias in observers and assessors. The more that these implicit details can be revealed, the clearer the path for the struggling learner, which will maximize the chance of success

3. **Communicating high standards** [66]: Again, this approach may seem counterintuitive, yet faculty can overcome their concerns and develop their own high standards for remediating learners across differences using deep empathic honesty, bravely offering the support required to change the educational trajectory for struggling learners, and taking heart in recognizing psychological defenses or projections when they arise. *"Mary, I have high standards for you and all the learners I work with. You have told me that you want to perform at a high level. I am committed to helping you get there."*

4. **Acknowledgment that bias exists in your organization**, often expressed through microaggressions. Begin the coaching relationship with *"I wish that bias didn't happen here. I'm asking your permission to check in with you about expressions of bias witnessed or that target you. No one should be alone with those experiences and experiences of bias interfere with performance."* When witnessing or presented with descriptions of microaggressions, proactively intervening or at the very least, debriefing the experience afterwards, represent necessary steps to preserve and deepen trust [18, 54, 55]

(continued)

Table 3.3 (continued)

5. **Recognition when stereotype threat goes both ways.** Stereotype threat becomes most salient when the subject cares about the outcome [66]. For coaches and leaders who have made a commitment to the success of all minoritized learners, finding themselves in a position to guide or pronounce judgments on struggling URHP learners compounds the stereotype threat of the coach/leader. Similar to how we approach learners: self-affirmation, structure, and high standards will help reduce the stereotype threat that may weigh on a faculty member

The Minority Taxes

On the clinical service, Mary spends extra time working with Black patients to counsel them in the morning. These patients are deeply grateful, saying that they trust her much more than other providers. Even though Mary tries to arrive earlier and earlier to complete her work before rounds, because of her commitment to her patients, she often arrives late to rounds and can appear clinically unprepared.

Because minoritized patients appear to gravitate toward URHP providers, educators must not only acknowledge but also encourage the connections that Mary develops, as well as solve the complex-variable equation to support her clinical training. If supervisors note Mary's strengths and then assign all patients of color on the service to Mary, this tokenism can exact an even greater "minority tax" on her time, energy, and emotional resources of URHP learners and faculty [20]. Institutions often underrecognize and undervalue these activities.

In addition, due to structural racism, URHP trainees are more likely to have personal experience with poverty, housing and food insecurity, and the criminal justice system compared with their majority counterparts; they may be very reluctant to share this information with people whom they do not yet trust [27]. Black medical students in the US also consistently carry more debt than Hispanic, Asian, and White peers [70]; those from underrepresented backgrounds, especially women, are more likely to have significant elder-care responsibilities [59].

Holding more than one marginalized identity magnifies both the complexities of navigating academic culture and the sense of isolation when a critical mass of individuals with similar intersecting identities is lacking. Mentors need to develop their own skills to be able to comfortably and knowledgeably ask about, explore, and empathize with a mentee's complex lived experiences. It is a tricky balance, though: eschewing reflexive avoidance, dismissal, minimization, or overidentification with their mentee's perspectives takes significant effort.

Recommendations: By making explicit what is otherwise covert, educators can specifically recognize the added value of racial concordance that URHP learners bring to minoritized patients, inquire directly about competing demands (Table 3.4), and acknowledge the presence and work toward the reduction of structural oppression (see next section).

Table 3.4 Sample questions to ask about learners' competing demands

"I wish that I didn't have to ask, but I will ask because I'm dedicated to your success. Do you feel that you've been treated differently? I have time to hear your thoughts"

"What other important demands on your time are you managing?"

"How is your living arrangement affecting your academic work?"

"Financial strains are common amongst health professions trainees. Do you have financial stressors you feel comfortable discussing with me?"

"What do you feel comfortable telling me about the mission you have to make this program better for others?"

"I wonder if you feel alone in that work"

"How much thought have you given to the implementation of your mission that might compete with the standards of the program?"

"What would support from our institution look like?"

Remediating Curricula and Systems

Naturally, many of the influences addressed above have origins in societal systems of oppression. Implicit bias, stereotype threat, and internalized oppression are not isolated from history, geopolitics, and other cultural forces. We have already discussed the perpetuation of implicit bias through cultural messaging, the awareness gap and reticence of faculty and supervisors to explicitly acknowledge their advantaged status(es) to URHP learners, the ongoing bias that drives stereotype threat and microaggressions and expressions of bias, and the minority tax that exaggerates social pressures on URHP trainees. These forces also deserve interventions at the systemic level.

Implicit bias: Institutional leaders and remediation coaches making decisions about Mary's progress may view her through the lenses of their own implicit biases. A programmatic approach to remediation can hold these numerous implicit biases in check. A cultural humility approach, however, also requires that we constantly review institutional perspectives for stubbornly opaque implicit bias [71]. Course content and assessment processes should be regularly reassessed for ingrained implicit bias. If a disproportionate number of minoritized learners underperform in a particular setting, systemic factors must be considered and mitigated. Institutional practices can also increase belonging and thereby prevent challenges in the learning climate that unduly affect minoritized learners. Examples include longitudinal faculty development with an equity focus, instituting and/or strengthening programs that integrate developing professional identities with underrepresented social identities: orientations to schools that emphasize inclusion, and affinity groups and/or leadership programs for URHP students [22, 72].

Just and equitable faculty representation and faculty development are also essential in creating a climate of equity. No matter how progressive institutional conversations are regarding equity, representation of URHP faculty and other leaders is vitally important. For example, the continued underrepresentation of Black, Latinx, and Indigenous RN students and faculty [73] sends a clear message to minority students and faculty

that structural barriers persist. Furthermore, merely plugging the leaky pipeline by prioritizing recruitment of URHP faculty alone is insufficient—institutions must also invest in minority tax-free support success for those faculty.

Location of self: Mentors tasked with giving modifying feedback often struggle with finding the right words when working with all students; perhaps especially when the learner identifies as a member of a marginalized group [74]. Though many acknowledge the existence of institutional biases, most faculty members also lack confidence in navigating conversations about racism, sexism, ableism, or anti-LGBTQ+ oppression in health professions education. A longitudinal narrative-based curriculum for faculty may increase comfort in discussions about race [75].

Stereotype threat and microaggressions: Counter-stereotypical examples should be emphasized in clinical vignettes and/or simulation exercises to provide students opportunities to recognize, practice, and habituate into anti-oppressive attitudes and behaviors. In addition, faculty need and deserve system-based interventions that address remediators' lack of confidence and anxiety about hosting crucial conversations. Institutions must spend time and resources to acknowledge and address the stereotype threat that affects faculty remediators and undermines performance, whether in the form of peer mentoring groups or formal trainings with experts in anti-oppression pedagogy.

Institutions should explicitly survey learners about their perceptions of racial climate, gender equity, and the presence or absence of faculty role models who share learners' identities. Learners, who are the experts on their own experiences in educational and healthcare systems, should be consulted often. Remediation faculty should consult campus surveys and equal employment opportunity complaints about systemic inequity to boost their knowledge of system strengths and weaknesses and inform their advocacy for mentees. In addition, institutional policies and rules must explicitly prohibit patients from discriminating against trainees, and these policies must be upheld and reinforced [76].

The minority taxes: The minority tax advantages faculty members from historically privileged positions, while holding minoritized mentors responsible for building relationships with learners who are disadvantaged because of notoriously challenging issues such as implicit bias, racial trauma, and stereotype threat. Institutions must first analyze patterns and then address situations where majority-identified faculty are "off the hook" when addressing the challenges of students who are members of historically marginalized groups. Institutions can ensure that "majoritized" coaches develop awareness of the needs and challenges of learners who identify with marginalized identities [77], while faculty from URHP backgrounds should be explicitly valued for advocacy and remediation they can bring to race-concordant relationships.

Remediation in the Twenty-First Century and Beyond

The Black Lives Matter and #metoo movements have catalyzed the publication of many articles on intrapersonal, interpersonal, and institutional forms of oppression, including racism and sexism, that affect patients, families, learners, and colleagues [78, 79]. Health professions faculty can and should avail themselves of the foundational knowledge about best practices in anti-oppression and culturally-sensitive pedagogy, supervision, and mentoring [73].

In this chapter, we have highlighted a case of a Black woman struggling to succeed. The issues of diversity in remediation clearly apply to a wide population of learners who hold marginalized identities and behaviors that may single them out for implicit bias on detection and reinforcement (for one of many possible examples: see Chap. 12 for neurodiverse learners).

The many recommendations included in this chapter range widely and may be time-consuming. We must act as humble exemplars, teachers, and allies to others. Ultimately, there are many knowledge gaps in this area of remediation work crying out for research and quality improvement. We will only be able to ultimately succeed if a critical mass of health educators, students, and patients (yes, everyone) recognizes these dynamics and makes tangible moves toward a culture of equity.

Acknowledgments Deepest thanks to Lynnea Mills, Maryann Chimhanda, Seward Rutkove, and the San Francisco VA DGIM Education Works in Progress group for commenting on earlier drafts of this chapter.

References

1. Institute of Medicine. Unequal treatment: confronting racial and ethnic disparities in health care. Washington, DC: The National Academies Press; 2003.
2. Saha S, Komaromy M, Koepsell TD, Bindman AB. Patient-physician racial concordance and the perceived quality and use of health care. Arch Intern Med. 1999;159:997–1004.
3. Laveist TA, Nuru-Jeter A. Is doctor-patient race concordance associated with greater satisfaction with care? J Health Soc Behav. 2002;43:296–306.
4. Shen MJ, Peterson EB, Costas-Muniz R, Hernandez MH, Jewell ST, Matsoukas K, Bylund CL. The effects of race and racial concordance on patient-physician communication: a systematic review of the literature. J Racial Ethnic Health Disparities. 2018;5: 117–40.
5. Morales DX, Grineski SE, Collins TW. Effects of mentor-mentee discordance on Latinx undergraduates' intent to pursue graduate school and research productivity. Ann N Y Acad Sci. 2021;1499:54–69.
6. Stegers-Jager KM, Steyerberg EW, Cohen-Schotanus J, Themmen AP. Ethnic disparities in undergraduate pre-clinical and clinical performance. Med Educ. 2012;46:575–85.
7. Bullock JL, Lai CJ, Lockspeiser T, et al. In pursuit of honors: a multi-institutional study of students' perceptions of clerkship evaluation and grading. Acad Med. 2019;94:S48–56.
8. Woolf K, Cave J, Greenhalgh T, Dacre J. Ethnic stereotypes and the underachievement of UK medical students from ethnic minorities. BMJ. 2008;337:a1220.
9. Rojek AE, Khanna R, Yim JWL, et al. Differences in narrative language in evaluations of medical students by gender and under-represented minority status. J Gen Intern Med. 2019;34:684–91.
10. Davis D, Dorsey JK, Franks RD, Sackett PR, Searcy CA, Zhao X. Do racial and ethnic group differences in performance on the MCAT exam reflect test bias? Acad Med. 2013;88:593–602.
11. Quinn DM, Cooc N. Science achievement gaps by gender and race/ethnicity in elementary and middle school: trends and predictors. Educ Res. 2015;44:336–46.
12. Orom H, Semalulu T, Underwood W 3rd. The social and learning environments experienced by under-represented minority medical students: a narrative review. Acad Med. 2013;88:1765–77.

13. Teherani A, Hauer KE, Fernandez A, King TE Jr, Lucey C. How small differences in assessed clinical performance amplify to large differences in grades and awards: a cascade with serious consequences for students underrepresented in medicine. Acad Med. 2018;93:1286–92.

14. Boatright D, Ross D, O'Connor P, Moore E, Nunez-Smith M. Racial disparities in medical student membership in the Alpha Omega Alpha Honor Society. JAMA Intern Med. 2017;177:659–65.

15. Lucey CR, Hauer KE, Boatright D, Fernandez A. Medical education's wicked problem: achieving equity in assessment for medical learners. Acad Med. 2020;95:S98–S108.

16. Jones CP. Levels of racism: a theoretic framework and a gardener's tale. Am J Public Health. 2000;90:1212–5.

17. Amodio DM, Devine PG. Stereotyping and evaluation in implicit race bias: evidence for independent constructs and unique effects on behavior. J Pers Soc Psychol. 2006;91:652–61.

18. Wittkower LD, Bryan JL, Asghar-Ali AA. A scoping review of recommendations and training to respond to patient microaggressions. Acad Psychiatry. 2022;46:627–39.

19. Sue DW, Capodilupo CM, Torino GC, Bucceri JM, Holder AM, Nadal KL, Esquilin M. Racial microaggressions in everyday life: implications for clinical practice. Am Psychol. 2007;62:271–86.

20. Rodríguez JE, Campbell KM, Pololi LH. Addressing disparities in academic medicine: what of the minority tax? BMC Med Ed. 2015;15:1–5.

21. Reicher S, Spears R, Haslam SA. The social identity approach in social psychology. In: Wetherell M, editor. The Sage handbook of identities. Thousand Oaks CA: SAGE Publications; 2010.

22. Bochatay N, Bajwa NM, Ju M, Appelbaum NP, van Schaik SM. Towards equitable learning environments for medical education: bias and the intersection of social identities. Med Educ. 2022;56:82–90.

23. Kahneman D. Thinking, fast and slow. New York: Farrar, Straus and Giroux; 2011.

24. Jacoby-Senghor DS, Stacey Sinclair J, Shelton N. A lesson in bias: the relationship between implicit racial bias and performance in pedagogical contexts. J Exp Soc Psychol. 2016;63:50–5.

25. McKown C, Weinstein RS. Teacher expectations, classroom context, and the achievement gap. J School Psychol. 2008;46:235–61.

26. Gorth DJ, Magee RG, Rosenberg SE, et al. Gender disparity in evaluation of internal medicine clerkship performance. JAMA Netw Open. 2021;4(7):e2115661.

27. Dugger RA, El-Sayed AM, Dogra A, Messina C, Bronson R, Galea S. The color of debt: racial disparities in anticipated medical student debt in the United States. PLoS One. 2013;8(9):e74693.

28. Sekaquaptewa D, Espinoza P, Thompson M, Vargas P, von Hippel W. Stereotypic explanatory bias: implicit stereotyping as a predictor of discrimination. J Exp Soc Psychol. 2003;39:75–82.

29. McConnell AR, Leibold JM. Relations between the implicit association test, explicit racial attitudes, and discriminatory behavior. J Exp Soc Psychol. 2001;37:435–42.

30. FitzGerald C, Hurst S. Implicit bias in healthcare professionals: a systematic review. BMC Med Ethics. 2017;18:19.

31. van Ryn M, Hardeman R, Phelan SM, Burgess DJ, Dovidio JF, Herrin J, Burke SE, Nelson DB, Perry S, Yeazel M, Przedworski JM. Medical school experiences associated with change in implicit racial bias among 3547 students: a medical student CHANGES study report. J Gen Intern Med. 2015;30:1748–56.

32. Dovidio JF. On the nature of contemporary prejudice: the third wave. J Soc Issues. 2001;57:829–49.

33. Dovidio JF, Penner LA, Albrecht TL, Norton WE, Gaertner SL, Shelton JN. Disparities and distrust: the implications of psychological processes for understanding racial disparities in health and health care. Soc Sci Med. 2008;67(3):478–86.

34. Nosek BA, Smyth FL, Hansen JJ, et al. Pervasiveness and correlates of implicit attitudes and stereotypes. Eur Rev Soc Psychol. 2007;18:36–88.

35. Galinsky AD, Moskowitz GB. Further ironies of suppression: stereotype and counterstereotype accessibility. J Exp Soc Psychol. 2007;43:833–41.

36. Stone J, Moskowitz GB. Non-conscious bias in medical decision making: what can be done to reduce it? Med Educ. 2011;45:768–76.

37. Byrne A, Tanesini A. Instilling new habits: addressing implicit bias in healthcare professionals. Adv Health Sci Educ. 2015;20:1255–62.

38. Dovidio JF, Kawakami K, Gaertner SL. Implicit and explicit prejudice and interracial interaction. J Pers Soc Psychol. 2002;82:62–8.

39. Gonzalez CM, Lypson ML, Sukhera J. Twelve tips for teaching implicit bias recognition and management. Med Teach. 2021;43:1368–73.

40. Reihl KM, Hurley RA, Taber KH. Neurobiology of implicit and explicit bias: implications for clinicians. J Neuropsychiatry Clin Neurosci. 2015;27:A6–253.

41. Moskowitz GB, Li P. Egalitarian goals trigger stereotype inhibition: a proactive form of stereotype control. J Exp Soc Psychol. 2011;47:103–16.

42. Devine PG, Forscher PS, Austin AJ, Cox WT. Long-term reduction in implicit race bias: a prejudice habit-breaking intervention. J Exp Soc Psychol. 2012;48:1267–78.

43. Wu D, Saint-Hilaire L, Pineda A, Hessler D, Saba GW, Salazar R, Olayiwola N. The efficacy of an anti-oppression curriculum for health professionals. Fam Med. 2019;51:22–30.

44. Lai CK, Skinner AL, Cooley E, Murrar S, Brauer M, Devos T, et al. Reducing implicit racial preferences: II. Intervention effectiveness across time. J Exp Psychol Gen. 2016;145:1001–16.

45. Sherman MD, Ricco J, Nelson SC, Nezhad SJ, Prasad S. Implicit bias training in a residency program: aiming for enduring effects. Fam Med. 2019;51:677–81.

46. Sukhera J, Watling CJ, Gonzalez CM. Implicit bias in health professions: from recognition to transformation. Acad Med. 2020;95:717–23.

47. Sukhera J, Wodzinski M, Teunissen PW, Lingard L, Watling C. Striving while accepting: exploring the relationship between identity and implicit bias recognition and management. Acad Med. 2018;93:S82–8.

48. Quinn DM. Identity concealment: multilevel predictors, moderators, and consequences. J Soc Issues. 2017;73:230–9.

49. Teherani A, Perez S, Muller-Juge V, Lupton K, Hauer KE. A narrative study of equity in clinical assessment through the antideficit lens. Acad Med. 2020;95:S121–30.

50. Watts-Jones TD. Location of self: opening the door to dialogue on intersectionality in the therapy process. Fam Process. 2010;49:405–20.

51. McDaniel SH, Beckman HB, Morse DS, Silberman J, Seaburn DB, Epstein RM. Physician self-disclosure in primary care visits: enough about you, what about me? Arch Intern Med. 2007;167:1321–6.

52. Edmondson AC, Lei Z. Psychological safety: the history, renaissance, and future of an interpersonal construct. Annu Rev Organ Psych Organ Behav. 2014;1:23–43.

53. Kim NY. Lining individuation and organizational identification: mediation through psychological safety. J Soc Psychol. 2020;160:216–35.

54. Wheeler DJ, Zapata J, Davis D, Chou C. Twelve tips for responding to microaggressions and overt discrimination: when the patient offends the learner. Med Teach. 2019;41:1112–7.

55. Bullock JL, O'Brien MT, Minhas PK, Fernandez A, Lupton KL, Hauer KE. No one size fits all: a qualitative study of clerkship medical students' perceptions of ideal supervisor responses to microaggressions. Acad Med. 2021;96:S71–80.

56. Steele CM, Aronson J. Stereotype threat and the intellectual test performance of African Americans. J Pers Soc Psychol. 1995;69:797–811.

57. Telio S, Ajjawi R, Regehr G. The "educational alliance" as a framework for reconceptualizing feedback in medical education. Acad Med. 2015;90:609–614.

58. Burgess DJ, Warren J, Phelan S, Dovidio J, van Ryn M. Stereotype threat and health disparities: what medical educators and future physicians need to know. J Gen Intern Med. 2010;25:S169–77.

59. Bullock JL, Lockspeiser T, Del Pino-Jones A, Richards R, Teherani A, Hauer KE. They don't see a lot of people my color: a mixed methods study of racial/ethnic stereotype threat among medical students on core clerkships. Acad Med. 2020;95:S58–66.

60. Patel R, Tarrant C, Bonas S, et al. The struggling student: a thematic analysis from the self-regulated learning perspective. Med Educ. 2015;49:417–26.

61. Kirtchuk D, Wells G, Levett T, Castledine C, de Visser R. Understanding the impact of academic difficulties among medical students: a scoping review. Med Educ. 2022;56:262–9.

62. Brooks KC. A silent curriculum. JAMA. 2020;323:1690–1.

63. Killeen OJ, Bridges L. Solving the silence. JAMA. 2018;320:1979–80.

64. Ackerman-Barger K, Jacobs NN. The microaggressions triangle model: a humanistic approach to navigating microaggressions in health professions schools. Acad Med. 2020;95:S28–32.

65. Anderson N, Lett E, Asabor EN, Hernandez AL, Nguemeni Tiako MJ, Johnson C, Montenegro RE, Rizzo TM, Latimore D, Nunez-Smith M, Boatright D. The association of microaggressions with depressive symptoms and institutional satisfaction among a national cohort of medical students. J Gen Intern Med. 2022;37:298–307.

66. Steele DM, Cohn-Vargas B. Identity safe classrooms. Thousand Oaks, CA: Corwin Press; 2013.

67. Bullock, personal communication.

68. Cohen GL, Steele CM, Ross LD. The mentor's dilemma: providing critical feedback across the racial divide. Pers Soc Psychol Bulletin. 1999;25:1302–18.

69. Hafferty FW. Beyond curriculum reform: confronting medicine's hidden curriculum. Acad Med. 1998;73:403–7.

70. Association of American Medical Colleges. Diversity in medicine: facts and figures. 2019. https://www.aamc.org/data-reports/workforce/interactive-data/figure-10-amountpremedical-education-debt-us-medical-school-matriculants-race/ethnicity-academic.

71. Vela MB, Erondu AI, Smith NA, Peek ME, Woodruff JN, Chin MH. Eliminating explicit and implicit biases in health care: evidence and research needs. Annu Rev Public Health. 2022;43:477–501.

72. Davis DLF, Tran-Taylor D, Imbert E, Wong JO, Chou CL. Start the way you want to finish: an intensive diversity, equity, inclusion orientation curriculum in undergraduate medical education. J Med Educ Curric Dev. 2021;8:23821205211000352.

73. Ferrell DK, DeCrane SK, Edwards N, Foli KJ, Tennant KF. Minority undergraduate nursing student success. J Cult Divers. 2016;23:3–11.

74. Croft A, Schmader T. The feedback withholding bias: minority students do not receive critical feedback from evaluators concerned about appearing racist. J Exp Soc Psychol. 2012;48:1139–44.

75. Holdren S, Iwai Y, Lenze NR, Weil AB, Randolph AM. A novel narrative medicine approach to DEI training for medical school faculty. Teach Learn Med. 2022:1–10. Epub ahead of print

76. AMA guidelines offer path to prevent discrimination in medicine | American Medical Association. ama-assn.org.

77. Najibi S, Carney PA, Thayer EK, Deiorio NM. Differences in coaching needs among underrepresented minority medical students. Fam Med. 2019;51:516–22.

78. Leonardo Z, Porter R. Pedagogy of fear: toward a Fanonian theory of "safety" in race dialogue. Race Ethnicity Educ. 2010;13:139–57.

79. Powell JA. Structural racism: building upon the insights of John Calmore. N C L Rev. 2008;86:791.

The Metacognitive Competency: Becoming a Master Adaptive Learner

4

Neva Howard and Martin Pusic

Introduction

Wyatt (he/him) had been an extremely successful undergraduate student with well-honed study and memorization skills. He focused his considerable intelligence on closely following the directions of professors and excelling on prescriptive assignments, with a major motivation to impress his teachers. But when he entered medical school, faced with the high volume of information, those strategies no longer worked, and he performed poorly on an exam for the first time in his life. His confidence fell. Unable to conceptualize why this happened, he did not take advantage of faculty or peer-led tutoring or seek other support. He worked harder but without altering his study strategies. He continued to fail and was required to enter a formal remediation process where he confronted the need to understand how he learns, how to adapt his learning to new situations, and how to reframe failure as part of an iterative improvement process.

All learners engage in cycles of learning; however, these cycles are generally reactive to the activities presented and are unplanned. Our experiences with learners who struggle demonstrate that surfacing, examining, and strengthening their frameworks for learning lead to long-lasting improvement in learning performance. For instance, before entering medical school, perhaps Wyatt had not been challenged enough to need these higher-order learning processes. Although he easily adjusted to the requirements of undergraduate education, he was unaware of how to use a more generalized learning process to adapt to all environments.

The Master Adaptive Learner (MAL) framework [1] integrates multiple underlying theories, such as learning curve theory [2], theory of expertise [3], theory of adaptive expertise [4], dual cognition theory [5, 6], mindset [7], and self-regulation theory [8], among others, to provide learners and educators with a shared view of the metacognitive and adaptive processes needed

N. Howard
University of Colorado School of Medicine, Aurora, CO, USA
e-mail: neva.howard@childrenscolorado.org

M. Pusic (✉)
Harvard Medical School, Boston, MA, USA
e-mail: martin.pusic@childrens.harvard.edu

to learn in health professions. The framework is similar to improvement frameworks, such as the PDSA cycle of quality improvement [9], Kolb's learning cycle rooted in constructivism [10], and the scientific method. The MAL Framework goes beyond these models by also considering the learning environment, the intrinsic qualities of learners, and the interaction of the learner with the broader organization [1].

MAL challenges learners to be aware of what learning strategies are needed for adaptation. Metacognition, defined in many ways, is colloquially referred to as "learning to learn" or "higher-order thinking skills." Practicing metacognition allows for control of one's own cognitive processes: not simply asking "how am I learning this?" but more specifically asking, "am I learning what I need to help the next patient?" [11]. This is great news for learners who struggle, as the framework helps identify specific areas of struggle and therefore guides remediation strategies [12].

In this chapter, we will describe the MAL framework and demonstrate how it can transform how all health professions trainees learn, guiding consistent improvement through coaching towards expertise, adaptability, and innovation. We will also explore the relationship between metacognition and the critical drivers of MAL: curiosity, motivation, mindset, and resilience.

The Master Adaptive Learner Framework

The MAL framework promotes a meta-cognitive, intentional perspective for health professions learning, including normalizing productive failure as an important strategy [13]. Figure 4.1 shows the MAL cycle as dynamic gears, including the planning phase, the learning phase, the assessment phase, and the adjustment phase [1]. MAL also considers the learning environment and the need for a coach to monitor the cycle. A coach is depicted metaphorically as a rheostat monitoring the learner's "batteries" of resilience, motivation, mindset, and curiosity.

The MAL framework explains how trainees and clinicians at all levels can improve or learn so that they can apply that learning to similar future situations. In a process known as *preparation for future learning*, a learner, ideally with the aid of an educator/coach, must invest time into learning the components of the framework. This means that in the early stages, the learner is productively double-tasked—learning the subject matter AND learning to learn. Thus, the going is initially slower than it might be otherwise; however, the learning-to-learn skills (metacognition, adaptability, approach to uncertainty) become ever more applicable moving forward, making subsequent learning easier and more effective [14].

The Planning Phase: Preparation for Future Learning

The usual entry point for the MAL process is the **planning** phase (Fig. 4.1), where a learner recognizes a gap in performance or knowledge and then determines the activities and resources they will use to close the gap. Common problems with the planning process can involve either an inability to recognize gaps or failure to create a credible plan using appropriate resources.

Recognizing gaps is complicated by weak self-assessment capacity. The literature shows that those with low ability are poor at self-assessment and tend to overestimate themselves. This cognitive bias (the "Dunning-Kruger effect") can necessitate reliance on external assessment at the beginning of the learning curve, often best mediated by a coach. With coached practice and improved self-assessment skills, our ability to recognize what we don't know can improve.

However, even with appropriate assessment abilities, planning can fail due to the inability to mobilize appropriate resources or methods. A learner may need a coach to help them engage in deliberate practice to push themselves to deeply understand a particular concept. Learners like Wyatt may previously never have broken down concepts into their component parts, deciding instead merely to re-read the material and memo-

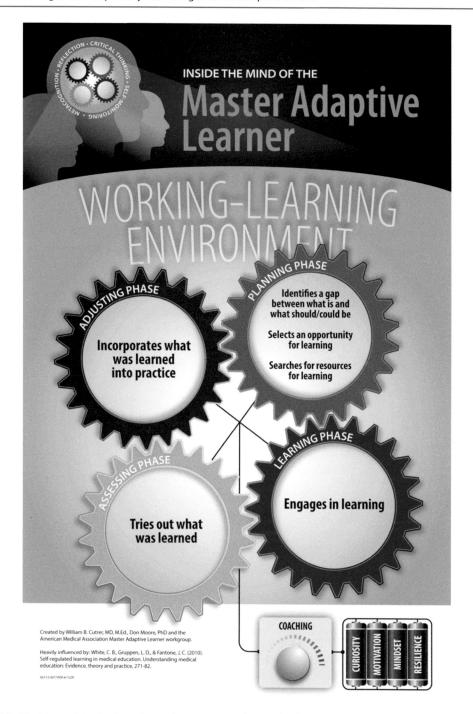

Fig. 4.1 The Master Adaptive Learning cycle is depicted as a set of four dependent gears, monitored by the coach at the bottom who moderates the driving batteries of curiosity, motivation, resilience, and mindset. All these processes occur within the learning environment. Used with permission [1]

rize superficial, easily-forgotten features or facts [15]. An effective coach can also conserve a learner's time. A novice such as Wyatt may need his coach to demonstrate evidence-based practices such as chunking the material and breaking down tasks [15]. Many trainees are unaware of the power of habits and how to harness their use for very successful learning [16].

In addition, many trainees fail to plan for the non-linearity of learning. The learning curve is a representation of the generally non-linear nature of progress or achievement over time. Consider Fig. 4.2, demonstrating the prototypical learning curve. At the beginning of a learning curve, on the left side, little progress in performance (y-axis) is seen initially. This is because the learner must become oriented to the task, spend time identifying resources, and learn how to best learn this subject matter.

Educators can work with all learners to foster a habit of adaptive expertise in early phases of learning [17]. For example, starting academic courses with authentic clinical problems and actively supporting reflective practice (sometimes with individual coaching) helps learners develop a tolerance for productive failure and uncertainty in clinical practice. Given that the health professions value supporting learner autonomy through graduated decreases, or fading in supervision, we must work hard to instill in our learners the self-coaching habits early in training.

The benefits of early investment in adaptive expertise development are hidden in the initial latent stages of the learning curve. However, this may be where remediation or coaching can have its greatest longer-term benefit. Early interventions have the potential to set the learner up for downstream learning success. In Table 4.1, we outline how a meta-cognitive approach can improve the conditions of learning all along the learning curve. We touch on these points in subsequent sections.

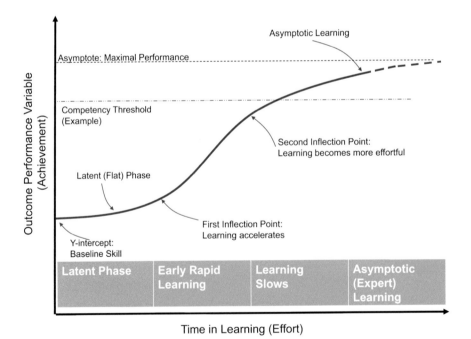

Fig. 4.2 Prototypical Learning Curve. A prototypical learning curve demonstrating how learning effort is related to learning outcomes. The implications of the successive phases are described in Table 4.1 and the accompanying text

Table 4.1 Opportunities for metacognitive intervention by phase of learning curve

Learning curve phase	Potential difficulties	Meta-cognitive question	Coaching/remediation
Latent phase	Inefficient orientation to the learning task	How can I quickly orient to a new learning situation?	Limit trial-and-error learning unless it is a productive struggle designed to promote future learning
	Suboptimal resources identified	What is an optimal resource?	Identify the best resources and why they are considered as such; critical appraisal.
	Lack of meta-cognition	How should I learn to learn?	Outline the learning path ahead, using the learning curve framework as organizing metaphor
	Inability to structure learning in terms of time or conditions	How do I best ration/prioritize my time?	Move from reactive to proactive time-planning
Early rapid learning	Intoxication by superficial approaches to learning	When should learning be rapid? When should it be desirably difficult?	Guide learning decisions based on longer-term retention rather than immediate gains
	Learning overly oriented to routinization	Is my goal routinized or adaptive expertise?	Create conditions for adaptive expertise including emphasis on deeper mechanisms, experience with variability, and productive failure
	Overconfidence (Dunning-Kruger effect)	How can I reliably assess my performance?	Calibrate the learner's insight into their performance with external measures
Inflection point—learning slows	Misinterpretation of slowing as achieving competency or mastery	I am not learning as quickly as I did before—how do I know when I'm done learning?	Explore what is meant by mastery in this domain, and across domains
Asymptotic learning	Misinterpretation of slowing of learning as a plateau where no further learning is occurring	What does expert learning look like?	Expert learning is slow, uncertain, and effortful. These features are to be celebrated, not avoided
	Fatalism as to the conditions of learning	How can I create the optimal conditions for expert learning?	Explain limits of Continuing Medical Education (CME) model; celebrate motivation, teamwork, curiosity, mindset, and resilience in learning

The Learning Phase: Aiming for Adaptive Expertise

There is explicit research evidence for how a learner should achieve their maximum potential [15]. Unfortunately, many learners inadvertently plan for the "illusion of knowing" with a preference for superficial and passive approaches: for example, reading, highlighting, and watching videos, without deeper reflection, to "efficiently" cover material. Furthermore, the ability to recognize more adaptive behaviors in oneself and know when to strategically apply them requires significant self-regulation and metacognition.

The core MAL concept for the **learning** phase is that a learner must become expert in their own learning by becoming familiar with the relevant core educational principles. Here we will highlight several of these—growth mindset, self-regulation, adaptive expertise—that are especially important to Master Adaptive Learning and how it is different from business as usual.

The metacognitive habit of leaning applied to challenging problems—rather than towards easier problems that display one's prowess—is a learned skill, characterized as the "growth mindset" [7]. Those who learn quickly without experiencing failure are generally worse off, as they do not develop the skill of rectifying failure [18]. In its cyclic nature, the MAL model proposes that, independent of intelligence and "so-called" talent [19], everyone needs an individualized approach for understanding their own learning.

Fundamentally, the difference between a novice and an expert is the degree to which the individual has developed self-regulatory behaviors that enable regular improvement. Self-regulation comprises a cyclical process reliant on self-efficacy, goal setting with self-observation, self-judgment, and self-reaction [8]. The process goes far beyond monitoring one's own tasks and into thoughts surrounding motivation and emotion [20]. While learners clearly must commit to self-regulation, teachers can also have a significant effect on their learners' self-regulation. Even career teachers may have difficulty conveying self-regulatory processes [21], suggesting that most teachers would benefit from professional development in modeling and coaching self-regulation [22]. Research has demonstrated that professional teachers can be taught these skills [23], with a large effect size both at the elementary level [24] and the collegiate level [25]. Whether

learner-initiated or facilitated by teachers, positive self-regulatory behaviors promote adaptation to different learning events and avoid maladaptive responses such as ruminating, focus on extrinsic motivators, and vacillating between different strategies [8].

Critical to becoming a MAL is the concept of **adaptive expertise.** In contrast to routine expertise [26], where extreme precision and efficiency are championed, adaptive expertise facilitates solving problems in novel ways, an inherently inefficient process [27]. This is not a dichotomous relationship: both routine expertise (efficient) and innovation (inefficient, tailored) are needed for the true adaptive expert (see Fig. 4.3). For example, a surgeon needs routine expertise to perform an uneventful procedure, but innovation to save a patient's life when a situation she has never seen before arises [28]. Thus, adaptive expertise is defined as a balance between innovation and efficiency, and knowing how to optimize the balance [14, 29]. To achieve this balance, the emphasis must shift from recognizing familiar

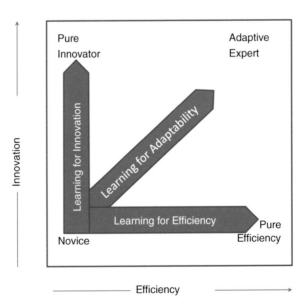

Fig. 4.3 Balancing efficiency in learning with the slow, deliberate learning for innovation necessary for all health professionals. This constant tension, induced by the health care environment's need for precision overlapping its need for constant problem solving, puts learners and experts in a state of always learning for adaptability. Research suggests that this requires very deliberate and time-intensive work by both the learner and coach [30]. Used with permission from [14]

situations in the current environment to adapting to the constantly changing environment.

There are two general approaches that a coach can take to guide a learner along the path of adaptive expertise: choosing problems that induce adaptive expertise and reinforcing adaptive approaches. Importantly, problems must include real-life ambiguity, allowing the learner to build not only an approach to the specific case under consideration, but also an approach to ambiguity. It is difficult to develop adaptive expertise based on a diet of clear-cut routinized cases. Case and practice variation have the beneficial effect of demonstrating the boundaries of adaptability. In approaching cases, highlighting deep underlying mechanisms is preferential to superficial recipes [29]. The coach can encourage the learner to voice their thought processes, thereby allowing them to clarify the learner's approach to a new problem. If the learner grasps at old scenarios to apply to the new, they must be consistently

coached longitudinally to become aware of and then eventually change this habit [14].

In Table 4.2, we compare "traditional learning models" with the adaptive expertise model and apply it to Wyatt's case [1].

We emphasize that this method moves learners from their more comfortable "zone of proximal development" [31] towards a more individualized curriculum with authentic settings and increased support. With the full support of a longitudinal coach and an environment where it is both psychologically and physically safe to fail, learners can take on much larger challenges than would be predicted in an unsupportive environment. This is different from traditional instruction for learning content (e.g., how to perform a lumbar puncture) and requires complementary coaching to support the development of self-regulated learning (e.g., how to adapt lumbar puncture skills in a patient with variant anatomy). As we are all consistently novices in some aspects

Table 4.2 Comparison of parameters of the traditional learning model and the adaptive expert. We have included ways that Wyatt could have been trained for adaptive expertise and avoided the harsh difference between his experiences in his undergraduate and medical school experiences

Parameter	Traditional learning model	Adaptive expertise	Improvements for Wyatt in the MAL framework
Emphasis	Learn well-known prototypes (illness scripts) efficiently	Develop expertise that can match any situation	*Wyatt experiences authentic clinical cases from day 1 of medical school, allowing him to learn how standardized illness scripts are applied in real clinical environments*
Unit of adaptation	Adapt environment to learner	Adapt learner to the environment	*Wyatt needs to move away from the safety of lectures and periodic multiple-choice exams. Ambiguous problems coupled with substantial metacognitive scaffolding would better prepare him for real clinical problems. This not only benefits struggling learners like Wyatt but trains every novice learner towards adaptive expertise*
Scaffolding	Keep learner in zone of proximal development [31]	Encourage learner to step out of comfort zone by emphasizing authentic complex challenges	*Learners need to have support not only for the content to be learned, but also for learning how to learn in difficult, uncertain contexts*
Progression	Progressively withdraw learning scaffolds or supports	Progressively add adaptive behaviors	*As time goes on, Wyatt can tolerate more uncertainty and more willingly adapt—but he needs to be challenged with increasing levels of ambiguity, likely with continuous, supportive coaching*
Endpoint	Fully withdraw scaffolds	None; continue long-term coaching for asymptotic improvement	*Wyatt assumes the identity of the Master Adaptive Learner: always striving to improve and learning to learn from the uncertainty inherent in clinical practice*

of our work as adaptive experts, the goal is to provide the support necessary to balance efficiency and adaptive behaviors to keep us in an "adaptability corridor" at all times [27, 32]. As we move towards self-directed learning and adaptive expertise, probably the single most important way to support the MAL cycle is to develop habits of self-assessment and feedback-seeking.

The Assessment Phase: Feedback Fuels the Self-Regulated Learner

The third phase of the MAL cycle is the **assessment** phase, wherein the learner candidly determines the success of their learning, asking three essential questions: "Have the goals I laid out been achieved?" "If I failed, can I learn from it?" "What information do I need to make this determination?"

Self-assessment can be painful, requiring relinquishing ego and perfectionism [33, 34]. Reframing this pain into metacognitive discipline may result in more productive habits and can transform one's identity [35, 36]. Seeking feedback is a habit that can be practiced [37]. Coaches and teachers can promote this habit in several concrete ways, including fostering a supportive environment that supports and celebrates learning from failure. With ample cognitive and emotional support, individuals can begin to see any failure as happening *for* them rather than *to* them [18]. In the face of failure, many learners have negative maladaptive thoughts, may become defensive and anxious, and may avoid feedback. By routinely and actively eliciting, empathizing with, and discussing learners' thoughts and feelings after failure, it may be possible to inculcate a productive habit of learning from failure, thereby fostering an individual's highest potential [38].

Teaching learners to seek feedback requires an environment infused with frequent data-rich assessments [39]. Professions are slowly shifting away from infrequent high-stakes summative assessments—mostly multiple-choice exams—towards more frequent but lower-stakes, multimethod assessments [40–42] that are timely and

constructed to help learners formulate future learning goals [4]. We recommend collecting multisource assessments in a portfolio [43] that is regularly and formatively reviewed with a coach who ensures that trainees reflect on their metacognition skills.

In our work with learners who struggle, educators must strive to model openness and non-defensive receipt of feedback. This requires admitting our own mistakes, acknowledging fallibility, and recognizing that we work in a fully interdependent environment. Demonstration of humility and introspection is associated with being a learner-centered educator [44]. These characteristics are also crucial to developing teamwork and quality improvement in the clinical realm and preventing medical errors [45]. Hosting effective feedback conversations takes training, time, and skill to execute because it is highly dependent on culture and context [46] (see Chap. 6).

> Using the MAL framework, we re-examined how Wyatt **planned** his learning, helping him to prioritize patient care rather than the next examination. As he engages in **learning**, we stressed the positive aspects of struggle in terms of depth and retention of learning. In **assessing** his learning, we noted development of the active habits of feedback-seeking and reflection. As Wyatt experienced more consistent success using these new approaches, he gradually rebuilt his confidence and began to inhabit his emerging medical professional identity formation.

The Adjustment Phase: Learning by Individuals as a Driver for Organizational Change

The first three phases of the MAL model, Planning, Learning, and Assessing, align with the precepts of Self-Regulated Learning, emphasizing individual improvement. The fourth **adjustment** phase considers how the individual intersects with the broader organization of people and resources around them [47]. The adjustment phase especially applies to learning by practicing clinicians, who can change the clinical microsystem around them and, by extension, influence the larger organization. But the adjustment phase also applies to the novice learner, highlighting the larger context of their individual learning. In fact, several organizational learning models (e.g., Senge's Five Disciplines [48]; Deliberately Developmental Organizations [49]) describe the expected mutual learning between the individual and the organization. Similarly, Rogers' Theory of Innovation Diffusion can be used to describe the variable capture of the hearts and minds of a population of learners—some being "early adopters," others as "laggards"—such that overall, an organization learns as its people do (Fig. 4.4). Remediation has its role to play in this process, not just in bringing "laggards" up to speed but also identifying and discussing critical issues raised in seemingly idiosyncratic stories to effect beneficial change for all.

All clinicians must find a balance between innovation and efficiency in their learning. Novices deserve support as they adjust to the clinical microsystem using new (to them), seemingly laborious, collaborative learning especially when compared to the highly efficient independent test-taking skills that may have dominated their prior experience with learning. The effective MAL appreciates their role in the larger learning trends that affect them [14]. This process of innovation becoming routine has been an underacknowledged, tacit aspect of clinical learning. In recent years, there is growing recognition that explicit consideration of the interaction of individuals with the larger system or organization can be beneficial for both. Whether labeled the "learning environment" [51], "clinical microsystem" [52], or health system science [53], all are applied manifestations of this adjustment phase between the individual and a larger structure.

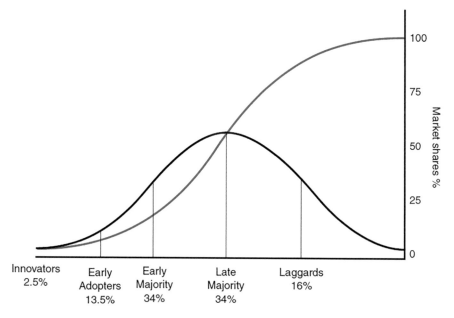

Fig. 4.4 The Rogers Innovation Curve approximates the first derivative of the learning curve suggesting that as a new technology or idea is taken up by a community, individuals vary in their propensity to adjust to their practice to the new method in a fashion that is approximately normally distributed (black curve). This adoption/adjustment process is a key driver of organizational learning (blue curve) [50]. In the Adjustment Phase of Master Adaptive Learning, the individual's relationship to larger learning trends is explicitly considered, to the benefit of both the individual and the organization. Taken with permission from [47]

Drivers of Metacognition and MAL: Curiosity, Motivation, Mindset, and Resilience

During medical school, Derek (he/him) spent much of his free time volunteering at a local free clinic. Prior to medical school, he had founded a very successful non-profit company that served low-income citizens. His compelling charisma and ability to tackle real-life problems, along with high incoming test scores and undergraduate grades, made him a desirable medical school candidate. He initially passed his medical school knowledge exams but had very little interest in the material. Over time, his engagement and performance on standardized exams started to falter, and his engagement during clerkships was low. Eventually, he failed a clinical clerkship. Derek came to remediation depressed and uncertain if he could succeed.

Focus on the critical drivers of metacognition and MAL—curiosity, intrinsic motivation, mindset, and resilience (depicted as batteries in Fig. 4.1)—can help learners perform better by strengthening metacognition and/or mitigating external factors. Because emotion drives self-regulation [20], external life stressors, structural racism, and threats to core identity can imperil our learners' success and the ability to engage in the MAL model (see Chap. 3). Stressors can also amplify feelings such as impostor syndrome and anxiety, common to many trainees. Derek's powerful "real-world" experience unfortunately did not prepare him emotionally or academically for the different challenges of medical school. The highly structured curriculum suppressed his innate curiosity and motivation. When he entered the more authentic practice of clerkships, depression overcame his resilience in the face of difficulty.

For learners who have fallen off the usual learning curve, the four MAL drivers move front and center. Unless those batteries are fueled, remediation attempts using the metacognitive lens necessary for the MAL process can fall flat. The coach (depicted as the rheostat, Fig. 4.1) must tune up their involvement in diagnosing these problems [54]. The MAL model suggests what a coach should pursue if learners disengage from the overall process. In remediation, Derek presented as a disinterested, minimally engaged medical student. However, a mentor recognized his potential and coached him (along with an appropriate referral for mental health support) to re-engage with the MAL process.

Curiosity drives the learner to notice a gap in understanding as an opportunity and, like the other MAL drivers, is considered both inherent and context-specific [39]. For Derek, the cognitive dissonance of fitting his identity into the medical world resulted in a maladaptive response to his learning environment. Reviving his curiosity required a multifaceted approach. Research demonstrates that curiosity is critical to the problem-solving process and necessary for empathy and humane practice in medicine [39]. Most medical curricula strive for efficiency and the necessity of a correct answer, which are known to diminish curiosity [55, 56]. Fortunately, many schools are moving towards problem-based and team-based learning, which promotes personal involvement and curiosity through exploring open-ended problems [57]. Furthermore, Derek was not finding the relevance he craved in medicine, dampening his curiosity. However, the cognitive dissonance he experienced in relating his identity as a resilient problem-solver to his medical studies offered a clue to a potentially successful remediation.

As the second driver of the MAL model, motivation fuels the impetus to initiate learning, set goals, and persevere to success, particularly in academic realms [58]. As the creative originator of a successful business Derek felt deep self-efficacy and autonomy, two important facets of intrinsic motivation [59], before medical school. He struggled with the extrinsic motivator of performance on multiple-choice exams. With coaching, he learned to rely more heavily on small-group work, where he excelled. He showed an advanced ability to tolerate the ambiguity of higher-level problem-solving, acquired in the uncertain realm of creating a successful business. This recognition renewed his interest and confidence in medical school. He then started to analyze his difficulty with multiple-choice exams, reframing it as a necessary challenge. Derek's previous experience fostered his implicit self-view that he could dig himself out of any hole and consistently improve. He fundamentally believed that he could work towards improvement, forged in the many small failures he consistently overcame in his previous career. With renewed motivation, he grew his belief that he could surmount this challenge through learning—relying on his robust growth mindset, the third driver of MAL.

Finally, Derek displayed the essence of resilience (see Chap. 18), the fourth driver of MAL, in adapting to his new environment despite significant adversity. A combination of coaching, small group problem-solving, and reflection enhances resilience [60]. Building on Derek's previously demonstrated resilience, these external interventions allowed him to recapture his identity as a problem solver and re-engage with the metacognitive practice of MAL. In fact, the very experience of struggle and remediation deepened his ability as a MAL, allowing his eventual success as a practicing physician.

Conclusion

Give someone a fish, and you feed them for a day. Teach them to fish, and you feed them for a lifetime – ascribed to Maimonides

We have described a framework rooted in sequential evidence-based learning processes governed by metacognition. The MAL process recognizes the struggle, planning, growth, and adaptation that we believe is the root of success not only in learning the health professions, but in *being* a health professional [14]. This process is not limited to "remediation" but rather applies to all learning, celebrating the struggle as core to how all human learning evolves.

While core knowledge and skills are the bedrock of effective clinical practice, we must now go further than previously expected and adapt to the changing clinical learning environment, where traditional learning models are only part of the equation. In fact, disparate uncoordinated approaches have never worked for the professional with a growth mindset, who needed to find ways to learn despite the formal curriculum. Recognizing the benefits of struggle—and learning how to learn—is a gift to all our learners.

References

1. Cutrer WB, Miller B, Pusic MV, Mejicano G, Mangrulkar RS, Gruppen LD, Hawkins RE, Skochelak SE, Moore DE Jr. Fostering the development of Master Adaptive Learners: a conceptual model to guide skill acquisition in medical education. Acad Med. 2017;92:70–5.
2. Thurstone L. The learning curve equation. Psychol. Review. 1919;34:278–86.
3. Ericsson KA, Krampe RT, Tesch-Römer C. The role of deliberate practice in the acquisition of expert performance. Psychol Rev. 1993;100:363–406.
4. Mylopoulos M, Brydges R, Woods NN, Manzone J, Schwartz DL. Preparation for future learning: a missing competency in health professions education? Med Educ. 2016;50:115–23.
5. Croskerry P. A universal model of diagnostic reasoning. Acad Med. 2009;84:1022–8.
6. Kahneman D. Thinking, fast and slow. New York: Farrar, Straus and Giroux; 2011.
7. Dweck CS. Growth. Br J Educ Psychol. 2015;85:242–5.
8. Zimmerman BJ. Self-regulated learning: theories, measures, and outcomes. In: International encyclopedia of the social & behavioral sciences. 2nd ed. Elsevier; 2015. p. 541–6.
9. Taylor MJ, McNicholas C, Nicolay C, Darzi A, Bell D, Reed JE. Systematic review of the application of the plan-do-study-act method to improve quality in healthcare. BMJ Qual Saf. 2014;23:290–8.
10. Kolb AY, Kolb DA. Learning styles and learning spaces: enhancing experiential learning in higher education. Acad Manag Learning Educ. 2005;4:193–212.
11. Kapp K, Thomas P. Which cognitive processes are involved in the Master Adaptive Learner? In: Cutrer W, Pusic M, editors. The Master Adaptive Learner. Philadelphia: Elsevier; 2020. p. 49–63.
12. Paunesku D, Walton GM, Romero C, Smith EN, Yeager DS, Dweck CS. Mind-set interventions are a scalable treatment for academic underachievement. Psychol Sci. 2015;2015(26):784–93.
13. Steenhof N, Woods NN, Van Gerven PWM, Mylopoulos M. Productive failure as an instructional approach to promote future learning. Adv Health Sci Educ. 2019;2019(24):739–49.

14. Pusic M, Cutrer W, Santen S. How does Master Adaptive Learning advance expertise? In: Cutrer WB, Pusic M, Gruppen LD, Hammoud M, Santen S, editors. The Master Adaptive Learner. Philadelphia: Elsevier; 2020. p. 10–8.

15. Brown PC, Roediger HL III, McDaniel MA. Make it stick: the science of successful learning. Cambridge, MA: The Belknap Press of Harvard University Press; 2014.

16. Duhigg C. The power of habit: why we do what we do in life and business. New York: Random House; 2013.

17. Mylopoulos M, Woods NN. When I say … adaptive expertise. Med Educ. 2017;51:685–6.

18. Kapur M. Productive failure. Cogn Instr. 2008;26:379–424.

19. Colvin G. Talent is overrated: what really separates world-class performers from everybody Else. New York: Portfolio/Penguin; 2008.

20. Lajoie SP, Gube M. Adaptive expertise in medical education: accelerating learning trajectories by fostering self-regulated learning. Med Teach. 2018;40:809–12.

21. Dignath C, Buettner G, Langfeldt HP. How can primary school students learn self-regulated learning strategies most effectively?. A meta-analysis on self-regulation training programmes. Educl research. Review. 2008;3:101–29.

22. ten Cate TJ, Kusurkar RA, Williams GC. How self-determination theory can assist our understanding of the teaching and learning processes in medical education. AMEE guide no. 59. Med Teach. 2011;33:961–73.

23. Ramsay CR, Grant AM, Wallace SA, Garthwaite PH, Monk AF, Russell IT. Statistical assessment of the learning curves of health technologies. Health Technol Assess. 2011;5:1–79.

24. Stoeger H, Ziegler A. Evaluation of a classroom based training to improve self-regulation in time management tasks during homework activities with fourth graders. Metacogn Learn. 2008;3:207–30.

25. Zimmerman B, Schunk D, editors. Handbook of self-regulation of learning and performance. New York: Routledge/Taylor & Francis Group; 2011.

26. Chi MTH, Feltovich PJ, Glaser R. Categorization and representation of physics problems by experts and novices. Cognitive Sci. 1981;5:121–52.

27. Schwartz DL, Bransford JD, Sears D. Efficiency and innovation in transfer. In: Mestre J, editor. Transfer of learning from a modern multidisciplinary perspective: efficiency and innovation in transfer. Greenwich, CT: Information Age Publishing; 2005.

28. Moulton CA, Regehr G, Lingard L, Merritt C, MacRae H. "Slowing down when you should": initiators and influences of the transition from the routine to the effortful. J Gastrointest Surg. 2010;14:1019–26.

29. Mylopoulos M, Kulasegaram K, Weyman K, Bernstein S, Martimianakis MA. Same but different: exploring mechanisms of learning in a longitudinal integrated clerkship. Acad Med. 2020;95:411–6.

30. Mylopoulos M, Regehr G. How student models of expertise and innovation impact the develop-ment of adaptive expertise in medicine. Med Educ. 2009;43:127–32.

31. Vygotsky L. Socio-cultural theory. Mind Society. 1978;6:52–8.

32. Pusic MV, Santen SA, Dekhtyar M, Poncelet AN, Roberts NK, Wilson-Delfosse AL, Cutrer WB. Learning to balance efficiency and innovation for optimal adaptive expertise. Med Teach. 2018;40:820–7.

33. Mann K, van der Vleuten C, Eva K, Armson H, Chesluk B, Dornan T, Holmboe E, Lockyer J, Loney E, Sargeant J. Tensions in informed self-assessment: how the desire for feedback and reticence to collect and use it can conflict. Acad Med. 2011;86:1120–7.

34. Sargeant J, Armson H, Chesluk B, Dornan T, Eva K, Holmboe E, van der Vleuten C. The processes and dimensions of informed self-assessment: a conceptual model. Acad Med. 2010;85:1212–20.

35. Duffy FD, Holmboe ES. Self-assessment in lifelong learning and improving performance in practice: physician know thyself. JAMA. 2006;296:1137–9.

36. Eva KW, Regehr G. Self-assessment in the health professions: a reformulation and research agenda. Acad Med. 2005;80:S46–54.

37. Croskerry P. The cognitive imperative: thinking about how we think. Acad Emerg Med. 2000;7:1223–331.

38. Deiorio NM, Carney PA, Kahl LE, Bonura EM, Juve AM. Coaching: a new model for academic and career achievement. Med Educ Online. 2016;2006(21):33480.

39. Dyche L, Epstein RM. Curiosity and medical education. Med Educ. 2011;45:663–8.

40. Driessen EW, van Tartwijk J, Overeem K, Vermunt JD, van der Vleuten CPM. Conditions for successful reflective use of portfolios in undergraduate medical education. Med Educ. 2005;39:1230–5.

41. West CP, Durning SJ, O'Brien BC, Coverdale JH, Roberts LW. The USMLE step 1 examination: can pass/fail make the grade? Acad Med. 2020;95:1287–9.

42. Chan T, Sebok-Syer S, Thoma B, Wise A, Sherbino J, Pusic M. Learning analytics in medical education assessment: the past, the present, and the future. AEM Educ Train. 2018;22:178–87.

43. Dannefer EF, Henson LC. The portfolio approach to competency-based assessment at the Cleveland Clinic Lerner College of Medicine. Acad Med. 2007;82:493–502.

44. Menachery EP, Knight AM, Kolodner K, Wright SM. Physician characteristics associated with proficiency in feedback skills. J Gen Intern Med. 2006;21:440–6.

45. Borrell-Carrió F, Epstein RM. Preventing errors in clinical practice: a call for self-awareness. Ann Fam Med. 2004;2:310–6.

46. Watling C, Driessen E, van der Vleuten CPM, Lingard L. Learning culture and feedback: an international study of medical athletes and musicians. Med Educ. 2014;48:713–23.

47. Pusic MV, Boutis K, Santen S, Cutrer W. How does master adaptive learning ensure optimal pathways to

clinical expertise? In: Cutrer WB, Pusic M, Gruppen LD, Hammoud M, Santen S, editors. The Master Adaptive Learner. Philadelphia: Elsevier; 2020. p. 174–92.

48. Senge P. The fifth discipline: the art and practice of the learning organization. 2nd ed. New York, NY: Random House; 2006.

49. Kegan R, Laskow LL. An everyone culture: becoming a deliberately developmental organization. Boston: Harvard Business Review Press; 2016.

50. Rogers EM, Adhikarya R. Diffusion of innovations: an up-to-date review and commentary. Ann Internat Commun Assoc. 1979;3:67–81.

51. Gruppen LD, Irby DM, Durning SJ, Maggio LA. Conceptualizing learning environments in the health professions. Acad Med. 2019;94:969–74.

52. Wong BM, Holmboe ES. Transforming the academic faculty perspective in graduate medical education to better align educational and clinical outcomes. Acad Med. 2016;91:473–9.

53. Gonzalo JD, Chang A, Dekhtyar M, Starr SR, Holmboe E, Wolpaw DR. Health systems science in medical education: unifying the components to catalyze transformation. Acad Med. 2020;95:1362–72.

54. Wolff M, Deiorio NM, Juve AM, Richardson J, Gazelle G, Moore M, Santen SA, Hammoud MM. Beyond advising and mentoring: competencies for coaching in medical education. Med Teach. 2021;43:1210–3.

55. Darley JM, Batson CD. "From Jerusalem to Jericho": a study of situational and dispositional variables in helping behavior. J Pers Soc Psychol. 1973;27:100–8.

56. Fitzgerald FT. Curiosity. Ann Intern Med. 1999;130:70–2.

57. Hidi S, Renninger K. The four-phase model of interest development. Educ Psychol. 2006;41:111–27.

58. Petri H. Motivation: theory, research and applications. 4th ed. Pacific Grove, CA: Brooks/Cole Publishing Company; 1996.

59. Deci EL, Ryan RM. Self-determination theory. In: Van Lange PAM, Kruglanski AW, Higgins ET, editors. Handbook of theories of social psychology: Volume 1. Newbury Park CA: Sage Publishing; 2012. p. 416–37.

60. Rogers D. Which educational interventions improve healthcare professionals' resilience? Med Teach. 2016;38:1236–41.

The Learner's Experience of Remediation

5

Lynnea Mills

Introduction

Dylan (he/him) is a first-year medical student who studied humanities as an undergraduate and does not have experience in the physical sciences beyond the premedical requirements. He has struggled on all of the multiple-choice exams thus far in medical school. His score on his first exam was one point above passing, and he failed the following two exams. Dylan attends all lectures, spends long hours studying, and makes use of all textbooks and recommended resources, but continues to get low scores.

In recent years, published work on remediation has grown significantly [1–5]. Much of this work centers around the identification of learners who struggle, methods to approach remediation planning, institutional policies for managing challenging remediation situations, and other "how-to's" for helping individuals like Dylan. There has been relatively little discussion of the learners' experience of remediation. While we should continue to study the techniques most likely to help Dylan improve his academic performance, we should also seek to appreciate how Dylan is affected by his test scores, how motivated he feels to change his approach, how invested he is in his future career, and why. Understanding the learner's lived experience of the process will greatly improve our ability to develop and individualize effective remediation interventions.

Being identified as "failing" or "behind" adds emotional challenges on top of the already-intense process of training to be a clinician. Going through a prescribed remediation process places additional burdens on learners, including spending time in remediation work outside their busy schedules, extending their schooling/training, delaying salary payments, or paying for courses or skill development. In this chapter, we explore what is already described in the remediation literature about learners' experiences, what we can extrapolate from work in other fields or contexts, and how we can use this information to move forward with more thoughtful and informed approaches.

What Learners Tell Us

We can summarize the findings of studies that describe learners' perspectives on remediation in three broad categories.

L. Mills (✉)
Department of Medicine, University of California, San Francisco, CA, USA
e-mail: lynnea.mills@ucsf.edu

Learners Prefer Active Remediation Approaches

Learners have described mixed feelings about the efficacy of remediation interventions. While some learners undergo remediation because it is required and do not perceive benefit, learners in multiple studies found the interventions helpful, ranging from improving preparation for clinical skills exams [6] to addressing gaps in prior training [7] and facilitating a transition from passive to active learning [8]. Experienced physicians reported experiencing significant practice change as a result of remediation, such as adjusting workload to decrease the risk of error [9]. Learners report a preference for small group activities and fieldwork [10], as well as simulation activities [11], for professionalism remediation. While these are early findings, we can conclude that learners appreciate active learning activities as part of a remediation plan.

Learners Recognize Skillful Remediation Coaches

Learners who recognize a need for growth desire a coach, rather than a cheerleader. They highly value remediation coaches who are honest and skillful facilitators [8], friendly but somewhat disciplinarian [12]. While it is likely that there is individual variability in what learners prefer, these few studies suggest they appreciate open and honest relationships with experienced remediation coaches who articulate high standards.

Learners Desire Attention to the Impact of Life Context and Emotions on the Remediation Process

Learners keenly feel and appreciate when explicit attention is placed on how their academic learning impacts their personal lives and emotions. In one study, learners felt that addressing personal life factors, in addition to focusing on specific skills, was essential to remediating low performance, and they would have preferred more attention to personal life factors and less focus on building knowledge [13]. Another study described a student who spoke of the need to "stop blaming myself and others and start blaming the process that I was using," as well as forming a positive identity around being "a repeater" [8]. (See below for more discussion of emotion, Chap. 4, and Epilogue.)

What Research Outside Remediation Tells Us

Several facets of the learners' experience are likely critical to remediation work.

Emotion

Emotion plays a significant role in learning. While emotion and cognition have historically been thought of as separate processes, we now understand them as complexly intertwined [14, 15]. For example, emotion mediates learners' ability to transition into the deeper conceptual understanding afforded by "threshold concepts," defined as core concepts that, once grasped, allow learners to instantly transform their thinking in a domain and enable deeper learning [16]. We also know that emotion directly impacts memory and cognitive performance during high-stakes work tasks; for example, anxiety and stress lead to impaired working memory and short-term recall but improved memory consolidation [17]. This is particularly salient in the health professions, where the work routinely involves high emotions.

Learners likely experience a range of intense emotions, both positive and negative, when faced with the need to remediate. Negative emotions such as shame [18] and fear [19] may lead to defensive reactions when learners are told they need remediation. However, anecdotally we know that positive emotions (e.g., relief, hope) may coexist, facilitating a learner's willingness to engage. In other areas of higher education, students who feel more positive emotions about learning are more likely to engage deeply with content than students who experience relatively more negative emotions [20]. In language learning, for instance, positive emotions facilitate uptake because they enable learners to open themselves to new perspectives [21]. Medical students, during their regular coursework, demonstrate an association between positive emotions and motivation to engage in learning [22]. Taken together, working to amplify positive emotions in remediation may improve learning. More research is needed to better understand how emotional reactions impact the outcomes of remediation.

Motivation and Feedback Responsiveness

Motivation has been explored extensively in health professions education (HPE), though infrequently in the remediation context. We do know that the source of motivation is important. HPE learners who are externally motivated (motivated by grades, desire to impress people, etc.) are less likely to do well in the remediation process than those who are internally motivated (motivated by a sense of altruism, mastery etc.) [23]. When learners have specific, personally meaningful goals that motivate them to invest academic effort, they are more likely to succeed when facing stumbling blocks like a disappointingly low performance [24]. Internal motivation and goal orientation also greatly impact learners' ability to receive and incorporate feedback, which is essential to remediation (see Chap. 4). Multiple studies in other disciplines, including management science, have investigated learner characteristics that influence feedback receptivity and uptake; these include the relationship with the feedback-giver, beliefs about the inherent value of feedback, self-awareness, and emotional regulation [25]. These factors likely also affect learners in health professions. A high degree of openness to feedback may imply that a learner has a growth mindset, which is presumed to be important to remediation (Chap. 4). Though recent meta-analyses have demonstrated that interventions to enhance growth mindset have

minimal impact on academic achievement [26], one key exception is "at-risk" learners (those with prior poor performance); in the remediation context, having a growth mindset likely enhances learners' ability to engage with the process and improve.

Insight/Accountability

Self-awareness is a key component of the self-regulatory process that allows learners to change their approaches and grow. Research indicates that this self-awareness, frequently referred to as "insight" in the remediation literature, is tied to, though distinct from, other metacognitive and emotional characteristics and processes described above. For example, without adequate insight into their struggles, even highly motivated learners are unlikely to make learning gains. We know that learners are often poor at self-assessing [27, 28], and research shows that underperforming learners tend to overestimate their performance [29]. This may manifest as confusion or surprise at objective measures of performance and may increase learners' difficulty in engaging with remediation. Outside of remediation, research shows that practicing physicians who struggle with an array of challenges, including medical errors and interpersonal conflict, often externalize responsibility for the struggle but see junior learners who do the same as lacking in insight [30]. Some scholars believe that lack of insight makes some learners, or at least some challenges, irremediable [31]. For professionalism lapses, lack of insight about the inappropriateness of the behavior and lack of taking responsibility is associated with greater rates of future lapses [32]. It is my personal experience that remediating learners who lack insight or accountability progress slowly.

Many successful remediation approaches depend on insight/self-awareness. For instance, approaches rooted in self-regulated learning theory, which emphasizes metacognitive processes that depend on self-awareness, show promise in remediation [33–35]. More work is needed in this area.

Academic Culture

The culture in which learners study or practice likely has significant impact on how they think and feel about their performance and help-seeking. The "summative assessment culture," in which learners perceive an emphasis on summative, rather than formative, assessment, creates an avoidance of failure [36]. In this culture, learners focus on passing assessments rather than developing their skills, and this behavior is exacerbated by interactions with others in the same culture [36]. This may mean learners reject information or feel bewildered when confronted with evidence of their low performance, heightening the emotions with which they approach remediation. This assessment culture also often shifts medical learners toward external motivation [24], which, as discussed above, can have further ramifications for their engagement and success with remediation. Similarly, an institutional "culture of excellence" emphasizes the academic strength of the community, making it harder for supervisors to give and for learners to receive modifying feedback [37], because it may seem to threaten the learner's identity as excellent. These cultural factors can significantly influence how learners perceive themselves and their expectations; therefore, these cultures likely significantly impede the success of growth processes like remediation.

Where Do We Go from Here?

The available evidence provides initial guidance for improving remediation by focusing on learners' experiences.

Normalizing/Destigmatizing the Process of Receiving Help

All clinical learning settings need to help members feel that receiving guidance on their performance is acceptable, normal, and even desirable. Normalizing the process of working deliberately and with assistance on one's skills would likely improve the success of remediation significantly [38]. *How* to destigmatize remediation is a more difficult question. Making intensive coaching and skill-building available to all learners, regardless of skill level, rather than just for those referred for remediation is one recommended approach. This emphasizes that everyone can improve and also decreases the stigma associated with receiving help. While there are cases in which efforts to destigmatize remediation actually worsen outcomes because learners may not appreciate the extent of their challenges [39], this can likely be mitigated through honest, data-driven coaching on learner skills.

A complementary approach might be to have respected role models openly seek help for themselves. For example, at my institution, a peer observation program helps faculty improve their skills while helping residents and students see that even their own attendings can welcome feedback and coaching. Seeing "high-performing" individuals, who they admire, seeking help may lower the barriers for all learners to seek and receive help.

How we frame and speak about remediation matters. Framing our offerings as supportive and meant to enhance learners' existing skills, rather than punitive, is likely to increase receptivity and engagement [40–43]. Taking this a step further, it may be time to stop using the word "remediation," which connotes correction of deficiencies or other noxious entities (given that, outside of education, remediation usually refers to removal of environmental toxins). In fact, the well-intentioned analogizing of clinical language to the learning setting (e.g., "diagnose" the learner) unnecessarily pathologizes learners. One proposed approach is to shift toward language common to athletic coaching situations, in which athletes' performance is described as not meeting a standard in relation to a particular event, but the athlete is not described globally as "deficient" or lacking [41].

An additional key to normalizing the process of receiving guidance is to decouple coaching from assessment. In many cases, the person or group assessing a learner's competence and progress is the same person or group overseeing the learner's remediation, creating a conflict of interest. For coaches and assessors to be completely separate reduces stress and enables learners to feel fully invested in learning and improvement, rather than simply jumping through an assessment hoop [38]. Even for clinicians post-training, who do not have routine workplace-based assessments, the roles of oversight and remediation are often linked. Institutional leaders often view remediation as a process of both fixing competency issues and alternately (or simultaneously) regulating behavior and performance for legal or policy purposes. This frame-shifting and lack of clear role delineation limit us from creating best practices for remediation [44] and likely also reinforce the misperception that remediation is punitive.

Time-variable education also promises to assist in normalizing both the process of help-seeking and the obvious but underappreciated idea that learners master content at different rates. Time-variability replaces the traditional time-delimited training period (e.g., 4 years for medical school) with a more flexible course that allows learners to progress at a rate that is most consistent with their skill development and personal life circumstances [45, 46]. Many institutions in the U.S. allow learners to pause or prolong their training in specific circumstances; making this option easier to access and treating it as a normal variation, rather than an exception or accommodation, would destigmatize students who take a time-variable approach to HPE. Even the way we label our learners can signal our expectations: it's common in the U.S. for students, immediately upon entering their training, to be cohorted with peers based on their expected graduation date (e.g., "Class of 2023"). A mentor of mine, who works at a time-variable medical training institution in the Netherlands, shared that, at his medical school, students are never described this way and are instead cohorted based on where they are in their current coursework, meaning students are much less likely to feel stigmatized if their trajectory varies from that of peers with whom they began school.

Gathering Information About Learners' Experiences

Many remediation programs begin with an intake process, wherein either the coach or another program representative speaks with the learner to understand the challenge and help set goals for the remediation work. This meeting may include an educational history and would likely further benefit from routinely incorporating additional questions targeted toward the learner's emotions and internal experiences (see Chap. 6). Answers to these questions can help the coach achieve a comprehensive sense of the learner's current state and assist both with providing support and tailoring the approach to the needs of the learner.

Explicitly Incorporating Emotion/Metacognition into Remediation Programs

We should consider how to help learners leverage adaptive emotions and mitigate maladaptive ones while implementing any remediation coaching program. We should be actively working to create programs that minimize shame, defensiveness, and similar emotions that learners experience [47]. We can also think about ways to cultivate insight within remediation programs, by asking learners to self-assess and then immediately afterward receive skilled feedback [48].

Bringing It All Together

Throughout the remainder of this book, you'll find evidence-based recommendations and practical guidance for coaching around a variety of skills, as well as information to help you think broadly about creating and managing remediation programs. At the center of all this work, of course, lies the learner. Further research will shed light on how best to incorporate the learner's perspective to improve remediation. Meanwhile, we can make explicit efforts to acknowledge and address the personal factors that impact learners, as well as working to normalize help-seeking behaviors and maximize metacognitive processes during remediation.

References

1. Boileau E, St-Onge C, Audetat M. Is there a way for clinical teachers to assist struggling learners? A synthetic review of the literature. Adv Med Educ Pract. 2017;8:89–97.
2. Chou CL, Kalet A, Joao Costa M, Cleland J, Winston K. Guidelines: the do's, don'ts and don't knows of remediation in medical education. Perspect Med Educ. 2019;8:322–38.
3. Heeneman S, Schut S. Meaningful mapping of remediation in longitudinal and developmental assessment models. Med Educ. 2020;54:866–75.
4. Shearer C, Bosma M, Bergin F, Sargeant J, Warren A. Remediation in Canadian medical residency programs: established and emerging best practices. Med Teach. 2019;41:28–35.
5. Warburton KM, Goren E, Dine CJ. Comprehensive assessment of struggling learners referred to a graduate medical education remediation program. J Graduate Medical Educ. 2017;9:763–7.
6. Myung SJ, Shin JS. Improvement of medical students' clinical performances after remediation program. Med Teach. 2012;34(4):338–9.
7. Swiggart W, Dewey C, Ghulyan M, Spickard AJ. Spanning a decade of physician boundary violations: are we improving? HEC Forum. 2016;28(2):129–40.
8. Winston KA, Van Der Vleuten CPM, Scherpbier AJJA. At-risk medical students: implications of students' voice for the theory and practice of remediation. Med Educ. 2010;44(10):1038–47.
9. Jolly J, Bowie P, Price J, Mason M, Dinwoodie M. Qualitative evaluation of an educational intervention to reduce medicolegal risks for medical doctors experiencing significantly more cases than their peers in the UK and Ireland. BMJ Open. 2018;8(4):e020838.
10. Findyartini A, Sudarsono NC. Remediating lapses in professionalism among undergraduate pre-clinical medical students in an Asian Institution: a multimodal approach. BMC Med Educ. 2018;18(1):88.
11. Guerrasio J, Aagaard EM. Long-term outcomes of a simulation-based remediation for residents and faculty with unprofessional behavior. J Grad Med Educ. 2018;10(6):693–7.
12. Winston KA, Van Der Vleuten CPM, Scherpbier AJJA. The role of the teacher in remediating at-risk medical students. Med Teach. 2012;34(11):e732–42.
13. Patel RS, Tarrant C, Bonas S, Shaw RL. Medical students' personal experience of high-stakes failure: case studies using interpretative phenomenological analysis. BMC Med Educ. 2015;15:86.
14. Pessoa L. On the relationship between emotion and cognition. Nat Rev Neurosci. 2008;9(2):148–58.
15. How emotions are made. Lisa Feldman Barrett. 2016. https://lisafeldmanbarrett.com/books/how-emotions-are-made/.
16. Irving G, Wright A, Hibbert P. Threshold concept learning: emotions and liminal space transitions. Manag Learn. 2019;50(3):355–73.
17. LeBlanc VR, McConnell MM, Monteiro SD. Predictable chaos: a review of the effects of emotions on attention, memory and decision making. Adv Health Sci Educ Theory Pract. 2015;20(1):265–82.
18. Bynum WE. Assessing for learner shame should be a routine part of remediation for unprofessional behavior. Acad Med. 2017;92(4):424.
19. Price T, Archer J. UK policy on doctor remediation: trajectories and challenges. J Contin Educ Heal Prof. 2017;37(3):207–11.
20. Trigwell K, Ellis RA, Han F. Relations between students' approaches to learning, experienced emotions and outcomes of learning. Stud High Educ. 2012;37(7):811–24.
21. MacIntyre P, Gregersen T. Emotions that facilitate language learning: the positive-broadening power of the imagination. Stud Second Lang Learn Teach. 2012;2(2):193–213.
22. Artino AR, La Rochelle JS, Durning SJ. Second-year medical students' motivational beliefs, emotions, and achievement. Med Educ. 2010;44(12):1203–12.
23. Thaxton RE, Jones WS, Hafferty FW, April CW, April MD, Self vs. Other focus: predicting professionalism remediation of emergency medicine residents. West. J Emerg Med. 2018;19(1):35–40.
24. Holland C. Critical review: medical students' motivation after failure. Adv Health Sci Educ Theory Pract. 2016;21(3):695–710.
25. Dahling JJ, Chau SL, O'Malley A. Correlates and consequences of feedback orientation in organizations. J Manag. 2012;38(2):531–46.
26. Sisk VF, Burgoyne AP, Sun J, Butler JL, Macnamara BN. To what extent and under which circumstances are growth mind-sets important to academic achievement? Two meta-analyses. Psychol Sci. 2018;29(4):549–71.
27. Chang A, Chou CL, Teherani A, Hauer KE. Clinical skills-related learning goals of senior medical students after performance feedback. Med Educ. 2011;45(9):878–85.
28. Dickson RP, Engelberg RA, Back AL, Ford DW, Curtis JR. Internal medicine trainee Self-assessments of end-of-life communication skills do not predict assessments of patients, families, or clinician-evaluators. J Palliat Med. 2012;15(4):418–26.
29. Srinivasan M, Hauer KE, Der-Martirosian C, Wilkes M, Gesundheit N. Does feedback matter? Practice-based learning for medical students after a multi-institutional clinical performance examination. Med Educ. 2007;41(9):857–65.
30. LaDonna KA, Ginsburg S, Watling C. Shifting and sharing: academic physicians' strategies for navigating underperformance and failure. Acad Med. 2018;93(11):1713–8.

31. Hays RB, Jolly BC, Caldon LJM, McCrorie P, McAvoy PA, McManus IC, et al. Is insight important? Measuring capacity to change performance. Med Educ. 2002;36(10):965–71.

32. Ainsworth MA, Szauter KM. Student response to reports of unprofessional behavior: assessing risk of subsequent professional problems in medical school. Vol. 23, Medical Education Online. Taylor & Francis Group; 2018. https://doaj.org.

33. Artino ARJ, Hemmer PA, Durning SJ. Using self-regulated learning theory to understand the beliefs, emotions, and behaviors of struggling medical students. Acad Med. 2011;86(10 Suppl):S35–8.

34. Sandars J, Cleary TJ. Self-regulation theory: applications to medical education: AMEE guide no. 58. Med Teach. 2011;33(11):875–86.

35. Andrews MA, Kelly WF, DeZee KJ. Why does this learner perform poorly on tests? Using self-regulated learning theory to diagnose the problem and implement solutions. Acad Med. 2018;93(4):612–5.

36. Harrison CJ, Könings KD, Schuwirth L, Wass V, van der Vleuten C. Barriers to the uptake and use of feedback in the context of summative assessment. Adv Health Sci Educ Theory Pract. 2015;20(1):229–45.

37. Ramani S, Könings KD, Mann KV, Pisarski EE, van der Vleuten CPM. About politeness, face, and feedback: exploring resident and faculty perceptions of how institutional feedback culture influences feedback practices. Acad Med. 2018;93(9):1348–58.

38. Kalet A, Chou CL, Ellaway RH. To fail is human: remediating remediation in medical education. Perspect Med Educ. 2017;6(6):418–24.

39. Deil-Amen R, Rosenbaum JE. The unintended consequences of stigma-free remediation. J Educ Sociol. 2002;75(3):249–68.

40. Cleland J, Cilliers F, van Schalkwyk S. The learning environment in remediation: a review. Clin Teach. 2018;15(1):13–8.

41. Bennion LD, Durning SJ, LaRochelle J, Yoon M, Schreiber-Gregory D, Reamy BV, et al. Untying the Gordian knot: remediation problems in medical schools that need remediation. BMC Med Educ. 2018;18(1):120.

42. Bourgeois-Law G, Teunissen PW, Regehr G. Remediation in practicing physicians: current and alternative conceptualizations. Acad Med. 2018;93:1638.

43. Kebaetse MB, Winston K. Physician remediation: accepting and working with complementary conceptualisations. Med Educ. 2019;53(3):210–1.

44. Bourgeois-Law G, Varpio L, Regehr G, Teunissen PW. Education or regulation? Exploring our underlying conceptualisations of remediation for practising physicians. Med Educ. 2018;53:276.

45. Carraccio C, Wolfsthal SD, Englander R, Ferentz K, Martin C. Shifting paradigms: from Flexner to competencies. Acad Med. 2002;77(5):361–7.

46. Frank JR, Snell LS, Cate OT, Holmboe ES, Carraccio C, Swing SR, et al. Competency-based medical education: theory to practice. Med Teach. 2010;32(8):638–45.

47. Chou CL, Chang A, Hauer KE. Remediation workshop for medical students in patient-doctor interaction skills. Med Educ. 2008;42(5):537.

48. Stirling K, Hogg G, Ker J, Anderson F, Hanslip J, Byrne D. Using simulation to support doctors in difficulty. Clin Teach. 2012;9(5):285–9.

A Stepwise Approach to Remediation for the Frontline Clinician-Educator

6

Archana Sridhar, Sara Rumrill, Calvin L. Chou, and Abigail Phillips

Introduction

This chapter seeks to provide clinician-educators with a framework for conducting remediation. We will first outline the overall process of remediation followed by a step-by-step process to intervene effectively with a clinical learner who struggles. In this chapter, we refer to the person undergoing remediation as the "learner" and to the educator tasked with remediation as the "coach." We use the term "coach" intentionally to signal that this educator's role is to guide learners by deepening their awareness and instilling motivation to enhance the growth of their knowledge and skills because it is their professional responsibility to do so.

We recommend remediating learners in four sequential phases, summarized in Box 6.1: *identification* of the learner and their struggles; *clarification* to determine the underlying reasons (including academic, nonacademic, individual, and curricular) for poor performance; a series of *interventions* to get the learner back on track; and *assessment*, of both the learner and the overall remediation process.

A. Sridhar (✉) · S. Rumrill · A. Phillips
Department of Medicine, Veterans Affairs Healthcare System, San Francisco, CA, USA
e-mail: archana.sridhar@ucsf.edu;
sara-megumi.rumrill@ucsf.edu;
abigail.phillips@ucsf.edu

C. L. Chou
Department of Medicine,
University of California, San Francisco, CA, USA

Veterans Affairs Healthcare System,
San Francisco, CA, USA
e-mail: calvin.chou@ucsf.edu

> **Box 6.1: Phases in the Remediation of the Learner Who Struggles**
>
> **Phase 1: Identification**
>
> - *Identify the area(s) where the learner exhibits inadequate performance*
> - *Acknowledge the learner's emotions, and commit to their success*
>
> **Phase 2: Clarification**
>
> - *Assess for systemic causes of suboptimal performance*
> - *Probe for individual factors that affect academic or clinical performance*
> - *Gather more information, directly observing the learner if at all possible*
>
> **Phase 3: Intervention**
>
> - *Collaboratively establish learning goals and choose assessment methods*
> - *Incorporate high-value interventions during remediation*

© The Author(s), under exclusive license to Springer Nature Switzerland AG 2023
A. Kalet, C. L. Chou (eds.), *Remediation in Medical Education*,
https://doi.org/10.1007/978-3-031-32404-8_6

Phase 4: Assessment

- *Assess the learner's progress*
- *Document all interventions, conversations, and progress*
- *Advocate for systemic change*

Phase 1: Identification

Identify the Area(s) Where the Learner Exhibits Inadequate Performance

Identification of the learner needing support typically occurs during the course or clinical assessments, whether formal (e.g., performance on examinations) or informal (e.g., observation on clinical rotations). Because of the complexity of clinical encounters, educators may identify a single or multiple competency area(s) of struggle. Initially, educators may have a vague sense that something is off-track or "not quite right" but may be unsure of how to proceed [1]. Subsequent sections, and Chaps. 7–16, will highlight various patterns of learner struggle. Alternatively, course or program directors may approach remediation coaches for expert guidance after pinpointing the domains of struggle.

Acknowledge the Learner's Emotions, and Commit to Their Success

In the first meeting with a learner who struggles, before delving into the business of remediation, we strongly recommend that the coach acknowledge and validate the learner's emotions. Learners who struggle seldom self-identify learning needs, and the need for remediation may come as a surprise [2, 3]. Understandably, their initial reaction is oftentimes negative, with shame predominating [4].

We suggest that the coach begin by briefly stating that it is their role to fully support the learner's growth and professional development, and clarifying that (ideally) this role is separate from making a high-stakes decision about the learner's standing in the educational program (see Chap. 2). The coach can then spend most of the remaining

Table 6.1 Examples of PEARLS© phrases to help build a safe, trusting coaching relationship

Sentiment communicated	Example phrases
Partnership	*"Let's work on this together"*
Empathy	*"I hear how unfair this feels to you"*
Apology	*"I am sorry that you are going through this alone"*
Respect	*"It takes a lot of courage to share this with me"*
Legitimization	*"Many students in your position would feel the same way"*
Support	*"I will do what I can to support you in developing your skills"*

time understanding the learner's emotions and perspectives around remediation. Often, learners will proactively express their emotions. If learners appear more guarded, it can be helpful for coaches to name an emotion they notice ("You seem upset about our meeting"), or to ask a direct question ("Many learners have emotions about undergoing a coaching process, and often they are negative emotions. How are you feeling, emotionally, about our meeting?"). In all cases, the goals are to listen much more than talk, and to avoid jumping into offering advice or technical solutions to the learner's struggles. While creating this space for the learner to voice their emotions may take significant time and energy, it helps the coach to better understand the learner's perspective, establishes trust, and encourages vulnerability and openness to feedback (see Chap. 5). Table 6.1 contains example phrases, using the PEARLS© framework for communication, that can help build a psychologically safe, trusting coaching relationship [5].

The second goal of the initial meeting is to work toward shifting the learner's perspective on remediation from a punitive intervention to a supportive, growth-oriented journey. After acknowledging the learner's emotional reactions, the coach may then help the learner articulate and clarify their core values and strengths on which to build. This appreciative approach to coaching redirects the focus of the conversation from the learner's failings toward building confidence that improvement is likely, thereby motivating the learner to participate productively in the process [6]. Evidence suggests that learners who invest themselves in remediation continue to derive benefits beyond the end of the remediation period [7].

At the conclusion of the initial meeting, we recommend that the coach outline next steps in the process. This includes frequency of meetings, responsibilities of the coach, and expectations of the learner. The coach should also discuss what can and cannot be kept confidential, and what they are ultimately obligated to report to those who will determine the consequences of the remediation.

Box 6.2 contains an example of an initial conversation between a learner and coach. In this vignette, the learner who struggles exhibits reactions commonly seen in trainees who are told they require remediation: denial, externalization, and defensiveness. Although the decision to remediate a learner is made after multiple clinical supervisors have raised performance concerns, this learner has only heard corrective feedback from one, further complicating the coach's task. Through supportive questioning, coaches can gradually help learners develop insight. Do not expect to accomplish this fully in one meeting: attending to the learner's emotions will be a recurrent theme throughout remediation.

Box 6.2: Example of an Initial Encounter Between a Coach and Learner Embarking on Remediation

Coach: *Good morning, Jake. You have been referred to me because your teachers report that you are struggling with organization and patient care skills. My goal is to try to help you achieve your own goals. I'd like to spend most of this meeting checking in with you about how you're feeling. Then, I'd like to end with what you can expect from me during this process. How does that sound?*

Learner: *Sure, that's fine.*

Coach: *Can I begin by asking you to talk about your understanding of why you were referred to me?*

Learner: *Well, I'm not sure I understand fully. My program director told me I needed remediation, which I think is pretty extreme, and honestly, I disagree. I know that my preceptor in clinic mentioned a lot of stuff to me that she was unhappy about,* but I feel that I get along well with other attendings, and no one else has said anything to me about how I'm doing.

Coach: *I hear how unexpected this news is for you.*

Learner: *Yeah. It also feels unfair and subjective.*

Coach: *I definitely see that you feel the process has been unfair. (brief pause) Tell me more about your interactions with your clinic preceptor.*

Learner: *Well, one day she sat me down after clinic and went through a patient note with me. She was pretty harsh and nit-picky about what I wrote. I think I get along really well with my patients and they like me a lot, so I was surprised by the conversation. I've felt really on edge when I precept with her—I think she hates me, or she's going through something personal and taking it out on me.*

Coach: *It sounds like you value your ability to establish rapport with your patients, and it was hard to hear her critical feedback.*

Learner: *Yeah. I mean, I understand what she was saying. I didn't provide a lot of differentials. And my note was disorganized. I've always had a problem with organization. And I'm just not as fast with writing notes as everyone else. But I don't think my notes are so bad that I need remediation.*

Coach: *You seem to have done a lot of thinking about this. Can you tell me more about what you meant when you said, "I've always had a problem with organization"?*

Learner: *Uh, yeah. Things have always taken me a little longer. Especially writing and focusing.*

Coach: *I see. How have you overcome this in the past?*

Learner: *It's never really been an issue until now. I think in medical school we only had to see one or two patients at a time, but now I'm seeing 5 or more patients in a half-day of clinic and on the wards. It's just* hard to get everything done on time. At the end of the day, my mind is buzzing about what I forgot to do, I can't sleep, and I'm even less focused the next day because I'm so sleep-deprived. I've been feeling really tired lately, but I figured that was just normal for residency.

Coach: *It sounds like it has been hard juggling all of the additional responsibilities on your plate. I am glad you told me about this. It takes a lot of courage to admit when things are hard. Are you dealing with this on your own?*

Learner: *I guess I haven't really told anyone about it until now. And every resident is sleep-deprived, so I figured what I was going through was normal.*

Coach: *I want to work with you so that you start to feel more successful in your work. You've already touched on this a bit, but what are some strengths that you currently bring to your work?*

Learner: *Well, like I said, I care a lot of about my patients. I think they see that, and I form good relationships with them.*

Coach: *It sounds like being able to provide empathic care to your patients is one of your core values. Showing empathy and building strong relationships with patients is an area where many doctors struggle. It's terrific that you already feel adept at this skill so early in your training.*

Learner: *Yes. It's why I wanted to be a doctor.*

Coach: *It is really important to keep this in mind when things get tough. Thank you for being open and honest about what you've been going through—now I have a better understanding of where you're coming from. Jake, let's work together to make sure you become the best doctor you can be. I'd like to give you a brief overview of what you can expect moving forward, okay?*

Phase 2: Clarification

The next three steps comprise the clarification phase of remediation. Multiple factors can contribute to suboptimal performance, including both systems-level considerations and circumstances unique to the individual learner. Table 6.2 summarizes these factors and suggests how a coach may elicit this information from a learner who struggles.

Assess for Systemic Causes of Sub-optimal Performance

Systems-level factors include implicit race and gender bias (see Chap. 3) or outright hostile work environments that result in the differential treatment of learners. For example, a training environment where men are given more opportunities to perform procedures compared to women, because of a prevailing belief that they are better at these types of activities or enjoy them more, may result in less procedural competence among women. In turn, women may internalize the message that they are less competent in procedures compared to men and avoid subsequent procedural opportunities, further widening the performance gap. Examples of this phenomenon, known as stereotype threat, clearly pervade the clinical learning environment. Faculty members and program leadership should continually monitor and assess for factors that contribute to or directly manifest as performance differences among learners.

By uncovering systems-level factors contributing to trainee performance, the remediation coach can be a powerful advocate for structural improvement in the academic learning environment. Systems-level contributors require thoughtful and comprehensive responses by academic leadership. Examples of structural improvements include curriculum revision, modification of assessment methods to eliminate bias, the institution of widespread faculty development, and/or modification of a working environment that is unsafe or harmful to learners.

Table 6.2 Factors affecting clinical performance

Factor	Examples of performance manifestation	Questions the coach may ask to elicit information about these factors
Systems-level factors affecting clinical performance		
Implicit bias Toxic work environment	Guardedness, passivity, helplessness, cynicism, apathy	*"I wish I didn't have to ask this question and that our learning environment was optimized for everyone. Have you ever felt like you have been treated differently or unfairly based on your gender, race, or other factors that are beyond your control?"* *"The culture of medicine has a long way to go as far as establishing an environment of diversity, equity, and inclusion. Faculty, staff, and peers can harbor implicit biases with negative effects on learners. Can you think of a situation where you were personally affected by implicit bias, micro-aggression, or discrimination?*
Individual factors affecting clinical performance		
Mental health		
Depression	Impaired motivation or concentration, tardiness, or inconsistent performance	*"Depression and anxiety are common among physicians and medical students. Our jobs are hard. I want to make sure I ask: do you think this applies to you?"*
Anxiety	Excessive stress around test-taking or when directly observed, such as when giving oral presentations	*"Sometimes people have difficulty with their emotions at work based on past experiences with trauma. Is this something that resonates with you?"* *"I'd like to ask you some more sensitive questions about your habits outside of work. Would that be okay with you?"*
Post-traumatic stress disorder (PTSD)	Impaired executive functioning and inconsistent clinical performance, emotional volatility	*"Lapses in professionalism are sometimes caused by a dependence on alcohol, opiates, or other substances. Is this something you struggle with, or have struggled with?"*
Substance use disorders	Absenteeism, tardiness, poor concentration at work, professionalism lapses	
Distraction or deprivation		
Sleep	Difficulty focusing at work, absenteeism, poor organizational skills, inconsistent performance, professionalism lapses	*"What are you managing outside of work?"* *"What are your stressors outside of work?"* *"Do you have access to food and a safe place to live? Do you run short of money by the end of the month? Do you ever feel unsafe at home or in school?"*
Economic stress		
Family responsibilities or interpersonal violence		
Disability and Difference		
Attention deficit disorder (ADD)	Poor organizational skills, difficulty following through on tasks	*"Do you feel you have to work harder than others organizing your day, responding to emails, and staying on track with tasks?"*
Autism-spectrum condition	Challenges with interpersonal communication	*"Do you feel you have to work harder than others to build rapport with patients and other staff members?"*
Dyslexia	Difficulty and slowness in processing written information	*"Do you struggle to convey your emotions or empathy to others?"*
Dyscalculia	Difficulty and slowness in interpreting and processing numerical data	*"Do you feel it takes you longer to process written information or numbers?"*

Probe for Individual Factors That Affect Academic or Clinical Performance

Factors affecting performance that are unique to the individual learner include life stressors, learning differences, and/or previously diagnosed or undiagnosed mental health conditions (see Chap. 17). These are prevalent in learners who struggle and frequently contribute to sub-optimal clinical performance [2]. Establishing a trusting relationship will increase the likelihood that a learner will share non-academic challenges affecting performance as early as in the first meeting with the coach. More often, however, these issues are revealed over time as trust in the coaching relationships builds.

Assessing for external factors helps the coach understand and work with the learner more effectively (see Chap. 2). Referring the learner to appropriate parties, such as program directors, learner wellness resources, or deans, can connect the learner with necessary accommodations and support during remediation, increasing their likelihood of academic success. In the case of suspected but undiagnosed learning differences, evaluation by a learning specialist is recommended (see Chap. 17). Learners struggling with substance use disorders or significant illness may need to be temporarily excused from clinical responsibilities to engage in treatment before returning to work or school.

It is important to note that coaches may unconsciously lower their expectations of learners after uncovering external factors. For example, a coach may be more willing to excuse performance lapses after hearing about a learner's past experiences with trauma or challenging life circumstances. While seemingly compassionate, this leniency bias may risk limiting the learner's professional growth in the long term. Coaches must be aware of this potential bias, seek advice from colleagues if needed, and attend to investing in the learner's success during remediation.

Gather More Information, Directly Observing the Learner If Possible

Coaches obtain data on learners' performance from a variety of sources. These include end-of-rotation global rating scales, informal "feed forward" comments by other faculty, incident reports, and test scores. These sources are helpful, but also have limitations: they may provide incomplete information, underreport or gloss over serious struggles, and be subject to bias [3, 8–10]. The medical education literature suggests that direct observation of the learner is the most effective way to understand their area of struggle [7, 11, 12]. We recommend evaluating the learner in more than one setting or context, including reviewing performance across different rotations through direct observation, written notes, and conferences. Direct observation clarifies and corroborates written documentation of the learner's performance and gives the coach a clearer and more authentic understanding of the learner's needs for future growth.

Having obtained and reviewed reliable performance data, the coach can identify which specific competency area or skill requires remediation. The Accreditation Council for Graduate Medical Education (ACGME) identifies six competency areas [13] for medical learners, which are summarized in Table 6.3. In a review of learners at all levels referred to a remediation program from 2006 to 2012, medical knowledge, patient care (specifically clinical reasoning), and professionalism were the most common competency areas requiring remediation [2].

Learners who struggle commonly have weaknesses in more than one domain [2], which can feel overwhelming for both the coach and learner. Initially, the coach and learner may choose to focus on remediating 1–2 competency areas at a time before building on additional skills. For example, a learner may struggle with medical knowledge, clinical reasoning, time management, and organization. The coach and learner may choose, in this scenario, to focus on improving medical knowledge and time management

Table 6.3 Description of the ACGME competency areas

ACGME competency area	Description
Medical knowledge	Basic understanding of illness scripts, pathophysiology, diagnostic testing, and therapeutic interventions
Patient care	Clinical skills such as history-taking, physical examination skills, procedural skills, clinical reasoning, and time management and organization
Interpersonal and communication skills	Ability to receive and communicate information meaningfully to patients, peers, and ancillary staff
Professionalism	Behaviors and attitudes including reliability, accepting responsibility for tasks, treating others with respect, and exhibiting integrity and honesty
Systems-based practice	Awareness of how to utilize the complex healthcare system to ensure safe and effective healthcare delivery, including attention to quality, safety, and transitions of care
Practice-based learning and improvement	Ability to receive feedback and data on performance and implement changes to improve one's practice over time

skills initially; subsequently, they can emphasize clinical reasoning skills. For other learners, focusing on a few areas simultaneously may allow for more rapid improvement in overall performance.

Phase 3: Intervention

Collaboratively Develop Learning Goals and Assessment Methods

Once the focus of remediation is clear, the next step is to collaborate with the learner to develop learning goals and create an Individualized Learning Plan (ILP). As discussed in Phase 1, we recommend that the coach begin this process by asking the learner to describe their strengths and

core values, and then inquiring about their hopes for future academic success. Ask the learner to articulate one learning goal in their own words, and then work with them to iteratively refine that goal to make it specific, measurable, attainable, relevant, and timebound ("SMART"). Through dialogue and active listening, the coach can encourage the learner to reflect on feedback they have previously received and choose learning goals that address the identified challenges. Guiding the learner to take ownership of their learning in this way helps build insight and self awareness (see Chap. 16). Taking time to define SMART goals enables assessment of progress and improvement.

After defining the learning goals, the coach must work with the learner to develop a plan and accountability for achieving them. The core question here is, "How will you know that you have achieved this goal?" Some competencies are relatively straightforward to assess. For example, one can assess medical knowledge through performance on knowledge tests or other methods of direct examination. Patient care competencies may be assessed by preceptor observation and evaluation. Other areas, such as professionalism, are trickier (see Chap. 14). It is good practice to collaboratively define appropriate forms of assessment early in the development of the remediation plan [14, 15]. Finally, it is important to have an honest and transparent discussion with the learner about the possible consequences if they do not achieve the goal within the specified time period.

When all of this has been completed—setting SMART goals, articulating the assessment method(s), and outlining potential outcomes—we recommend that the coach share the content of the conversation with the learner in writing, preferably in the form of an ILP. This ensures that there is clarity and transparency between the coach and learner about the remediation process. It also provides documentation that programs and institutions must track to demonstrate learner readiness for graduation and independent prac-

Table 6.4 Components of an Individualized Learning Plan (ILP), with examples of learning goals and assessment methods

| Area requiring remediation | Examples of collaborating on the learning goal | | | Examples of assessment methods |
	Initial learner-generated learning goal	What data indicate that this should be my learning goal?	SMART learning goal after refining with coach	How will we know if my goal is achieved by the end of remediation?
Medical knowledge	*I will improve my medical knowledge*	*Low examination scores on board exams. Clinic preceptor noted lack of knowledge on the management of diabetes and hypertension on my evaluation.*	*I will be able to describe the presentation, diagnosis, and management of common conditions encountered in a primary care clinic (list included).*	*I will improve my score in the General Medicine section of the in-training exam to the 50th percentile. My 3 clinic preceptors will evaluate my medical knowledge at the end of remediation and will attest to my knowledge of chronic disease management.*
Time management and organization (patient care)	*I will be able to care for 8 patients in the wards*	*My senior resident has to take over my presentations on rounds because I do not have data available. Recent evaluation stated that "I could not be relied on to complete tasks without reminders."*	*I will be able to collect vital signs, labs, and examine 8 patients before rounds. I will be able to complete notes and tasks by 5 pm each day. I will not require reminders to complete tasks.*	*I will have notes done and leave the hospital by 5 pm at least 75% of the time. Evaluations by clinical supervisors at the end of the remediation period will attest to my preparedness on rounds and the fact that I do not require reminders to complete tasks.*
Clinical reasoning (patient care)	*I will provide well-reasoned clinical management for patients I see on the wards and in clinic*	*Feedback on the quality of my assessment and plans from clinic and recent wards rotation.*	*I will include at least three diagnoses on my differential for each new problem on my in-patient history and physicals. I will explain my thought process for the differential diagnosis I provide.*	*Evaluation by clinical supervisors, who will review my notes and evaluate the clinical reasoning in my assessment and plans on a rubric.*

tice (see Chaps. 20, 26, 29). Table 6.4 highlights the main components of an ILP, describing the process of creating learning goals and determining assessment methods.

Incorporate High-Value Interventions During Remediation

Each remediation plan should be individualized and meaningfully designed to help the learner achieve the specific learning goals they have identified. While subsequent chapters in this book will describe interventions aimed at remediating specific competency areas, we recommend including the following high-value practices in all successful remediation plans.

Meet Regularly with the Learner

Remediation is a time-intensive endeavor. To be effective, a coach must ensure that they have the time and capability to sincerely commit themselves to the learner's success. In one study, learners who struggled required, on average, close to 20 hours of dedicated faculty time during remediation [2]. Some learners will require more time and support than others. Because learners may struggle with insight, time management, initiative, and the stigma of remediation, the coach may need to organize the first few meetings rather than relying on the learner to initiate them. But once scheduled, the content of the meetings should be co-owned by the coach and learner. They should focus on reviewing and refining individualized learning goals, giving high-quality feedback, and improving skills in self-regulated learning.

Encourage Self-Regulated Learning Skills

Learners who struggle may use maladaptive coping strategies when they encounter challenges. They are more likely to externalize reasons for failure, attribute their lack of success to factors that are unchangeable and therefore not worth addressing (e.g., "I'm just not a good test-taker"), or spend more time using the same ineffective study strategies rather than adopting new behaviors to achieve greater success. Coaches can reset these tendencies by framing failure as normal and an opportunity to reflect, make changes, and build new skills. According to self-regulated learning (SRL) theory, this approach empowers learners to build self-efficacy, a strong internalized sense of confidence in their ability to achieve success (see Chap. 4).

SRL is defined as a cyclical process where learners engage in specific goal-directed thoughts and behaviors, self-monitor their progress, and adapt their actions based on reflection to achieve individual learning goals [16]. There are three phases in which the cycle unfolds: (1) before ("forethought"), (2) during ("performance"), and (3) after ("self-reflection"). Table 6.5 describes the major activities that occur in each of the phases.

Each SRL phase contains several key processes. Table 6.6 defines these processes and also contains questions the coach can ask to promote meaningful dialogue around goal-setting and adaptive behavior change relevant to each process [17]. Effective coaches engage learners in these cycles by doing a lot of curious (rather than

Table 6.5 Self-Regulated Learning (SRL) phases and associated activities

SRL phase	Activities
Before ("forethought")	Goal setting, planning specific steps towards achieving a goal. The preparation and motivation required to act
During ("performance")	Actual actions and real-time monitoring and modifications that are executed based on the planned strategy established in the "forethought" phase
After ("self-reflection")	Review of the "performance" phase and description of the changes made to the original strategy to ensure the initial goal was achieved

interrogative) questioning. This entails reflecting the content and emotion of what the learner says without prematurely sharing the coach's own critique, analysis, or anecdotes, and encouraging the learner to uncover individual goals, self-monitor progress, and make adaptive changes. The theoretical underpinning for these processes is outlined in detail in Chap. 4.

Building the learner's self-efficacy, defined as an intrinsic sense of confidence that they can achieve a task and overcome challenges, is central to SRL. The coach may assess self-efficacy during the "before" phase and again during the "after" phase of the SRL cycle for comparison.

Provide High-Quality Feedback

We believe that framing feedback conversations in the SRL model helps learners develop internal motivation and lifelong skills in performance improvement that apply well beyond the remediation period. Effective feedback is an essential component of remediation. Leaders in medical education often lament that direct and accurate feedback is seldom given to learners who struggle by frontline clinician-educators who supervise them [3, 18]. To mitigate the perceived severity of their judgment, supervisors may gloss over or talk around areas of concern while overemphasizing positive comments [19]. Some supervisors choose not to give undesirable feed-

Table 6.6 Self-Regulated Learning (SRL) phases and processes, with examples of questions and responses the coach may pose to the learner to encourage reflection and provide feedback (adapted from [17])

SRL phase	SRL process	Definition of process	Example questions the coach may ask the learner to assess the process	Goal of feedback	Example responses the coach may pose to the learner in a feedback discussion
Before	Goal-setting	Steps towards achieving the desired goal should be specific and measurable	*"What learning goals do you have in mind to help you…"*	Ensure goals are SMART (specific, measurable, attainable, relevant, time-bound)	*"Let's discuss ways to make this goal more specific and measurable."*
	Strategic planning	Specific strategies or techniques (such as memorization of procedures) to help learners monitor and regulate their progression through the task	*"What do you think are the next steps needed to accomplish…"*	Encourage learners to create strategies and organize a plan for their goals	*"I noticed you might be skipping a few steps towards goal A. Let's discuss how we can fill in those gaps."*
During	Self-monitoring	Adapting and changing their strategies by constantly checking in on their progress towards achieving their desired goals	*"What are your thoughts about what you tried?"*	Encourage learners to think about their progress	*"You mentioned to me that you felt hesitant, because you weren't sure if your strategy would be effective in this scenario. Let's discuss how we can adjust your strategy for future cases."*
After	Self-evaluation	Critical reflection and incorporation of feedback through writing or question-asking to improve future performance	*"What happened that made you feel that it was successful/ unsuccessful?"*	Prompt learners to think about what outcomes they desire for their goals	*"Do you think you have performed well thus far or have you made any mistakes?"*
	Attribution beliefs	Learner's specific beliefs about the causes of their performance (e.g., ability to identify and acknowledge their own mistakes instead of blaming factors outside of their control)	*"Why do you think that you could not achieve…"*	Encourage learners to reflect on their own efforts, abilities, and mistakes	*"Based on what you told me, I would recommend thinking about how to improve the ability to…"*
	Adaptive changes	Learner's ability to adjust their approach during real-time tasks to improve their performance. Best utilized after a poor performance	*"What do you need to do to become successful on your next attempt?"*	Encourage learners to think about changing their strategy	*"What would you have done differently if you had to try again? Why would you choose to do that differently?"*
Before and after	Self-efficacy	The extent to which an individual feels confident about whether they can achieve a task	*"How confident are you in doing…"*	Identify baseline confidence to compare after intervention	*"Let's come up with a plan to increase your confidence moving forward."*

back altogether, instead directing concerns to third parties. In the end, what is heard by the learner may not accurately reflect the true assessment of their performance. These tendencies, grounded in the understandable desire to avoid uncomfortable conversations, hinder successful course correction and remediation. This section describes a framework to help the clinician-educator host effective feedback conversations with all learners, whether they struggle or not [20].

Set Up for Success

Much of the work in establishing a safe environment for difficult conversations has already occurred at the beginning of remediation (Phases 1–2). For meaningful feedback to occur, the coach must create a safe space where the learner expects to hear feedback, reflect on their performance, and collaborate on future performance goals. Coaches should share these objectives with the learner in advance of or at the outset of each meeting. In addition, coaches should optimize the meeting time so that learners can candidly engage in a thoughtful conversation. A trainee who has just worked a 24-hour shift or is grappling with a traumatic day on clinical service is almost certainly unable to engage in a productive feedback conversation. While it is impossible to control for all the factors that may adversely affect the emotional state of both the learner and coach prior to a feedback meeting, certain factors, such as sleep and time, can be addressed to ensure a productive session.

Observe the Learner

As mentioned above, direct observation of the learner is the most effective method of acquiring knowledge of their performance. Coaches should conduct observations with close attention to the specific learning goals or competency areas requiring remediation. We recommend paying particular attention to, and if possible, scribing, specific behaviors or reactions that the observer

sees or hears. This helps to minimize subjectivity when hosting the feedback conversation and reduces the risk of the learner perceiving the feedback as unfair, subjective, or judgmental. As human beings, it is impossible not to create judgments from observations. Our strong recommendation is for coaches to use information about feelings or inferences as starting points for deeper reflection and analysis about what specific behaviors created those judgments [21].

In practice, coaches may not have time to directly observe learners on a regular basis and may instead rely on written documentation submitted by other clinical supervisors. In this scenario, it is important that the narrative comments submitted to the coach are behaviorally specific, accurate descriptions of observations rather than interpretations of the learner's intentions. The potential for bias and subjectivity in using such proxy data can be mitigated by committing to widespread faculty development on feedback and narrative evaluation at your institution (see Chap. 19).

Ask for the Learner's Self-Assessment, Initially Focusing on What They Did Effectively

After the observation, the coach may prompt the learner to reflect on their performance. When discussing written documentation submitted by another supervisor, ask the learner to read the comments and offer their reflections or perspective. To elicit critical reflection, we recommend asking *specific* questions of the learner. Clinical supervisors commonly ask, "How do you think that went?" This type of open-ended question risks veering the feedback conversation off the focus of learning. Specific questions targeted at the competency area requiring remediation promote better reflection and discussion.

Learners who have internalized the message that they are substandard performers may choose to discuss only the negative aspects of performance. In these situations, it is useful to re-direct them to recall parts of the encounter that they did effectively. Helping them articulate strengths promotes greater self-confidence. Confident learners are more likely to be motivated to improve their practice over time.

After drawing out these initial reflections, the coach may then ask the learner to reflect on specific aspects of their performance that can be improved. Box 6.3 contains examples of such guiding questions.

Box 6.3: Examples of Specific Questions a Coach Can Ask to Elicit the Learner's Reflection and Self-Assessment

Example 1:

One of the goals we set at our last meeting was to improve the quality of your clinical assessments on rounds, with a particular focus on the 'one-liner' or summary statement. What do you think you did effectively today with respect to this?

What do you want to do differently tomorrow on rounds?

Example 2:

Can we debrief about the family meeting you led?

What are some communication techniques that you used that seemed to work?

Can you recall moments that could have gone better?

What could you have done differently during those moments?

Respond with Reflection and Empathy

It is tempting, after hearing the learner's perspective and assessment of their performance, to respond immediately with either affirming or disagreeing statements. This is especially true if the coach has strong opinions about the observation that are discordant with the learner's perception. Before sharing your own views, however, we recommend that the coach pause and take a moment to convey to the learner that their perspective has been understood. This is done by summarizing what you have heard in your own words, even if you do not share their view of events:

> *I am hearing that you felt you needed to call out the nurse for not checking vital signs when the patient arrived on the surgical ward. I am also hearing that you were concerned for the patient's safety and felt that other members of the interprofessional team were not.*
>
> *I am hearing that you felt that the situation was not set up for you to perform at your best. I'm sorry about that.*

Empathic statements, using the PEARLS© framework (see Table 6.1) are useful communication tools in this step. Note that these phrases are used to give space for the learner's emotions and acknowledge their perspective but do not necessarily agree with that perspective: reflection does not necessarily indicate concurrence. If the learner feels that the coach has heard them, then they are more likely to listen to modifying or corrective suggestions. However, this approach is not merely a strategy to entrap the learner. Importantly, these empathic statements must be authentic. Being authentic requires that the coach be exquisitely aware of their own feelings and reactions and actively seek to have positive regard for the learner as a person even when feeling critical of the learner's performance, behavior, or attitude. The ability to achieve this authentic "stance" is a skill that can be cultivated through practice with feedback and reflection and should be a goal of faculty development (Chap. 19).

Share Your Assessment and Thoughts

Reinforcing Feedback: When it is time to provide your feedback, it may be tempting to try to "fix all the problems" that you note. Strongly resist this urge! We recommend first providing reinforcing feedback, and plenty of it, for two reasons. First, reinforcing feedback provides validation and mitigates the learner's internalized conviction that they are in a permanent state of "struggling" or "failing." Second, focusing early on what the learner did effectively generates additional trust, strengthens the relationship, and contributes to a positive learning climate [22].

As with responses to the learner's perspectives in the preceding section, reinforcing feedback must be specific and sincere to be useful. A general laudatory remark (such as "strong work") is less effective than naming specific behaviors to maintain competent performance (such as "I saw in your note how you prioritized your differential diagnosis and clearly documented your clinical reasoning."). Acknowledging progress on learner-identified areas of struggle is especially meaningful in promoting behavior change (for example, "I know you are working on conveying empathy in your communication. During that family meeting I noticed you repeating the patient's words back to her. It's clear to me that the patient felt connected to you as a result. Congratulations on the progress you have made.")

The ideal ratio of reinforcing feedback to modifying feedback is higher than many think. In general, people are more accustomed to providing corrective comments rather than reinforcing ones. Coaches must work hard to overcome this tendency. This can initially be hard to do, but effective coaches work hard to develop this skill.

Modifying feedback is necessary for course-correction and is given with the intent to improve the learner's performance. When communicating modifying feedback, coaches must convey that their intent is supportive. Ask permission to share your observations and thoughts—this gesture indicates respect for the learner and softens the inherently hierarchical nature of the relationship. The coach can also preface the feedback by reaffirming their commitment to helping the learner achieve the professional goals they set at the beginning of remediation, encouraging greater buy-in for what you have to say.

When sharing modifying feedback, we recommend stating specific behaviors rather than vague or general impressions, starting with impartial observations and using them to ground your suggestions. As with any skill, preparation and deliberative practice in communication are key. Table 6.7 contains examples of modifying feedback in a variety of scenarios. The italicized text denotes the coach's nonjudgmental observations.

Table 6.7 Examples of modifying feedback for learners who struggle in specific clinical skill areas

Area requiring feedback	Example of communicating corrective feedback
Oral presentations	"With your permission, can I share some observations with you? *I observed that with your first patient, you had written down her vital signs, physical examination, and lab results on a piece of paper and presented them smoothly. When the time came for your assessment and plan, you spoke off the top of your head and seemed to search for the right words to convey your thoughts coherently.* You appeared to be less prepared with your thoughts on the assessment and plan section of your presentation. I suspect your team may have interpreted this unpreparedness as a lack of medical knowledge and clinical reasoning skills"
Interpersonal communication	"Can I tell you what I noticed? *When you spoke to the patient on how bad smoking is for his health and then listed all the complications of tobacco in detail, he looked away, sighed, and rubbed his forehead.* It looked to me like he had disengaged, and I'm concerned that he did not internalize what you said. I imagine that this was not your intent"
Professionalism	"I fully recognize the stress while the patient was decompensating, and I know what a caring and competent clinician you aspire to be. *I noticed that when you gave the nurse orders during the code, you raised your voice and used a clipped tone. I noted that the nurse left the room in tears.* I am concerned that the tone you used had a negative effect on collegiality and teamwork in the intensive care unit. I worry about its potential to adversely affect patient safety, which I know is something you care deeply about"

Italicized = coach's observations; Underlined = coach's assessment/thoughts

The underlined text contains the coach's editorial comments based on those observations.

The examples in Table 6.7 contain statements that give the learner validation and the benefit of the doubt ("I imagine this was not your intent")

and reinforce the learner's core values ("I know you care deeply about patient safety"). This approach works well with learners who are highly sensitive to modifying feedback. You may find that fewer validating statements are necessary for learners who are more receptive to modifying feedback.

Collaborate on Improvement Strategies

Once the learner has heard and reflected on the feedback, the coach should prompt them to think about what they can do to course-correct. Through iterative questioning, the coach can encourage the learner to come up with specific strategies to improve their performance and set short-term performance goals to be visited at subsequent meetings. Learners who can articulate their own action plan are more likely to follow through with it. Box 6.4 contains a vignette in which a coach encourages a learner to develop an improvement strategy, using one of the modifying feedback examples from Table 6.7.

Box 6.4: Example Conversation Between a Learner and Coach Collaborating on Improvement Strategies

Coach: *With your permission, may I share some observations with you? (pause)*

(Learner nods.)

I observed that with your first patient, you had written down her vital signs, physical examination, and lab results on a piece of paper and presented them smoothly. When the time came for your assessment and plan, you spoke off the top of your head and seemed to search for the right words to convey your thoughts coherently. You appeared to be less prepared with your thoughts on the assessment and plan section of your presentation. I'm afraid your team may have interpreted this unpreparedness as a lack of medical knowledge and clinical reasoning skills.

Learner: *I know. I was really embarrassed during rounds. I just don't know why I can't come up with an assessment and plan the way the other interns can. It's so easy for them. Why is it so hard for me?*

Coach: *You clearly demonstrated today that you can easily present vital signs and lab results. Why do you think the assessment and plan portion was more challenging for you?*

Learner: *I think I get performance anxiety. When I'm in front of all those people, my brain stops and I'm not able to get the words out right. I stutter and sound disorganized.*

Coach: *I see. Can you think of something you can do to overcome your performance anxiety? I am confident that you can be successful in this, as you appeared quite calm and confident during the first part of your presentation.*

Learner: *Well, if I'm reading something off a piece of paper like I did with the vital signs I'm less likely to trip up over my words. Maybe I can spend some time before rounds writing out the words I will say for the assessment and plan so that I have something to look at if my mind goes blank on rounds.*

Coach: *Writing out your assessment and plan on paper so that you have a chance to prepare coherent thoughts—this sounds like a promising strategy. It will require you to spend more time preparing for rounds.*

Learner: *That's true.*

Coach: *When do you think you can start to implement this plan?*

Learner: *Probably as early as tomorrow.*

Coach: *That's terrific. Can we check in at the end of rounds tomorrow? I would like to follow up with you to see how this plan is working.*

Phase 4: Assessment of the Learner's Progress

Coaches must continuously assess for progress during remediation. After the learner articulates a plan for improvement, the coach should ensure there is a plan for follow-through. This is an essential, yet often overlooked, step in feedback. We recommend that the coach follow up with the learner at the next meeting about their successes and challenges in implementing the improvement strategy articulated at the prior meeting, as alluded to in the vignette contained in Box 6.4. The coach may also choose to perform a repeat observation or follow up with the learner's clinical supervisors to assess for progress. Formative assessment is defined as a series of ongoing analyses of a learner's progress. In formative assessment during remediation, the coach determines whether they must adjust the remediation plan to keep the learner on track. Important components include continuing direct observations of the learner, acquiring information about the learner's performance from other supervisors, and encouraging the learner to reflect on their progress and areas of ongoing struggle. **It is essential to document the content of each meeting** (including learning goals, what was accomplished, and next steps) so that the coach and learner can keep track of progress. This practice ensures transparency and accountability for the learner during remediation and provides clear data for ultimate arbiters to make decisions (Chap. 29). In addition, coaches should communicate to leadership any systems-level factors uncovered in the remediation process for programmatic change (Table 6.2).

Summative assessment recaps the learner's progress at the end of remediation and what the coach reports back to the arbiters of remediation—the academic deans, clinical competency committees, and/or program directors. If the expectations for performance and the summative assessment of progress are clearly established at the outset of remediation (see Phase 3), the arbitration of remediation should be straightforward for both the learner and the arbiters. While it

helps for the remediation coach to attend the arbitration process to provide information and prepare to help the learner with the outcome, we recommend that the coach not have voting power during the arbitration process, as this may compromise the relationship of trust with the learner during remediation.

Many learners who struggle will continue to benefit from mentorship beyond the end of remediation. Maintaining a coaching relationship with the learner is invaluable for their professional well-being and subsequent skill development. This can be done by either the coach who was involved in the formal remediation process or by another faculty member who has a longitudinal relationship with the learner.

Conclusion

Many clinician-educators, chief residents, and faculty members become de facto remediation coaches of learners who struggle. The task requires reflection, diligence, and deliberate communication, and is an essential component of medical education. If done attentively and compassionately, the coach has the potential to change a learner's trajectory for the remainder of their career.

References

1. Boileau E, St-Onge C, Audetat M. Is there a way for clinical teachers to assist struggling learners? A synthetic review of the literature. Adv Med Educ Pract. 2017;8:89–97.
2. Guerrasio J, Garrity M, Aagaard E. Learner deficits and academic outcomes of medical students, residents, fellows, and attending physicians referred to a remediation program, 2006-2012. Acad Med. 2014;89:352–8.
3. Yao D, Wright S. National survey of internal medicine residency program directors regarding problem resident. JAMA. 2000;284:1099–104.
4. Bynum WE IV, Varpio L, Lagoo J, Teunissen PW. "I'm unworthy of being in this space": the origins of shame in medical students. Med Educ. 2021;55:185–97.
5. Clark WD, Russell M. Skill set two: skills that build trust. In: Chou CL, Cooley L, editors. Communication Rx. New York: McGraw Hill; 2017.

6. White MK, Chou CL. Appreciative coaching: "I want to be known as the clinician who…" in Chou CL, Cooley L, eds. Communication Rx. New York: McGraw Hill; 2017.

7. Coelho C, Zahra D, Ali K, Tredwin C. To accept or decline academic remediation: what difference does it make? Med Teach. 2019;41(7):824–9.

8. Holmboe E, et al. Faculty development in assessment: the missing link in competency-based medical education. Acad Med. 2011;86:460–7.

9. Kogan J, Holmboe E, Hauer K. Tools for direct observation and assessment of clinical skills of medical trainees: a systematic review. JAMA. 2009;302:1316–26.

10. Papadakis M, et al. Disciplinary action by medical boards and prior behavior in medical school. N Engl J Med. 2005;353:2673–82.

11. Weller JM, et al. Can I leave the theatre? A key to more reliable workplace-based assessment. Br J Anaesth. 2014;112(6):1083–91.

12. Chou CL, et al. Guidelines: the do's, don'ts and don't knows of remediation in medical education. Perspect Med Educ. 2019;8:322–38.

13. The Accreditation Council of Graduate Medical Education. www.acgme.org.

14. Cleland J, et al. The remediation challenge: theoretical and methodological insights from a systematic review. Med Educ. 2013;47:242–51.

15. Hauer K, et al. Remediation of the deficiencies of physicians across the continuum from medical school to practice: a thematic review of the literature. Acad Med. 2009;84:1822–32.

16. Sandars J, Clear T. Self-regulation theory: applications to medical education: AMEE guide no. 58. Med Teach. 2011;31(11):875–86.

17. Leggett H, Sandars J, Roberts T. Twelve tips on how to provide self-regulated learning (SRL) enhanced feedback on clinical performance. Med Teach. 2017;41:147–51.

18. Yao D, Wright S. The challenge of problem residents. J Gen Intern Med. 2001;16:486–92.

19. Scarff C, et al. Keeping mum in clinical supervision: private thoughts and public judgments. Med Educ. 2019;53:133–42.

20. Kalet A, Chou CL. Remediation in medical education: a mid-course correction. New York: Springer; 2014.

21. Senge PM. The fifth discipline: the art and practice of the learning organization. New York: Doubleday/Currency; 1990.

22. Ramani S, Krackov S. Twelve tips for giving feedback effectively in the clinical learning environment. Med Teach. 2012;34:787–91.

Part II

Remediation by Competency

"They Need to Read More": Helping Trainees Who Struggle with Knowledge Base

7

Jeannette Guerrasio, Bau P. Tran, and Kalman Winston

Introduction

A distinctive feature of health professions education is the need to learn enormous amounts of information. While modern learners can quickly access information electronically, they still require solid foundational knowledge to perform effectively and efficiently as health professionals. Often, trainees struggle with the volume of facts they need to commit to memory. Trainees performing below their potential must develop new, more rigorous learning strategies; in fact, such learners request support for their study skills [1]. We will follow the remediation framework listed in Chap. 6 to guide the reader through effective means of providing support to these learners.

Identification

Insufficient knowledge is prevalent among students who struggle; at one medical school, 42% of students referred to a remediation program and 60% of residents placed on probation had a medical knowledge gap [2, 3]. Certainly, learners who consistently score poorly on assessments of their knowledge base, such as high-stakes standardized examinations [4], likely have needs for support in this area (see Clarification section, below).

In clinical practice, we believe that insufficient knowledge is "over-diagnosed" by educators who have some sensitivity but lack specificity in identifying remediation issues. Many students told by clinical supervisors to "read more" have adequate foundational knowledge. They can recall facts, but they lack understanding of the implications of and interrelationships between facts, have disorganized memory coding (i.e., retrievability), are unable to apply knowledge in the context of clinical reasoning (Chap. 10), or suffer from performance anxiety, or inadequate interpersonal communication (Chap. 13). Therefore, to provide effective support, educators must consider remediation strategies that go beyond simply needing to "read more."

J. Guerrasio
Medicine Within Reach, PLLC, Denver, CO, USA
e-mail: jeannette@coloradocme.com

B. P. Tran (✉)
Department of Physician Assistant Studies,
University of Texas Southwestern, Dallas, TX, USA
e-mail: bau.tran@utsouthwestern.edu

K. Winston
Cambridge University, Cambridge, UK
e-mail: kaw82@medschl.cam.ac.uk

Clarification

Sam (they/them) is getting ready to start their third year of medical school, which marks the start of their clinical clerkship rotations. They twice failed their Step 1 United States Medical Licensing Examination (USMLE), the first of three that assess factual and applied medical knowledge, and passed it on the third attempt. They are interested in improving their test scores, as they will have to take USMLE Steps 2 and 3, as well as clinical science subject examinations.

To create a targeted remediation plan, it is essential to elucidate the underlying causes of knowledge gaps. Reviewing the trainee's academic record or asking if they passed all prior standardized exams may help differentiate medical knowledge gaps from other areas of struggle. Answers to the following questions (Box 7.1) can paint a comprehensive picture of the learner's challenges with exams. Chapter 17 also provides an in-depth treatment of detecting, diagnosing, and managing learning differences and disabilities.

Box 7.1: Questions to Clarify Underlying Reasons for Knowledge Gaps
- Why did the learner think they struggled with this exam?
- Has the learner's performance on exams been consistent?
- How did the learner score on other standardized exams such as the Scholastic Aptitude Test (SAT) for college admissions, Graduate Record Exam (GRE) for graduate school admissions, Medical College Admission Test (MCAT) for medical college admissions, or the USMLE compared to peers?
    - Was the learner's performance consistent across all components of the assessments, or did the learner score low in one area and high in others?
    - Is the learner's knowledge gap global or related to a specific topic or set of topics?
- Can the learner identify a point in time when their performance significantly worsened?
    - If so, what factors contributed to this low performance (i.e., study habits, personal issues, change in context, etc.)?
- What approaches have the learner been using to study? Is the learner able to describe their study habits in detail?
- Trainees studying or practicing in a foreign country may struggle with language barriers that require them to spend extra time and effort to comprehend language and/or translate complex technical material [5, 6]—does that apply to the learner?
- Has the learner been previously diagnosed with one or more learning disabilities?
    - If so, does the learner have effective strategies to address their challenges? is the learner able to advocate for reasonable accommodations? Are more needed? (see Chap. 17)
- What demands on the learner's time outside of the classroom may influence their ability to perform?

Upon further questioning, Sam reports doing well on the SAT, placing in the 95th percentile of all college-bound high school students in the US. The total MCAT score places them in the 80th percentile of US medical school applicants. Sam's scores are not unlike their high-achieving peers. Sam scored just about average on most pre-clerkship exams.

Apart from one's cognitive abilities, individual characteristics also influence learning and performance [7], including openness, conscientiousness, dependability, curiosity, intellectual engagement, growth mindset, and grit [8–11]. Every learner requires individualized strategies to maximize success. Common issues in learners who struggle with knowledge base include performance vs. mastery orientation (seeking to master the material rather than merely score well on an exam), lack of effective and efficient study skills, slow language processing, underlying learning disabilities, and physical or mental illness.

If the knowledge gap is limited to one or two topic areas, subject-specific remediation will likely be straightforward. Those who procrastinate and work to avoid appearing incompetent are most likely to underperform [12]. Increasing learners' awareness of this performance orientation and asking them to reflect on their own experiences may help motivate them to change their behavior and attitudes toward learning [13]. Engaging them in conversations about how clinicians must develop lifelong learning skills and a mastery orientation may also help motivate them to change ineffective study habits (see Chap. 4).

Learners who spend sufficient time studying but do not apply cognitively and behaviorally active learning strategies (e.g., rereading the same textbook many times rather than summarizing the material into briefer study tools) may benefit greatly from study skills coaching (see "Study Skills Interventions" below). In addition, if the learner has a previously diagnosed learning disability, their experience with accommodations (e.g., extra time for exams, use of a calculator for calculations, or computer for writing) may provide straightforward study skill guidance [8]. Study skills coaches can help students with learning disabilities adjust to new learning environments (see Chap. 17).

For other learners reporting that they have always been "bad test takers," or had an injury or illness that resulted in a change in performance, cognitive or neuropsychological evaluation can identify new or undiagnosed learning disabilities resulting from physical or mental illness. Signs of a longstanding underlying learning disability include prior difficulties in school, difficulty understanding and following instructions, trouble remembering what someone just told them, difficulty distinguishing right from left, difficulty identifying words or a tendency to reverse letters, words, or numbers, lack in physical coordination, easily losing or misplacing items, or difficulty understanding the concept of time [14]. Other clues that neuropsychological testing is indicated include history of head trauma, failure to achieve developmental milestones as a child, such as delayed language development, hearing or visual deficits, exposure to drugs, alcohol, or maternal illness *in utero,* exposure to chemicals, toxins, or heavy metals, tics, seizure disorders, substance abuse, strokes, and psychiatric disorders.

Trainees who learn in settings where their native language is not used often notice that it takes them longer to complete exams and to read and process information compared with their peers. This slow reading rate may also be seen in native speakers ("slow processors"). Often such students undergo testing and can receive time accommodations on written tests. Students with a slow reading rate can partially overcome this gap through training by completing large volumes of practice test questions under timed conditions. Normalizing these issues by having other trainees or faculty with similar struggles share their experiences can be very helpful.

Intervention

Many adult learners who struggle believe that putting more time into familiar, previously successful study strategies will improve their performance ("I just need to read more"). These trainees require external support to encourage them to master new, more efficient strategies [15–18]. In conducting medical knowledge remediation programs, we create opportunities for learners to learn new study strategies to improve lifelong knowledge acquisition through cycles of effortful practice, tailored feedback, and self-reflection. These are key components of deliberate practice critical to developing expertise [19, 20] (see Chap. 4). After describing evidence-based strategies that can support all learning, we describe remediation tailored to three commonly encountered issues that interfere with knowledge gain: ineffective study skills, distraction, and anxiety with low self-confidence.

Evidence-Based Learning Strategies

When asked to discuss their study strategies, Sam admits that because the grading policy is pass/fail, they stopped going to class once they felt confident passing the courses. Instead, they sleep until noon, attend mandatory small group sessions in the afternoon, and watch video recordings of the lectures from home in the evenings, often at double speed. Starting 2 days before an exam, they repeatedly review lecture notes and textbook chapters, taking brief breaks to eat and sleep. They feel that this "healthier" approach provides more control over their time and energy.

Health professions schools often have different expectations for self-regulated learning compared with students' prior learning contexts [21]. Sam's "pump and dump" (also known as "binge and purge" or "brute force") study strategy is an inefficient means of knowledge acquisition and is among the least effective in producing future recall and application of that information to new problems. Curricular structures that heavily weigh one or two comprehensive knowledge-based exams foster these ineffective approaches. The learning science literature provides evidence-based strategies that facilitate durable learning and long-term retention by using (1) spaced practice, (2) interleaving, (3) elaboration, (4) concrete examples, (5) dual coding, and (6) retrieval prac-

Table 7.1 Learning strategies and approach to incorporation

Step 1. Organized study sessions (distributed learning) [24, 25] into a regimented schedule that allows learners, over a defined time frame, to apportion their study activities	
Spaced practice [23, 26, 27]	Encourages the frequent review of small blocks of information/topics at regular intervals over time
Interleaving [22, 23, 28]	Scaffolds multiple problems or topics within a single study session, in addition to shifting the order of topics reviewed
Step 2. Meaningful study time [29]—deepens understanding of the topic	
Elaborative interrogation or elaboration [22]	Uses a higher-order questioning strategy that enables the learner to triangulate existing knowledge with new knowledge to promote a deeper understanding of topics and concepts—understanding the "how" and "why"
Concrete examples [30, 31]	Applying abstract concepts to real-life examples or specific relatable experiences
Dual coding [23, 31]	Verbal and visual information are combined
Step 3. Knowledge check—engaging long-term memory	
Retrieval practice [32–34]	Recalling learned information from long-term memory via low stakes, weekly formative quizzes, accompanied by summative open-ended question exams; alternatively, in a "cover the options" approach, students answer multiple-choice questions after reading the stem rather using the listed response options to arrive at the best answer

tice [22, 23]. Table 7.1 summarizes each learning strategy and an approach to incorporation into self-regulated learning.

Regrettably, learners often perceive that these approaches are less effective because they slow down learning and require more effort. Curriculum structures that clump similar content and assessment approaches, and which do not test material cumulatively, reinforce this study behavior. Alerting learners to these effective learning strategies can encourage more self-regulated learning through using them. Additionally, faculty must appreciate the mechanisms to fully support their use in curricular planning and evaluation to maximize knowledge acquisition and retention.

Study Skills Interventions

On clinical rotations, Sam is unable to answer basic fact-based questions in several different content domains. Their clinical supervisors report that their knowledge gaps are global and not related to any disease, organ system, or specialty of medicine. Sam reports that they haven't had as much time to study on their current rotation nor purchased the text recommended by the clerkship director. In the past week, the supervisor suggested Sam read about the mechanisms of action of the medications used for the treatment of congestive heart failure, but they haven't yet.

For a student like Sam, it is critical to create a highly structured remediation process. Such trainees need explicit guidance to emphasize high-yield material and the appropriate depth of learning. It is imperative to make specific recommendations with strict timelines and to clearly warn the learner that the process can require frequent meetings with a supervisor and an extended amount of time.

Time Management

Time management is essential to successful demonstration of knowledge and improves exam scores. A disciplined study structure, including timelines as noted above, underscores the overall importance of time management and deemphasizes the use of cramming strategies [35]. Many students who are easily distracted struggle to manage their time during an exam, either rushing through questions due to their underlying impulsivity or becoming distracted, leaving insufficient time to finish. Knowing the testing format, the number of sections and questions per section, the types of questions being asked, and how much time they will have for each section is critical to manage time effectively. For some tests, a breakdown of topics is also helpful, as it will direct the learner to study the highest-yield topics first. Practice exams, flashcards, or sample questions from reputable testing banks, are widely available [36, 37].

We work with the learner to develop a specific study schedule, including the number of pages to read and short answer practice questions to complete daily and weekly. We give specific reading assignments with source and page numbers (e.g., "Internal Medicine Essentials for Clerkship Students, pages 75-99") rather than leaving this up to the student by saying, "read about cirrhosis." If possible, we correlate readings with clinical activities and make specific assignments for the student to do before, during, or after an educational experience. This way, we use distributed learning to model effective ways to blend background and just-in-time reading with experiential learning. Taking regular planned breaks ("joy breaks") also increases learners' retentive ability [38]. Finally, learners should reflect on how well the study calendar worked each week and adapt as necessary for subsequent weeks.

Study Skills Coaching

Study skills coaching is readily available in many academic communities. Even if the individual coach has no prior experience working with professional school students, most can work effectively in consultation with an experienced clinician-educator. Learners have better outcomes with experienced coaches who are more likely to engage their learners with challenging models of facilitating learning, take a dialogic stance that encourages more collaborative discussions, diagnose cognitive errors, and use effective tactics such as taking metacognitive time-outs and making crosslinks between various curricular content (interleaving) [39]. Initially, we carefully choose the material that directly relates to course or clerkship objectives, targets the appropriate level of learning, and is manageable to complete during the time available. In doing so, the student learns to read with increased focus.

In addition to time management skills (see above), learners should take written notes as they read and summarize each section or teaching session in writing, identifying the major themes, important facts, and take-home points of figures, tables, and cases [40]. For students who routinely cram for exams, it is important to encourage them to actively learn the material in depth to facilitate long-term retention and clinical application. As they read about a patient case, learners should be encouraged to use elaborative interrogation, going beyond answering the "what and how" questions (e.g., treatment options for gout and how to administer them) and asking "why" questions (e.g., mechanisms of action, and conditions for using certain treatments instead of others). Additionally, it can be helpful to the learner to create their own mnemonics, visual maps, charts, pictures, and algorithms from the extracted material. They should log remaining questions about the material and discuss these questions with their study coach, clinical or course supervisors, or in study groups with their peers [8, 41]. Innovative technology is available to assist students with difficulty "capturing" information in writing (see Chap. 17).

Lastly, allow learners to reflect on new study methods. What have been the pros and cons of having such a strict study schedule with weekly quizzes? What have they noticed about the effect on their performance? Do they now have more to add to patient or education discussions, and can they follow those discussions better? Ideally, this intensive process will result in the trainee's ability to link her enhanced effort with higher achievement [40].

Remediation Roles and Practices

Though working with trained study skills coaches is optimal, competent peers or near-peers can function as tutors. Peers most capable of providing this support need not be the highest performers: success in developing more effective study habits predicts success in peer coaching. Faculty educators should concentrate on identifying students who need help, structuring and monitoring the remediation process, and participating in making summary judgments about a student's success in remediation. As content experts, educators must also clarify any knowledge gaps. We recommend

that content experts avoid merely telling information to students who struggle and instead facilitate trainees' learning by reviewing the practice questions the learner answered incorrectly, drilling down to reveal why the learner stumbled.

A faculty coach should ask the trainee to rephrase the question to demonstrate understanding of the assessed concept and encourage the learner to explain why the given answer is correct and the incorrect answers are wrong. Then, educators can work with the learner to identify keywords and concepts to help develop the ability to distinguish salient information from distracting facts. Encouraging the learner to write their own multiple-choice questions on a challenging topic actively engages the student in encoding, retrieving, and applying the information to authentic scenarios [42]. Some course directors routinely have students write test questions as a study strategy.

Self-Regulation

Students should identify their most productive time of day for studying and monitor relevant issues such as how much sleep they receive and require; use of caffeine, over-the-counter medications, and prescription medications; and the role of exercise and study location (e.g., students with ADHD paradoxically prefer public locations such as coffee houses rather than being isolated) in helping them attend to studying. A medical or psychiatric evaluation may be warranted for medication recommendations and sleep problems. Sleep disorders and undertreated mental illness affect alertness and efficient use of time. Specific distractors and interruptions should be identified and eliminated to make study time more efficient and productive [40]. The student may need advice on confronting their family members' and friends' wishes and expectations to preserve the necessary amount of protected study time.

Taking Advantage of Aural and Visual Learning

Audio recording a summary of the student's study notes and listening to the recordings on their way to work, while walking the dog, or working out at the gym is a strategy that helps students with language fluency. The repetition involved in making and listening to such recordings takes advantage of the multimedia effect of processing information using dual channels, both verbally (spoken and written words) and visually (pictures) [43]. The resultant solidification and retention of the material will help decrease anxiety and increase confidence walking into writing exams and other evaluative assessments. Box 7.2 summarizes these and other strategies to support learners' study skills.

Developing self-awareness and a repertoire of strategies can ensure that trainees achieve their goals and meet competency standards. In addition to all the strategies discussed above, a mentor can advise students on how to establish healthy boundaries with others, locate study space, relinquish nonacademic tasks and responsibilities to preserve protected study time, and provide the student permission and support to sustain the courage needed to explore and optimize study techniques.

Box 7.2: Study Skills Support
- Help the students develop a study schedule.
- Encourage openness, conscientiousness, dependability, individual curiosity, intellectual engagement, and mastery of the material.
- Warn against procrastination and effort and time invested in appearing competent.
- Instruct the students to focus on learning and understanding, as well as application and analysis, rather than just remembering or memorizing.
- Encourage the students to take written notes on reading, attend teaching and group study sessions, and create diagrams, charts, and maps.
- Encourage students to learn the language and vocabulary of medicine by going back to basic definitions and discussing questions that arise while studying with a knowledgeable other.

- Identify the most productive time of day for studying.
- Find efficient, protected time, and an appropriate space to study.
- Get at least 6 h of sleep per night.
- Develop a routine exercise regimen.
- Limit caffeine and use medication appropriately.
- Consider having the student audio record their notes or a summary of their notes and listen to the recordings.

Distracted Learners

Ann (she/her) has been referred for knowledge remediation because her exam scores have consistently been in the bottom quintile of her class. She says she has always been a "bad test taker" but is adamant that her knowledge base is comparable to her peers, as demonstrated on clinical performance evaluations.

Ann spends 2 h every evening reading and completing practice questions. When asked for more detail, she admits to only being able to complete 2–5 pages of reading per night and about 2 or 3 practice questions. She finally admits that she carries the diagnosis of Attention Deficit Hyperactivity Disorder (ADHD) and that because she feared being stigmatized, she has not requested testing accommodations or sought treatment.

ADHD is one of the most common learning disorders seen in health professions students. While not associated with intelligence, it is associated with poor attention, impulsivity, distractibility, restlessness, impaired organization and time management, and procrastination [44, 45]. These features impact both knowledge acquisition and test-taking as demands of the curriculum increase. While both males and females are affected by ADHD, females are diagnosed at a lower rate [46, 47] (see Chap. 17).

Without support, these students cannot get through an adequate proportion of material during their study time and retain less of it compared to their peers. With earlier diagnosis of learning difficulties and more effective interventions for learners with ADHD, increasingly, students are arriving at professional school with a much more sophisticated understanding of their situations and are better prepared to strategize effectively and advocate for their own learning needs. The prognosis for students like Ann is good if competent study skills coaching is available. This includes focusing on organizing study material, transforming from passive to active study strategies, and learning strict time management techniques. It is important to determine if supportive medication treatment is appropriate.

Training for Test-Taking

Practice answering test questions improves performance [8, 29, 34, 48–51]. Practice exams should closely simulate the actual test environment, including timing and the number, format, and types of test questions. Learners should practice answering the easier, more straightforward questions first, then complete the remaining, more complex questions rather than answering questions in order. They should be cautioned to avoid careless errors by not rushing through the exam. On the other hand, for non-computer adaptive testing, if a question takes more than 4–5 min, they should move along to the next question. During the final 2 min of the allotted time, have the learner fill in answers to the unanswered questions: they should not leave any questions blank [36, 37]. High performers on the USMLE Step exams typically read one review book series entirely from start to finish, *at least* once, then study their notes and complete 1500 questions. An alternative focused strategy is to complete 2500 questions, thoroughly review the explanations for each answer, and look up topics they did not perform well on [52].

For case-based or long-format questions, a helpful technique is to read the stem question at the very end of the passage first, review the answer choices, and then go back and read the entire case. Understanding the question allows the learner to identify relevant facts or key features from all the information commonly provided in these question types. This ability, which maximizes the use of our limited working memory, is called *saliency determination*, and can be honed with practice. Explicitly enhancing saliency determination is particularly useful for learners with ADHD [53].

Another technique involves helping learners to switch perspectives on a question, also known as *cognitive flexibility*. Some learners prefer to view the world through a big picture lens; others tend to initially see each tree first rather than the whole forest. Both are necessary. If the learner is struggling with a question or concept, have them try looking at it from both views. Likewise, some learners focus more on concrete information, details, and facts, while others work better with abstract concepts and theories. It is essential for learners to understand their preferred approach and be able to switch perspectives. This perspective-switching may help distracted learners attend longer and therefore improve performance.

For multiple-choice test questions, instruct the student to look at all the answer choices, eliminating the incorrect choices and choosing from the remaining ones [36, 37]. A learner who consistently narrows the answers down to two or more choices may lack the specificity of knowledge and needs to focus their study time on acquiring more details, in addition to understanding the big picture. Alternatively, such challenges may indicate an underlying learning difference (see Chap. 17).

Using these techniques on practice questions and exams will help provide the learner with feedback on the progression of their knowledge, the effectiveness of different study and test-taking strategies, and optimal pacing for studying and completing exam questions. Practice test data should be monitored to provide feedback on the effectiveness of study and testing strategies. Such learning should be noted and reinforced until better strategies become habitual. Box 7.3 summarizes tips for preparing for and taking exams.

Box 7.3: Advice for Preparing For and Taking Tests

• Make liberal use of practice tests and questions.
• When studying from practice questions:

– If you consistently narrow the answers down to two or more choices, you lack the specificity of knowledge in that domain. Read more with intent.
– Make sure you can rephrase questions, explain why the given answer is correct and the incorrect answers are wrong, and identify and define the keywords.
– Analyze and monitor the reasons why you get practice questions wrong. A knowledge gap? Why didn't you know this material? Not enough time spent? Did you misread the question? Get discouraged or anxious? Document lessons learned and follow up on specific learning issues.
– Track practice scores and document lessons learned.
– Learn to manage time during exams.
– Take practice tests in an environment that simulates the testing environment.
– Review lessons learned about test-taking before the exam.

• Be familiar with the test format and content.
• When taking the test:

– Keep track of how long it takes to complete a certain number of questions.
– Practice answering the easiest questions first.
– Do not rush through any one question.
– If a question is taking more than 4–5 min, move on.

– During the final 2 min of the time period, fill in answers to the unanswered questions.
– For long-format questions read the end of the passage and response options first.
– Consider each test question from both the big picture and the detailed view.

Learners with Anxiety and Low Confidence

Juan (he/him) admits that taking tests is extremely anxiety-provoking. His anxiety slows him down, and he starts thinking in his native language, Spanish. Juan calls the school's education specialist to help him prepare for USMLE Step 1. He is no longer confident that he will ever pass the test or graduate from medical school. In the past, Juan consistently scored in the bottom 10% on exams and has had to repeat one course each of the past 2 years. Juan has been reading and re-reading the suggested board preparation text books and question banks for the past year, in parallel to his classroom courses. He has never been evaluated for a learning disability and has never sought testing accommodations. He lives with his family to reduce the cost of his education. While they are extremely supportive of his study time and proud that he is the first member of his family to attend graduate school, Juan doesn't have private study space and is expected to and wants to engage with them frequently.

Chronic anxiety has been consistently associated with poor performance on cognitive assessments [54, 55]; however, the nature of this correlation is not well-understood. Multiple factors likely contribute to reducing cognitive resources, thus causing cognitive overload. Furthermore, numerous forces conspire against learners whose backgrounds include disadvantaged learning environments and/or identities that are stereotyped as lower performing in scientific fields (see Chap. 3). Once in professional schools, such learners are less likely to use academic support services [56]; stereotype threat can lead to a consistent exam performance decrement ([57]; see Chap. 3); and confidence, which correlates with better test performance, may be lacking [58]. In fact, being identified as "struggling" is likely to reduce confidence. The cycle continues as learners who lack confidence avoid challenging situations, such as courses, study groups, and higher-level discussions [59–61].

The main remediation strategies for learners with anxiety, low confidence levels, and chronic low scores include fine-tuning study skills, increasing preparation for exams, and repetition. One strategy is to encourage learners like Juan to take written notes in English as he reads and attends teaching sessions, which can build confidence in English language fluency and the new medical vocabulary. In addition, study groups help learners who lack awareness of their knowledge gaps [62]. In groups, learners can see alternative explanations and solutions to patient cases and medical questions, develop a sense of group identity, and feel supported [39, 63, 64]. An advanced group will be able to give each other feedback and begin to self-regulate their learning.

Assessment

> **Sam's story:**
> *Sam works closely with a mentor who helps them design a study schedule. Initially, Sam is disgruntled at having to take weekly quizzes. However, Sam soon notices an improvement in knowledge base and in overall performance. This in turn enables deeper, more satisfying,*

and enjoyable engagement on rounds and with patient care. They even received the second highest score on their Internal Medicine subject exams.

> **Ann's story:**
> *Ann sought counseling and pharmacologic treatment for ADHD. She incorporated visual maps and algorithms while reading, making her studying more efficient, interactive, and interesting. She no longer needs to stay up all night to get through required material and now wakes up early in the morning to run for 45 min before work. Overall, she is feeling less burnt out and has passed all exams.*

> **Juan's story:**
> *Juan is frustrated that he must study more than his peers. However, the time and repetition are paying off. For Juan, taking notes, recording his voice explaining concepts, and listening to the recordings on his way to work have been helpful. He has begun sharing his struggles with a few of his classmates and has found them supportive. They have been available to discuss concepts with him to reinforce his learning, and he has found the confidence to engage more with the resident and faculty members on his teams. With the help of his family, he was able to create a quiet space to study at home, and they encouraged him to spend time in the local public library. Juan took a month off clinical rotations to concentrate on practice questions prior to USMLE Step 2, which paid off. He was able to complete all questions and received an average score.*

There are several programmatic ways in which health professions schools can decrease the need for knowledge base remediation. Best curriculum design practices incorporate learning strategies listed in Table 7.1 and introductory classes on study, cognitive, and metacognitive skills [65, 66]; these strategies are beneficial for all students. Institutions should provide ready availability to question banks, highest-yield reading materials, and academic support resources [67], including a pool of learners and faculty who are skillful tutors and good role models. Finally, after analyzing available data to predict at-risk students, schools should plan interventions to support them.

Conclusion

While it is common for health professions educators to be concerned about a learner's knowledge base, few have a sophisticated toolbox of effective remediation strategies. Based on our experience and the literature, we have illustrated evidence-based and road-tested effective remediation strategies for the most typical trainee scenarios [68]. We hope that this chapter encourages an optimistic embrace of individually tailored and closely supervised remediation based on deliberate practice, which is effortful, challenging, and supported by multiple sources of feedback and requires metacognitive awareness through self-reflection.

References

1. Olmesdahl PJ. The establishment of student needs: an important internal factor affecting course outcome. Med Teach. 1999;21:174–9.
2. Guerrasio J, Garrity MJ, Aagaard EM. Learner deficits and academic outcomes of medical students, residents, fellows, and attending physicians referred to a remediation program, 2006-2012. Acad Med. 2014;89:352–8.
3. Guerrasio J, Brooks E, Rumack C, Christensen A, Aagaard EM. Association of characteristics, deficits, and outcomes of residents placed on probation at one institution, 2002-2012. Acad Med. 2016;91:382–7.
4. Hoffman KI. The USMLE, the NBME subject examinations, and assessment of individual academic achievement. Acad Med. 1993;68:740–7.
5. Edwards-Capello A, Silbert-Flagg J. Academic dismissal from a baccalaureate nursing program: the student's perspective. Nurse Educ Today. 2021;104:104996.
6. Zhen L, Heath MA, Jackson AP, Kawika Allan GE, Fisher L, Chan P. Acculturation experiences of Chinese international students who attend American universities. Prof Psychol Res Pract. 2017;48:11–21.
7. Beier ME, Campbell M, Crook AE. Developing and demonstrating knowledge: ability and non-ability determinants of learning and performance. Intelligence. 2010;38:179–86.
8. Swan Sein A, Dathatri S, Bates TA. Twelve tips on guiding preparation for both high-stakes exams and long-term learning. Med Teach. 2021;43:518–23.
9. Barrick MR, Mount MK. The big five personality dimensions and job performance: a meta-analysis. Pers Psychol. 1991;44:1–26.
10. Beier ME, Ackerman PL. Current-events knowledge in adults: an investigation of age, intelligence, and nonability determinants. Psychol Aging. 2001;16:615–28.
11. Colquitt JA, LePine JA, Noe RA. Toward an integrative theory of training motivation: a meta-analytic path analysis of 20 years of research. J Appl Psychol. 2000;85:678–707.
12. Artino AR Jr, Dong T, DeZee KJ, Gilliland WR, Waechter DM, Cruess D, Durning SJ. Achievement goal structures and self-regulated learning: relationships and changes in medical school. Acad Med. 2012;87:1375–81.
13. Winston K. Core concepts in remediation: lessons learned from a 6-year case study. Med Sci Educ. 2015;25:307–15.
14. American Academy of Child and Adolescent Psychiatry. Children with learning disabilities. Facts for Families; 2011. p. 2. http://www.aacap.org/page. ww?section=facts_for_Families&name=Children_ with_Learning_Disabilities.
15. Loyens SMM, Rikers RMJP, Schmidt HG. The impact of students' conceptions of constructivist assumptions on academic achievement and drop-out. Stud High Educ. 2007;32:581–602.
16. Sayer M, Chaput De Saintonge M, Evans D, Wood D. Support for students with academic difficulties: support for students with academic difficulties. Med Educ. 2002;36:643–50.
17. Mattick K, Knight L. High-quality learning: harder to achieve than we think? Med Educ. 2007;41:638–44.
18. Audétat MC, Laurin S, Dory V. Remediation for struggling learners: putting an end to 'more of the same': commentaries. Med Educ. 2013;47:230–1.
19. Hauer KE, Ciccone A, Henzel TR, Katsufrakis P, Miller SH, Norcross WA, Papadakis MA, Irby DM. Remediation of the deficiencies of physicians across the continuum from medical school to practice: a thematic review of the literature. Acad Med. 2009;84:1822–32.
20. Gladwell M. Outliers: the story of success. New York: Little Brown; 2008.
21. Dresel M, Schmitz B, Schober B, Spiel C, Ziegler A, Engelshalk T, Jostl G, Klug J, Roth A, Wimmer B, Steuer G. Competencies for successful self-regulated learning in higher education: structural model and

indications drawn from expert interviews. Stud High Educ. 2015;40:454–70.

22. Wlodarczyk S, Muller-Juge V, Hauer KE, Tong MS, Ransohoff A, Boscardin C. Assessment to optimize learning strategies: a qualitative study of student and faculty perceptions. Teach Learn Med. 2021;33:245–57.

23. Nebel C. Considerations for applying six strategies for effective learning to instruction. Med Sci Educ. 2020;30:9–10.

24. Benjamin AS, Tullis J. What makes distributed practice effective? Cogn Psychol. 2010;61:228–47.

25. Dunlosky J, Rawson KA, Marsh EJ, Nathan MJ, Willingham DT. Improving students' learning with effective learning techniques: promising directions from cognitive and educational psychology: promising directions from cognitive and educational psychology. Psychol Sci Public Interest. 2013;14:4–58.

26. Dunlosky J, Rawson KA. Practice tests, spaced practice, and successive relearning: tips for classroom use and for guiding students' learning. Scholarsh Teach Learn Psychol. 2015;1:72–8.

27. Cutting MF, Saks NS. Twelve tips for utilizing principles of learning to support medical education. Med Teach. 2012;34:20–4.

28. Platt MP, Davis EM, Grundfast K, Grillone G. Early detection of factual knowledge deficiency and remediation in otolaryngology residency education: early detection of knowledge deficiency. Laryngoscope. 2014;124:E309–11.

29. Pashler H, Bain PM, Bottge BA, Graesser A, Koedinger K, McDaniel M, Metcalfe J. Organizing instruction and study to improve student learning. IES practice guide. Washington, DC: Institute of Education Sciences; 2007.

30. Gick ML, Holyoak KJ. Schema induction and analogical transfer. Cogn Psychol. 1983;15(1):1–38.

31. Weinstein Y, Madan CR, Sumeracki MA. Teaching the science of learning. Cogn Res Princ Implic. 2018;3:2.

32. Roediger HL III, Putnam AL, Smith MA. Ten benefits of testing and their applications to educational practice. In: Mestre JP, Ross BH, editors. The psychology of learning and motivation: cognition in education. Elsevier; 2011. p. 1–36.

33. Roediger HL 3rd, Butler AC. The critical role of retrieval practice in long-term retention. Trends Cogn Sci. 2011;15:20–7.

34. Larsen DP, Butler AC, Roediger HL 3rd. Test-enhanced learning in medical education. Med Educ. 2008;42:959–66.

35. Vrugt A, Oort FJ. Metacognition, achievement goals, study strategies and academic achievement: pathways to achievement. Metacogn Learn. 2008;3:123–46.

36. Cutts J, Campbell M, Gotlib L, Oman D, Oman R, Wallace JS. MCAT. New York: Barron's; 2011.

37. Magliore K. Cracking the AP biology exam. 2011 Ed. New York: Random House, Inc.; 2010.

38. Shreffler J, Huecker M, Martin L, Sawning S, The S, Shaw MA, Mittel O, Holthouser A. Strategies to combat burnout during intense studying: utilization

39. Winston KA, Van Der Vleuten CPM, Scherpbier AJJA. Remediation of at-risk medical students: theory in action. BMC Med Educ. 2013;13:132.

40. Connelly J, Forsyth PB. The study skills guide: essential strategies for smart students. Philadelphia: Kogan Page; 2010.

41. Kebaetse MB, Kebaetse M, Mokone GG, Nkomazana O, Mogodi M, Wright J, Park E. Learning support interventions for year 1 medical students: a review of the literature. Med Educ. 2018;52:263–73.

42. Winston KA, Van Der Vleuten CPM, Scherpbier AJJA. An investigation into the design and effectiveness of a mandatory cognitive skills programme for at-risk medical students. Med Teach. 2010;32:236–43.

43. Mayer RE. Cognitive theory of multimedia learning. In: The Cambridge handbook of multimedia learning. Cambridge University Press; 2014. p. 43–71.

44. Hosterman JA, Shannon DP, Sondheimer HM. American Association of American Medical Colleges. Medical students with disabilities: resources to enhance accessibility. Washington, DC: Association of American Medical Colleges; 2010.

45. American Psychiatric Association. Diagnostic and statistical manual of mental disorders: DSM-IV. 4th ed. Washington DC: American Psychiatric Association; 1994.

46. Arnold LE. Sex differences in ADHD: conference summary. J Abnorm Child Psychol. 1996;24:555–69.

47. Gaub M, Carlson CL. Gender differences in ADHD: a meta-analysis and critical review. J Am Acad Child Adolesc Psychiatry. 1997;36:1036–45.

48. Thalheimer W. The learning benefits of questions. 2003. https://www.worklearn-ing.com/wp-content/uploads/2017/10/learning-benefits-of-questions-2014-v2.0.pdf.

49. Gibbs G, Simpson C. Conditions under which assessment supports students' learning. Learning and teaching in High Educ. 2005;1:3–31. http://eprints.glos.ac.uk/id/eprint/3609. Accessed 27 Sept 2022.

50. Sivagnanam G, Saraswathi S, Rajasekaran A. Student-led objective tutorial (SLOT) in medical education. Med Educ Online. 2006;11:4610.

51. Marcell M. Effectiveness of regular online quizzing in increasing class participation and preparation. Int J Scholarsh Teach Learn. 2008;2:7.

52. Guerrasio J. Teaching those who need us Most: remediation of the struggling medical learner. Irwin, PA: Association for Hospital Medical Education; 2013.

53. Kelly DP, Levine MD. A neurodevelopmental approach to differences in learning. In: Fine AH, Kotkin R, editors. Therapist's guide to learning and attention disorders. Elsevier Science; 2003. p. 87–108.

54. Ackerman PL, Heggestad ED. Intelligence, personality, and interests: evidence for overlapping traits. Psychol Bull. 1997;121:219–45.

55. Hembree R. Correlates, causes, effects, and treatment of test anxiety. Rev Educ Res. 1988;58:47–77.

56. Toretsky C, Mutha S, Coffman J. Breaking barriers for underrepresented minorities in the health professions. Retrieved from Healthforce Center at UCSF Website. 2008. https://healthforce.ucsf.edu/publications/breaking-barriers-underrepresented-minorities-health-professions.

57. Steele CM. Whistling Vivaldi and other clues to how stereotypes affect us. New York: W. W. Norton and Company; 2010.

58. Elliott R. Tests, abilities, race and conflict. Intelligence. 1988;12:333–50.

59. Fenollar P, Román S, Cuestas PJ. University students' academic performance: an integrative conceptual framework and empirical analysis. Br J Educ Psychol. 2007;77:873–91.

60. Malau-Aduli BS, Page W, Cooling N, Turner R. Impact of self-efficacy beliefs on short- and long-term academic improvements for underperforming medical students. Am J Educ Res. 2013;1:168–76.

61. Stegers-Jager KM, Cohen-Schotanus J, Themmen APN. Motivation, learning strategies, participation and medical school performance: motivation, learning strategies and participation. Med Educ. 2012;46:678–88.

62. Kruger J, Dunning D. Unskilled and unaware of how difficulties in recognizing incompetence lead to inflated self-assessments. J Pers Soc Psychol. 1999;77:1121–34.

63. Volet S, Vauras M, Salonen P. Self- and social regulation in learning contexts: an integrative perspective. Educ Psychol. 2009;44:215–26.

64. Hmelo-Silver CE, Barrows HS. Facilitating collaborative knowledge building. Cogn Instr. 2008;26:48–94.

65. Flavell JH. Metacognition and cognitive monitoring: a new area of cognitive–developmental inquiry. Am Psychol. 1979;34:906–11.

66. Mevarech ZR, Amrany C. Immediate and delayed effects of meta-cognitive instruction on regulation of cognition and mathematics achievement. Metacogn Learn. 2008;3:147–57.

67. Saks NS, Karl S. Academic support services in U.S. and Canadian medical schools. Med Educ. Online. 2004;9:4348.

68. Horton C, Polek C, Hardie TL. The relationship between enhanced remediation and NCLEX success. Teach Learn Nurs. 2012;7:146–51.

Remediation of Physical Examination Skills

8

Tahlia Spector, Cha-Chi Fung, and Ronald Olson

Observe, record, tabulate, communicate. Use your five senses. Learn to see, learn to hear, learn to feel, learn to smell, and know that by practice alone you can become expert.–Sir William Osler

Introduction

Novice clinicians demonstrate a range of physical examination (PE) skill levels. Learners' approaches to and facility with the PE are influenced by many factors, ranging from knowledge and application of physiology and pathophysiology to personal biases, perceptions, and sensory or physical disabilities, to curricular design differences during pre-clinical and clinical years, to workplace-based experiences (including the "hidden curriculum"). In this chapter, we will briefly name and define

common areas where learners struggle with PE skills, describe methods to identify learners needing remediation, describe potential tools that can be used in remediation, and finally, revisit each of the domains with an illustrative case and specific remediation strategies.[*] Notably, there is usually some overlap between domains, and learners often struggle in more than one domain.

Many would argue that the focus and structure of performing PEs both in health professional schools and in clinical practice has changed over the past decade. The need for routine annual PEs has largely been questioned (as evidenced by Medicare no longer paying for this evaluation), and many practicing clinicians have deprioritized aspects of the PE. Simultaneously, over 88% of medical schools have begun teaching ultrasound in some capacity in the pre-clerkship years, some with a robust point-of-care ultrasound (POCUS) curriculum, which allows direct visualization of pathology previously only surmised [1]. Some programs provide learners with handheld ultrasound machines from day one, seamlessly supplementing and altering fundamental PE teaching. While POCUS enables a bedside "look under the skin" and has the potential to positively impact learning in many ways [2, 3], it can introduce additional

T. Spector (✉)
Department of Emergency Medicine,
David Geffen School of Medicine, University of California, Los Angeles, CA, USA
e-mail: tspector@ucla.edu

C.-C. Fung
Department of Clinical Medical Education, Keck School of Medicine, University of Southern California, Los Angeles, CA, USA
e-mail: chachi.fung@med.usc.edu

R. Olson
Department of Family Medicine, Keck School of Medicine, University of Southern California, Los Angeles, CA, USA
e-mail: ronald.olson@med.usc.edu

[*]Editor's note: We refer the reader to the first edition of this book for detailed cases where the authors describe remediation techniques for many of the struggles listed here.

© The Author(s), under exclusive license to Springer Nature Switzerland AG 2023
A. Kalet, C. L. Chou (eds.), *Remediation in Medical Education*,
https://doi.org/10.1007/978-3-031-32404-8_8

challenges as well. Depending on relative expectations of POCUS mastery, remediation of this modality may also be required.

We will use the four-phase framework from Chap. 6 to frame a remediation process for both general PE skills and POCUS, the latter being an additional tool in a clinician's PE toolbox. Moreover, because POCUS allows for real time visualization of anatomy, faculty can use it during remediation to clarify elements of PEs, even if learners lack significant POCUS experience or knowledge. This more basic and limited use of POCUS has the secondary benefit of exposing the learner to this valuable adjunct to PE if not yet embedded in the curriculum.

Identification

Chris is a clerkship student assessing a patient with atherosclerotic disease who had gnawing back pain. The patient's drape fell off, exposing the patient's undergarment. Without explaining to the patient what was about to happen, Chris palpated below the umbilicus to a depth of about 1 cm, checking for an enlarged pulsating aorta. Not palpating in the correct location, nor at the correct depth, nor with the correct technique, in a patient who was unable to relax abdominal musculature due to the discomfort of being exposed, Chris did not detect the obvious enlarged pulsating mass. Moreover, during the rest of the exam, Chris seemed unaware of the patient's discomfort and did not reposition the drape leaving the patient partially exposed.

Common Domains Where Learners Struggle with PE and POCUS Skills

1. **Basic motor and technical skills**
2. **Experience and medical knowledge**
3. **Interaction**
4. **Clinical reasoning**

1. **Struggles with motor/technical skills** are typically readily observable. Common examples are when a trainee palpates the abdomen at insufficient depth or incorrect location, produces inadequate percussion tones on pulmonary or abdominal exam, or has misdirected or incorrectly placed the ultrasound probe.

   These struggles may be attributable to learning lapses or may indicate more complex educational systems issues. Technical best practices when conducting the PE (for example, auscultating the lungs from one side to the other in at least six places) is taught in classroom settings, on peers or standardized patients. This method, though efficient and least disruptive to busy clinical practice, separates the relevance of PE skills from actual clinical contexts; therefore, novices often have a limited ability to select which techniques should be applied to which patients and to interpret the significance of PE findings such as percussion or auscultation sounds until more immersive clinical exposure. A seasoned clinician, for example, would auscultate the lungs differently in a patient suspected of having a pneumothorax compared with one suspected of being in heart failure. In addition, learners quickly adopt poor habits, such as listening to the heart and lungs through the patient's gown, from supervisors on clinical rotations. Faculty conducting remediation should be aware that this hidden curriculum about the PE can thwart their educational efforts.

2. Learners with **experiential/medical knowledge struggles** may exhibit aptitude in performing pertinent exams on patients presenting with certain chief concerns, but not others. Alternatively, they may not know how to perform a health maintenance examination, seeking evidence of complications in a patient with chronic illness. Similarly, they may be unable to discern subtle differences between disease entities (for example, mistakenly identifying the dry "Velcro" crackles of interstitial lung disease for rales of congestive heart failure). In a POCUS curriculum, these students lack skill or experience using this modality. Unless accompanied by other struggles, this

scenario can be a simple teaching opportunity to expand a learner's experience and/or knowledge base. (See Chap. 7 for further details on remediating medical knowledge.)

3. **Interactional struggles** manifest when learners fail to establish trust, ensure patient comfort and privacy, gain patient cooperation and collaboration in PE maneuvers, and communicate PE findings. Illustrative behaviors include forgetting to wash their hands (or the ultrasound probe), improperly draping the patient, displaying overt awkwardness when performing aspects of the PE, omitting explanations about maneuvers they perform, and not recognizing a patient's pain during a maneuver. Occasionally, a learner's personal hygiene (e.g., halitosis, body odor, unlaundered clothes) is objectionable to patients and contributes to patient discomfort and lack of cooperation. In the case of patients who have experienced previous physical assault or psychological trauma, poor performance may even contribute to or trigger anxiety. It has been estimated that nearly 70% of adults in the USA have experienced some type of traumatic event, with higher estimates in historically marginalized populations [4]. Therefore, every physical exam should be done in a way that ensures safety, informed patient choice, collaboration, trust, and empowerment. (See Chap. 12 for remediating struggles in interpersonal communication.)

4. **Clinical reasoning** struggles may represent the most challenging scenario, as there are multiple steps in the clinical reasoning process (see Chap. 9 for details). Even when the comprehensive physical exam is taught effectively and a learner knows and is able to demonstrate how to perform specific maneuvers technically, they may lack the ability to select the relevant focused physical exam elements to perform in the context of a patient's presenting situation. In other words, they know "how" to do the exam but not "when" to do the exam [5]. Often, learners struggle to identify how the physical exam helps narrow and prioritize a differential diagnosis.

Clarification

Referred for remediation, Chris met with a coach. In the initial meeting, the coach explored the issues underlying the poor performance and discovered that, in addition to a poor understanding of the anatomy and physiology of the aorta and its branches, Chris avoided deep abdominal palpation for fear of hurting the patient. On further discussion, this fear of causing patient discomfort was a recurrent problem across many elements of Chris's PE.

Ideally, experienced clinician educators would observe learners conduct comprehensive patient encounters in actual clinical settings, offer detailed feedback, and identify PE skills-related struggles in clinical reasoning, knowledge, and/ or skill. Unfortunately, this is rarely logistically possible [6]. Instead, most learners' skills are assessed through conference room-based clinical rounds, where groups of clinicians hear patient case presentations that include reports of PE findings [7]. Though efficient from the perspective of clinical patient care, this approach makes it challenging for clinicians to accurately identify learners' needs and domains for improvement in PE skills. Without direct observation, we cannot assess the accuracy of PE findings obtained by a learner. For example, when told that the "neuro exam was unremarkable," it is unclear which of the many components of the exam were performed and if they were conducted or interpreted accurately. If the learner reports diminished reflexes, is this to be interpreted as due to a neurological problem, or were the reflexes poorly elicited by the learner? Perhaps the learner didn't hear a heart murmur but was "coached" about its presence by a resident. Perhaps the learner was unable to address patient comfort and attain full cooperation when performing sensitive exam maneuvers. Therefore, conference room rounds are not an effective environment in which to assess a learner's PE skills, and ultimately, these inaccuracies can significantly compromise clinical reasoning and patient management plans. A powerful, longstanding debate over the value of the PE compared with "paraclinical" or laboratory and imaging modalities to obtain similar information has negatively impacted the rigor of and emphasis placed on teaching this material [8, 9]. Direct observation, focused teaching, and assessment of the PE, especially in patients with actual rather than simulated disease, can counter the loss of these skills to the benefit of clinical excellence, patient safety, and improved patient outcomes.

Despite the logistical constraints posed by an increasingly busy clinical practice setting, several structured opportunities, all of which require direct observation by experienced clinical educators, allow for clarification of learner struggles with PE skills:

- **"Bedside Teaching"**: Largely informal educational sessions where patients, teachers, and learners collaborate to provide opportunities for learners to demonstrate, both technically and interactionally, their ability to perform PE and POCUS maneuvers and discern notable findings.
- **Semi-formal patient interactions** (e.g., Clinical Evaluation Exercise—CEX, Mini-CEX (3), or BSCO—Brief Structured Clinical Observations): Structured opportunities to observe a learner perform specific components of a clinical encounter and are flexible in terms of the setting and time. Multiple observations are necessary when using these tools to achieve an acceptable level of accuracy in assessing a learner's performance [10].
- **Formally structured skills courses/workshops:** Highly structured learning experiences designed to teach specific skills (for example, cardiopulmonary or musculoskeletal examination techniques or POCUS), usually incorporating standardized or real patients in small group settings, and providing ample opportunities for direct observation of learner performance.
- **Formal testing** (e.g., OSCE—Objective Structured Clinical Examinations [11] using standardized patients): Important assessment tools where faculty have the opportunity to observe a single student across multiple clinical encounters or stations, as well as observing multiple students conducting the same standardized patient encounter. Coaches can therefore calibrate feedback to the learner's training level by explicitly designing encounters to enable identification of struggles in clinical reasoning, knowledge, and skills. In addition, trained and highly calibrated standardized patients can provide structured checklist-based feedback on their experience of the learner's interactional skills and other components of the encounter, including the PE. Because these exercises require significant resources, they often have limited utility and do not replace the need for real-world clinical learning settings [12, 13]. However, especially if they are videotaped, OSCEs can provide objective information about learner performance. Faculty can review performance with learners who struggle, encourage learner self-reflection, and prescribe individualized remediation plans [14–16].

Certain struggles (e.g., technical skills and interactional elements) may be obvious after simple observations. Others, especially clinical reasoning, must be ascertained through a more thorough process, for example, probing questioning that leads the learner to recall and critique the thought process behind why they chose to examine the patient a certain way, how they interpreted the information obtained, and what they might do differently in future cases (see Chap. 9 for further details).

To elucidate both the scope of the struggle and the degree of learner insight, we have relied on asynchronous faculty precepted video review. In this process, the learner reviews a video of their encounter with a standardized patient and self-assesses by completing a checklist designed to create awareness of best practices for both the technical and interactional aspects of the physical exam. Following this self-assessment, the learner and faculty coach review the videotape together, and the faculty proposes a series of questions aimed at impelling reflection on the integration of the physical exam with clinical reasoning [17].

Reflective Questions to Ask in the Clarification Phase

1. After completing your history, what are the top 3–5 disease processes in your differential diagnosis in order of likelihood?
2. What are the disease processes you are most concerned about that need to be ruled out?
3. What do you think is going on at this point in the encounter?
4. What pertinent positive or negative PE findings were you looking for or would you look for now?
5. If you were to perform the physical exam again based on this differential, describe what you would do.
6. If POCUS is to be used, what anatomical structure would be scanned?
7. What examination findings would support or refute your hypothesis?
8. I see that you listened to the [heart]. What were you listening for? How would you change the exam to find what you are looking for?
9. What do you think is the best position for the patient to be in to elicit that finding? Why?

Intervention

To address knowledge and technical skills struggles, we directed Chris to choose between several books and online resources that highlight the technical skills required to evaluate abdominal structures and suggested selecting learning one specific technique per day, followed by deliberate practice of that technique on every patient seen clinically that day. We required Chris to briefly document each practice case, including a description of the PE findings and interpretation of the information in the context of the clinical case. We encouraged Chris to add a new

technique daily until Chris conducted and documented comprehensive abdominal exams on a few patients a day. In addition, we guided Chris to visualize each patient's anatomy using POCUS: the location of the abdominal aorta and bifurcation, to assess the width of the aorta, and to observe the pulsations before repalpating.

Book and Video Suggestions:

- Physical examination textbooks: Bates' Physical Examination and History Taking [18] or DeGowin's Diagnostic Examination [19]
- Online videos or real-life/real-time demonstration of correct exam techniques: Bates' Physical Examination Videos provided as part of the textbook package; UCSD Practical Guide to Clinical Medicine [20]
- Online videos of examination of abdominal aorta (for example: https://www.youtube.com/watch?v=2MO3en1D_w8)
- Online videos of basic ultrasound techniques
- Online videos of the eFAST examination (Extended Focus Assessment with Ultrasonography in Trauma) or other specific exams
- Using the ultrasound probe to examine geometric models (e.g., cylinders) to understand how orientation of the probe affects the image

To address the interactional component, we had Chris practice performing non-invasive physical exam maneuvers with friends, family members, or colleagues, requesting detailed feedback on Chris's ability to address draping and privacy, to explain actions before performing them, and to share the "findings" without utilizing medical jargon. Then we asked Chris to demonstrate how to drape and ensure patient privacy. We also arranged to have Chris experience being the patient for near peers practicing abdominal exams and asked Chris to reflect on how various approaches contributed to Chris's own degree of comfort.

Learners require individualized remediation strategies, depending on their needs and domain(s) in which they struggle. Strategies that incorporate hands-on, practical, and interactive activities are more effective than reading and shadowing alone [21]. To address knowledge gaps, preparatory reading is required before starting interactive case-based exercises that promote application of acquired knowledge [22].

- **Real-Time Remediation:** We find it highly efficient and meaningful to take learners to a patient's bedside to demonstrate correct PE and POCUS techniques, discuss underlying physiological rationale for those techniques, and to teach PE pearls (e.g., how to examine a ticklish patient). When more in-depth teaching is needed, or discussion of a topic that is very personal for the student is likely, bedside teaching may be inappropriate.
- **Independent study/self-directed learning exercises** to establish the necessary fundamental knowledge base and clinical reasoning include:
  - Listing differential diagnoses for certain chief complaints based on age, gender (if relevant), and possibly co-morbidities in the order of most common and most dangerous
  - Creating charts that discriminate which exam findings are consistent with or help discern between different but similar diseases
  - Considering what examination would be required in a patient with various chief complaints—can be done as an exercise on a simulated patient (either role play with another learner or on paper)
  - Considering what examination should be performed in a well-person visit when the

patient has various underlying medical problems. This is usually a two-step process: first, identification of the possible complications of a disease process, followed by demonstration of an exam to look for pathology
  - Reading parts of a PE skills textbook or watching videos that elucidate appropriately and correctly performed PE and POCUS maneuvers. Texts that are organized on cases or chief complaints rather than by organ system may have the added benefit of modeling more accurate and complete examinations
- Many of these activities can be done alone or in small study groups. We also often pair these cognitive exercises with other experiential activities (for example, practice interactions with standardized or real patients).
- **Clinical activities focused on PE skills** specific to learners' struggles can be incorporated as part of a regular clinical rotation. Examples include: (1) practice systematizing approaches to the history and physical exams; (2) practice creating an appropriate differential diagnosis that includes dangerous entities, asking specific questions to rule these in or out and then performing an exam that supports/refutes these entities in the differential; (3) repetition with feedback to increase speed and flow of the encounters to improve patient comfort while maintaining accuracy; (4) practice announcing to patients what exam will be performed and verbalizing the findings; and (5) practice performing certain examinations [e.g., ophthalmological or cardiovascular exam, POCUS of the heart, lungs, or kidneys] on each patient to improve technique.
- **Organized group activities/courses** have been designed for medical students on fundamental or advanced clerkships specifically to address struggles identified either via a structured curriculum or faculty teaching at the bedside. These activities, though faculty-intensive, are often very well-attended and appreciated.

  - Advanced diagnostic skills courses using real patients with chronic but stable medical problems to appreciate the subtleties of the physical exam.

- Engagement in teaching pre-clerkship students [23]
- Hypothesis-Driven PE workshops that use standardized patients who act out specific clinical presentations and guide learners through the reasoning process by conducting a focused PE [24, 25]
- Evidence-based PE workshops, using the Rational Clinical Examination series from the *Journal of the American Medical Association,* [26] to help recap basic PE skills and enable learning of the highest-yield disease-specific PE maneuvers [23]
- POCUS workshops and courses for skill improvement and visualization of structures to enhance physical exam technique

Assessment

Reassessment, using any of the strategies used for primary assessment at pre-determined intervals, is critical to determine the success of any remediation. It is helpful if the evaluator is aware of the specific struggle(s) focused on in the remediation, through sharing of the remediation plan or direct conversation with the learner. It is critical for the learner to take a high degree of responsibility for self-monitoring of progress, since doing so constitutes the basis for the lifelong, self-directed learning skills needed to maintain clinical competence.

Finally, on a systems level, curriculum leaders responsible for educating students on the physical exam must monitor remediation activities for emerging patterns as a matter of program evaluation. If multiple learners struggle in a given area, the curriculum, rather than the learners, may need revision and supplementation with additional education and/or skill-building.

Conclusion

We have named four distinct domains where learners struggle with PE: motor/technical skills,

knowledge or experience, interaction, and clinical reasoning. Most learners requiring remediation demonstrate a combination of struggles; therefore, remediation strategies must be individualized for best results. Though PE skills remediation typically occurs during routine clinical learning at a patient's bedside and uses role modeling to impel learners toward deliberate practice, a range of strategies, including the use of structured and standardized simulations and workshops, should always be considered. Depending on the resources available and students' individual needs, remediation can be enhanced by utilizing technology such as digitally enhanced or multi-headed teaching stethoscopes, POCUS, simultaneous cardiac echo, among others. It is also helpful to keep handy a catalog of vetted learning resources such as YouTube videos of examination skills. Early identification of student struggles, use of diverse remediation strategies targeted to learner needs, and regular progress monitoring represent the core steps in supporting learner proficiency in the PE.

There remain significant logistical constraints in the remediation process that need to be addressed. Curricula and faculty skills and attitudes must be continually monitored to ensure effective teaching of PE skills. Faculty clinicians with exemplary PE and coaching skills also must have time and resources available to engage with learners. In these ways, we believe that most learners will attain the skills to be both excellent clinicians and capable teachers for future generations.

References

1. AAMC Curriculum reports: ultrasound use at US and Canadian medical schools. 2020. https://www.aamc.org/data-reports/curriculum-reports/interactive-data/ultrasound-use-us-and-canadian-medical-schools. Accessed 29 Dec 2022.
2. So S, Patel RM, Orebaugh SL. Ultrasound imaging in medical student education: impact on learning anatomy and physical diagnosis. Anat Sci Educ. 2017;10:176–89. https://doi.org/10.1002/ase.1630.
3. Hoppmann RA, Rao VV, Bell F, et al. The evolution of an integrated ultrasound curriculum (iUSC) for medical students: 9-year experience. Crit Ultrasound J. 2015;7(1):18. https://doi.org/10.1186/s13089-015-0035-3.

4. TraumaInformedcare.chcs.org. Understanding the effects of trauma on health fact sheet. 2017. Accessed 29 Dec 2022.

5. Wilkerson L, Lee M. Assessing physical examination skills of senior medical students: knowing how versus knowing when. Acad Med. 2003;78:S30–2.

6. Herbers JE Jr, Noel GL, Cooper GS, Harvey J, Pangaro LN, Weaver MJ. How accurate are faculty evaluations of clinical competence? J Gen Intern Med. 1989;4:202–8.

7. Kassebaum DG, Eaglen RH. Shortcomings in the evaluation of students' clinical skills and behaviors in medical school. Acad Med. 1999;74:842–9.

8. Harwick L, Cleland J, Kitto S. Sending messages: how faculty influence professional teaching and learning. Med Teach. 2017;39:987–94.

9. Faustinella F, Jacobs R. The decline of clinical skills: a challenge for medical schools. Int J Med Educ. 2018;9:195–7.

10. Norcini JJ, Blank LL, Duffy FD, Fortna GS. The mini-CEX: a method for assessing clinical skills. Ann Intern Med. Mar 18 2003;138:476–81.

11. Harden RM. What is an OSCE? Med Teach. 1988;10(1):19–22.

12. Barman A. Critiques on the objective structured clinical examination. Ann Acad Med Singap. 2005;34(8):478–82.

13. Frye AW, Richards BF, Philp EB, Philp JR. Is it worth it? A look at the costs and benefits of an OSCE for second-year medical students. Med Teach. 1989;11:291–3.

14. Chang A, Chou CL, Teherani A, Hauer KE. Clinical skills-related learning goals of senior medical students after performance feedback. Med Educ. 2011;45:878–85.

15. Dornan T, Scherpbier A, Boshuizen H. Towards valid measures of self-directed clinical learning. Med Educ. 2003;37:983–91.

16. Sargeant J, Eva KW, Armson H, et al. Features of assessment learners use to make informed self-assessments of clinical performance. Med Educ. 2011;45:636–47.

17. Saxena V, O'Sullivan PS, Teherani A, Irby DM, Hauer KE. Remediation techniques for student performance problems after a comprehensive clinical skills assessment. Acad Med. 2009;84:669–76.

18. Bickley LS. Bates' guide to physical examination and history taking. 11th ed. Walters Kluwer Health/Lippincott Williams & Wilkins; 2013.

19. DeGowin RLB, D. D. DeGowin's diagnostic examination. 9th ed. The McGraw-Hill Companies, Inc.; 2009.

20. Goldberg C. A practice guide to clinical medicine. 2009. http://meded.ucsd.edu/clinicalmed/. Accessed 29 Dec 2022.

21. Clark REV, A. Transfer of training principles for instructional design. Educ Technol Res Dev. 1985;33(2):113–23.

22. Perkins DNS, G. Transfer of learning. International encyclopedia of education. 2nd ed. Oxford, England: Pergamon Press; 1992.

23. Chou CL. Physical examination teaching curriculum for senior medical students. Med Educ. 2005;39:1151.

24. Nishigori H, Masuda K, Kikukawa M, et al. A model teaching session for the hypothesis-driven physical examination. Med Teach. 2011;33:410–7.

25. Yudkowsky R, Otaki J, Lowenstein T, Riddle J, Nishigori H, Bordage G. A hypothesis-driven physical examination learning and assessment procedure for medical students: initial validity evidence. Med Educ. 2009;43:729–40.

26. Simel DL, Rennie D, eds. The Rational Clinical Examination: Evidence-Based Clinical Diagnosis. New York: McGraw Hill Medical, 2008. https://jamanetwork.com/collections/6257/the-rational-clinical-examination.

Assessment and Remediation of Clinical Reasoning

9

Andrew S. Parsons and Karen M. Warburton

Introduction

Ethan (he/him), a second-year internal medicine resident, is called to meet with the program director, Dr. Ramirez (she/her), to discuss concerns about his clinical performance. Dr. Ramirez alerts Ethan that senior residents and faculty have raised concerns in their written evaluations about his clinical decision-making. Select comments include: "cannot tell a story," "struggles when things are complex, or when the service is busy," "cannot put the pieces together," and "has tunnel vision at times." One evaluator did note that he "can make an accurate decision when given all of the data."

Clinical reasoning is a term used to describe the processes of making a diagnosis and managing a patient [1]. Learners can struggle with one or both of these components, commonly referred to as diagnostic reasoning and management reasoning [2]. Effective remediation of learners who struggle with clinical reasoning includes timely identification, global and targeted appraisal, coaching, and continuing evaluation and assessment. The goal of this process is to ensure patient safety and move the learner toward consistent expert performance. National organizations and landmark publications, such as The National Academy of Sciences' "Improving Diagnosis in Healthcare," have called for enhanced teaching of clinical reasoning to reduce clinical errors [3]. Unfortunately, the rate of diagnostic and management error is difficult to determine in the routine assessment of individual trainees. Clinical evaluators may lack the skills necessary to assess the clinical reasoning of their learners, limiting intervention efforts. Once identified, dedicated coaching and deliberate practice are the most effective means of moving these learners toward expert performance [4, 5]. However, effective clinical reasoning remediation requires significant time investment by both coach and learner [6]. In addition, learner buy-in is essential to a successful remediation process. We follow many of the steps listed in Chap. 6; the first steps in this process are asking the learner about their perspective, empathizing with what they almost assuredly see as a predicament, and drawing out the learner's perspective on their own plight.

A. S. Parsons (✉)
Departments of Medicine and Public Health, University of Virginia School of Medicine, Charlottesville, VA, USA
e-mail: Asp5c@virginia.edu

K. M. Warburton
Department of Medicine, University of Virginia School of Medicine, Charlottesville, VA, USA
e-mail: Kmw2g@virginia.edu

Identification

Dr. Ramirez: *Ethan, do these comments resonate with your experience?*

Ethan: *It's definitely not the first time I've been given feedback like this, but I am not exactly sure what is going on. I felt that I was improving in these areas as an intern, but now that I have more responsibility, I am struggling with my decision-making.*

Dr. Ramirez: *I know this can be hard, and I hear that this is not a shock to you. If we can figure out where exactly you're struggling, we can tackle these problems together.*

Ethan: *Sometimes I'm just not sure what is wrong with my patients, and which steps I should take next, especially with the more complex patients. Maybe I just need to read more? I always did well in medical school.*

Struggles with clinical reasoning can be difficult to recognize and are often "misdiagnosed" as struggles either with fund of knowledge or organization and efficiency ([7]; see Chaps. 7, 11). Clinical reasoning is not recognized as a distinct clinical competency by the Accreditation Council for Graduate Medical Education (ACGME), and thus data on the prevalence of struggles with clinical reasoning are often not captured in surveys about learners who struggle [8–10]. According to reports from two centralized remediation programs across the continuum of medical education, clinical reasoning was identified in 25–45% of learners who struggled [5, 11].

Struggles with clinical reasoning can impact performance in many ways. Learners may have trouble with patient presentations or making clinical decisions. Table 9.1 includes some common

Table 9.1 Commonly used phrases to describe the learner struggling with clinical reasoning

Presentations are disorganized and often miss important details
Easily overwhelmed with complex patients
Can't see the forest for the trees
Can't connect the dots
Struggles to prioritize a differential diagnosis
Can't call a consult
Handoffs don't convey the important information
Can't structure an admission (or clinic visit) efficiently
Can't triage a task list
Can't tell sick versus not sick
Anchors, or demonstrates premature closure

descriptive phrases used to describe the learner struggling with clinical reasoning.

Often, the evaluator recognizes that a learner is struggling, but cannot quite pinpoint the problem. Learners who make confusing, disorganized, or inaccurate case presentations or write disappointedly inadequate clinical notes are worrisome because they potentially endanger patient safety. Clinical reasoning is a complex cognitive process, dependent on, but not limited to, adequate fund of knowledge. Because many clinical supervisors may lack a framework for analyzing clinical reasoning struggles, they are less likely to effectively coach learners to improve clinical reasoning. Moreover, we often do not spend enough time directly observing our learners' clinical skills and are therefore left to infer a great deal about their performance from how they answer factual questions on rounds or in conference. Many learners struggling with clinical reasoning are reflexively advised to "read more."

Ethan's case is typical of learners who struggle with clinical reasoning. Based on test scores, his knowledge base is sound. However, his performance drops during clinical encounters that require a structured approach and application of knowledge.

Clarification: Global and Targeted Appraisal of the Learner Struggling with Clinical Reasoning

Further conversation between Ethan and Dr. Ramirez revealed that Ethan's performance on standardized tests was good to average. He remembers struggling on Observed Structured Clinical Examinations in medical school. Dr. Ramirez determines that Ethan struggles to apply knowledge to the clinical environment and refers him to Dr. Williams, a clinical reasoning remediation coach.

Global Appraisal

Effective remediation hinges on accurate determination of specific performance gaps, which is best accomplished with a systematic review of the learner's performance in the current and, when available, prior program(s). As described in Chap. 6, a comprehensive investigation includes talking with the learner about underlying causes of unsatisfactory clinical performance such as impairment, performance anxiety, or burnout [11]. It is important to review educational history for evidence of primary struggles with medical knowledge; after all, one needs to know the alphabet to spell. Signs consistent with clinical reasoning struggles include failure in one or more objective structured clinical examinations (OSCEs) in medical school; average or above average standardized knowledge test scores coupled with consistently low scores in clinical performance; and comments from clinical rotations (Table 9.1). We recommend that the remediation coach attempt to speak directly with a few clinical educators who have worked with the learner across clinical

contexts. And, as described in Chap. 7, knowledge can be assessed by asking direct, factual questions during direct observation of the learner's performance in the clinical learning environment, or through discussing cases in a coach's office.

Targeted Appraisal

If global appraisal leads to the determination that the learner's struggle is predominantly related to clinical reasoning, the next step is a targeted appraisal [5]. The goal of targeted appraisal is to identify strengths and challenges along the clinical reasoning pathway. It is important to determine if the primary struggle is ineffective diagnostic or management reasoning by a thorough review of clinical evaluation data. In fact, clinical evaluation data are critical because they add context to the targeted assessment which can limited by case specificity and a learner's content knowledge. For the purposes of appraisal of clinical reasoning, it is useful to simplify and consider diagnosis and management as a linear pathway, starting with diagnostic reasoning and then basing management strategies on that diagnosis (although in practice, there is a dynamic and iterative relationship between the two). A clinician must always reconsider the diagnosis as new information emerges from the patient's response to treatment and the evolution of the clinical predicament.

For learners who struggle with diagnosis, the initial objective is to further specify an area to support along the following diagnostic reasoning pathway: hypothesis generation; data collection; problem representation; refinement of hypotheses; and development of working diagnosis (script selection). We suggest using a seven-step, case-based approach (Fig. 9.1) that incorporates these steps.

The coach provides the learner with the initial clinical case information (patient age, gender) and the chief complaint in the patient's own words.

Coaching prompt:

Step 1: Based on this information, generate hypotheses (broad differential diagnosis) using both non-analytic (pattern recognition) and analytic methods (anatomical, systems based, or pathophysiology based; be sure to incorporate pre-test probability).

Coaching Probes:

Which analytical approach would work best for this case and why?

Step 2: Based on the broad differential you created, what questions do you want to ask this patient? Keep in mind that we are working towards a hypothesis driven approach to history taking. In other words, the differential guides data gathering.

The learner is provided further history of present illness in response to their questions.

Step 3: Based on this information, how would you manipulate and reprioritize the differential?

Coaching Probes:

Do you recognize any patterns?

Use pretest (prior) probability to prioritize your differential diagnoses.

The learner is provided history and review of systems.

Step 4: Based on your updated differential, select which physical examination data you would like to receive and why.

The learner is provided with pertinent physical examination findings in response to their questions.

Step 5: Create a problem representation, a 1-2 sentence summary of the pertinent information you have learned to this point. A problem representation has three components: demographics/risk factors, tempo, and syndrome(s). Use semantic qualifiers to change from the patient's voice to medical terminology. Keep in mind that a major purpose of the problem representation is to refine and narrow your initially broad differential diagnosis.

Step 6: Which illness scripts are prompted by your problem representation? Remember, an illness script has three components: epidemiology (who gets the condition and when), pathophysiology, and clinical presentation (signs and symptoms).

Step 7: Reprioritize the differential diagnosis with an emphasis on identifying a working diagnosis.

Fig. 9.1 Case-based identification of struggles with diagnostic reasoning: a seven-step appraisal. Use this case-based appraisal method to identify areas to support along the diagnostic reasoning pathway. It is critical to use this approach across a range of clinical cases and include varying contextual factors

Hypothesis Generation

The diagnostic reasoning process begins with the development of a broad list of potential diagnoses based on a limited set of key pieces of information from the chief complaint and patient demographics. This list of hypotheses is generated using two well-described cognitive systems of decision-making. Dual-process theory summarizes a vast cognitive psychology evidence base and provides a robust framework for understanding clinical reasoning [12]. The dual-process theory describes two systems that are relatively independent but work together, enabling a physician to reason rapidly and deliberately. System 1 is non-analytical, intuitive, and efficient [13]. The basic clinical reasoning skill in System 1 is pattern recognition. System 1 thinking is most obvious when an experienced physician immediately recognizes a well-established illness script when presented with a patient presentation. In contrast, System 2 is an analytical process. It is slow, deliberative, conscious application of an analytical approach to arrive at a diagnosis [13]. Which system is activated depends on the clinician's prior experience with a given clinical presentation, and their ability to activate the appropriate illness script [14]. To avoid mistakes, experts consciously toggle between systems, confirming a diagnosis they reached quickly through System 1 by applying System 2 reasoning to the case [15]. Novices also use both systems; however, given their limited experience, their System 1 is likely to be less accurate, and they are more likely than experts to anchor on a final diagnosis based on their initial thoughts. Because of this, inexperienced clinicians are at risk of prematurely committing to a diagnosis with inadequate information.

Data Gathering

Data gathering involves asking questions about the patient's history (see Chap. 7), performing the physical examination (see Chap. 8), and collecting initial laboratory and imaging results. Consideration of diagnostic hypotheses prior to data gathering, termed hypothesis-driven data gathering, improves diagnostic accuracy [16].

Problem Representation and Illness Scripts

The problem representation is a an abstraction of the important features of a case using paired, opposing descriptive terms referred to as semantic qualifiers [17]. When in the form of a verbalized or written summary statement, the problem representation is commonly referred to as the "one-liner" and is used to summarize patient cases when clinicians communicate with each other (oral presentations on rounds, handoffs, progress notes, calling consults). When done correctly, formulating problem representations

strengthens clinical reasoning [18, 19] by activating or accessing illness scripts, or mental representations (schemas) from the clinician's long-term memory. Illness scripts, which usually include key risk factors, pathophysiology, and clinical presentation, reflect the clinician's organized stored knowledge of a given disease [14, 20]. With experience and attention to accuracy, learners should enhance their illness scripts to better estimate the likelihood of a diagnosis when a clinical feature is present or absent [21].

The ability to formulate an effective problem representation is a fundamental skill and one that, for many learners, needs to be taught explicitly. Difficulties with problem representation can manifest in many ways. For example, a learner may be unable to provide effective handoffs of care, as observed in their "sign-out" to other providers. Other signs of gaps in this domain are struggles with succinct and accurate presentations, calling consults, or managing more than one complex patient. Evaluators may comment that these learners lack an understanding of the big picture with their patients, or "just don't get it."

Management Reasoning

Cook et al. recently defined management reasoning as "the process of making decisions about patient management, including choices about treatment, follow-up visits, further testing, and allocation of limited resources" [2]. They also identified some key differences between diagnostic and management reasoning. For instance, diagnostic reasoning is a classification task of assigning a single diagnosis, operates independently of context, and does not require patient interaction. In contrast, management reasoning is a task involving shared decision-making and monitoring, can include multiple solutions, depends on context (e.g., patient, provider, and system preferences), and requires patient communication [2]. Diagnostic reasoning likely ends with activation of a management script, the first step in management reasoning. Like illness scripts, management scripts are activated in real time in response to encountering a clinical problem [22]. Once a management script is activated (accessed, recalled, retrieved) for a given condition, clinicians can then select actions (i.e., laboratory, imaging, procedures, consultants, medications, monitoring, etc.) based on the needs of a specific patient and the current situation. This process, termed management option selection [22], requires the learner to estimate the harms and benefits of each intervention, taking patient preferences into account. Though the evidence base supporting our understanding of management reasoning is less robust than that for diagnostic reasoning, the two processes are highly analogous, and the literature is growing.

Intervention: Coaching Clinical Reasoning

Setting: Ethan's first meeting with Dr. Williams (she/her), the clinical reasoning coach

Dr. Williams: *Ethan, I look forward to working with you on this. Let's begin by setting some specific goals. Then I will introduce you to a standardized approach to clinical reasoning, which will give us a shared language we can use to talk about and work on clinical reasoning and clinical decision-making.*

Once the targeted appraisal is complete, coaching should begin with a discussion of expectations and goals to obtain a commitment from the learner, because successful clinical reasoning coaching is time-intensive and requires deliberate practice. As clinical reasoning may be a new language to the learner, an explicit discussion of the reasoning processes should follow closely after the initial appraisal. The discussion should include an introduction or review of key clinical reasoning terms. The learner should be informed that the coaching process will include working through segmented cases and clinical reasoning exercises, employing frequent "stops" to determine the reasoning behind the learner's decisions. Some learners find this

approach needlessly theoretical and must be convinced that the ability to think critically and reflect on their own thought processes is critical to development of strong clinical reasoning (see Chap. 4).

The coach and learner together should design a remediation strategy that employs exercises (Fig. 9.2) targeted to the identified area requiring support [23–25]. Because successful clinical reasoning depends on context, coaching must include a substantial number of cases across a broad array of clinical conditions. We suggest that coaching encounters begin with simple, typical presentations of common problems that progressively increase in complexity [26, 27]. The coach should give the learner cases with varied chief complaints and demographic information. The coach's approach, based on the reasoning level of the learner, should provide scaffolding for the learner, at first being very structured and supportive even to the point of sharing a detailed "worked example" if needed, and then fading back as the learner becomes more self-sufficient (see Chap. 19, cognitive apprenticeship). The coach should aim to create a safe atmosphere where the learner can develop strong self-regulatory skills, metacognition, and reflective practice (see Chaps. 4, 15).

Hypothesis Generation (Fig. 9.2, Purple Gear)

Dr. Williams: *From the cases we have worked through together so far, I notice that you do not always begin by creating a broad differential diagnosis.*

Ethan: *Yes, I didn't feel like I had enough information. I usually go see the patient right away, collect all the information I can, and then think about what may be causing the patient's symptoms. At times, I come out of the patient's room feeling confused and disorganized.*

Dr. Williams: *Can you tell me more about what you mean by disorganized?*

Ethan: *Yes. I feel overwhelmed, especially when the patient is critically ill.*

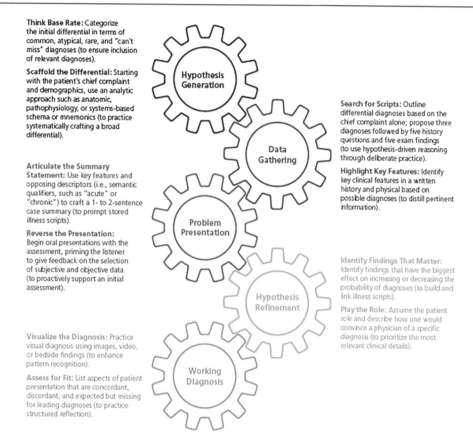

Think Base Rate: Categorize the initial differential in terms of common, atypical, rare, and "can't miss" diagnoses (to ensure inclusion of relevant diagnoses).

Scaffold the Differential: Starting with the patient's chief complaint and demographics, use an analytic approach such as anatomic, pathophysiology, or systems-based schema or mnemonics (to practice systematically crafting a broad differential).

Articulate the Summary Statement: Use key features and opposing descriptors (i.e., semantic qualifiers, such as "acute" or "chronic") to craft a 1- to 2-sentence case summary (to prompt stored illness scripts).

Reverse the Presentation: Begin oral presentations with the assessment, priming the listener to give feedback on the selection of subjective and objective data (to proactively support an initial assessment).

Visualize the Diagnosis: Practice visual diagnosis using images, video, or bedside findings (to enhance pattern recognition).

Assess for Fit: List aspects of patient presentation that are concordant, discordant, and expected but missing for leading diagnoses (to practice structured reflection).

Search for Scripts: Outline differential diagnoses based on the chief complaint alone; propose three diagnoses followed by five history questions and five exam findings (to use hypothesis-driven reasoning through deliberate practice).

Highlight Key Features: Identify key clinical features in a written history and physical based on possible diagnoses (to distill pertinent information).

Identify Findings That Matter: Identify findings that have the biggest effect on increasing or decreasing the probability of diagnoses (to build and link illness scripts).

Play the Role: Assume the patient role and describe how one would convince a physician of a specific diagnosis (to prioritize the most relevant clinical details).

Hypothesis Generation

Data Gathering

Problem Presentation

Hypothesis Refinement

Working Diagnosis

Fig. 9.2 Targeted strategies to coach struggles with diagnostic reasoning. The process begins with hypothesis generation and ends with a working diagnosis. Each component of the process has two recommended coaching exercises [23–25]. Adapted with permission

Ethan struggles to generate potential diagnoses with limited information and distinguish between concerning and less concerning diagnoses. With limited information, and usually limited experience, the learner must rely on System 2 to build or broaden their initial list of hypotheses. Learners can use frameworks or organizing scaffolds (Fig. 9.2, purple gear), to systematically approach this process. Because clinical information can be retrieved and manipulated as a single item within the working memory, the use of frameworks to develop schemas may help learners manage their cognitive load [28, 29]. As certain frameworks may be more appropriate for a given chief complaint, we recommend use of one or more of the following frameworks [27]. We guide the learner toward the appropriate framework through repetitive case-based application and have provided some guidance below.

Schema 1: Pre-test Probability

Consider the probability or likelihood of suspected diseases, based on their prevalence before any diagnostic tests are conducted (also referred to as base rate or prior-probability), specific to a given patient from a particular population. Common diseases are common, and rare diseases are rare. It is important to encourage the learner to routinely familiarize themselves with the epidemiology of the geographic locale and understand how referral filters and recency or availability effects may bias their judgement on what is most likely in a particular clinical setting. We encourage use of this framework for all cases.

Example: While a complaint of chronic cough is usually post-nasal drip, reactive airway disease, or gastroesophageal reflex, during a viral pandemic, adjustments in prior probability need to be carefully considered.

Schema 2: Anatomical

Consider the organs and surrounding structures in a given location and what can go wrong with each. We encourage use of this framework for localized complaints such as pain, redness, swelling, or other signs of inflammation.

Example: For a complaint of chest pain, think of anatomical features in the chest (skin, muscles, ribs, mediastinum, heart, lungs, spine, and associated bony structures) as well as the few instances where this is potentially confusing because pain may be referred from elsewhere.

Schema 3: Pathophysiology

Consider the physiological processes of disease leading to the chief complaint. We encourage use of this framework for isolated abnormal vital signs, laboratory values, or imaging findings.

Example: For an abnormally elevated creatinine level in outpatient clinic, think of pre-renal, intrinsic, and post-renal causes.

Schema 4: Systems

Consider various organ systems and disease processes in each. We encourage use of this framework for nonspecific complaints such as fatigue, weight loss, and fever.

Example: For a complaint of unintentional weight loss in a refugee patient

Neurological—Depression, eating disorder, laxative abuse
Gastrointestinal—Malabsorption, dental disease
Endocrine—Thyroid disease, diabetes mellitus
Neoplastic—Many forms of cancers
Infectious—Tapeworm, dysentery
Vascular—Ischemic bowel disease
Social—Poverty, isolation

Schema 5: Worst-Case Scenario

Consider specific conditions that can lead to significant morbidity or death, or are time-urgent. These are "cannot-miss" diagnoses. We encourage use of this framework for all cases, while emphasizing that inappropriate consideration of such diagnoses can, in some cases, lead to over-testing.

Example: For a complaint of acute shortness of breath, consider pulmonary embolism, decompensated heart failure, and myocardial infarction.

Data Gathering (Fig. 9.2, Pink Gear)

Dr. Williams: *Now that you have a framework for generating a broad differential diagnosis, let's work through some more cases.*

Dr. Williams: *Great question. As we discussed, clinical reasoning is a complex process. Efficiency and accuracy come with practice in developing hypotheses to guide our data gathering. Let's work on that.*

Ethan: *I have been told that I take a long time to see patients. This approach might make it worse. How do the attendings always seem to know what questions to ask to get to the heart of the matter quickly?*

Students are generally taught how to take a comprehensive patient history using a structured approach (i.e., chief complaint, history of present illness, past medical history, etc.). However, learners may struggle to adapt and refine their history-taking based on a given patient's clinical presentation. To improve hypothesis-driven data gathering, learners need dedicated case-based coaching and deliberate practice. We recommend a "search for scripts" exercise (Fig. 9.2, pink gear) where the learner is provided a specific chief complaint, asked to generate a differential diagnosis, and then asked to propose 3–5 history items and 3–5 physical exam findings that would be expected for each item on the differential [23–25, 29]. This exercise forces the learner to consider differentiating and distinguishing features of each diagnosis. The coach should ask the learner to compare and contrast key features of each diagnosis. This exercise should be repeated for multiple chief complaints. Additionally, coaches should employ an exercise known as "highlight key features" (Fig. 9.2, pink gear) [23–25, 29]. In this exercise, a learner is provided comprehensive written H&Ps for unfamiliar patients. The learner is asked to literally highlight key features of the history and physical exam while reading the note from beginning to end. This exercise asks the learner to identify differentiating and distinguishing features of a case while simultaneously considering multiple diagnoses.

Problem Representation (Fig. 9.2, Orange Gear)

> Ethan: *I still receive some pushback from other services when calling consults. Maybe I am not communicating effectively?*
>
> Dr. Williams: *It sounds like you may struggle with problem representation.*

Successful development of an accurate and concise problem representation is reliant upon a strong repository of illness scripts in the learner's long-term memory and a solid base of biomedical knowledge [17]. There are several targeted exercises for learners who struggle with problem representation. We recommend "reversing the presentation" [23–25, 29], a technique in which the learner begins the oral presentation at what is typically expected at the end, with the assessment to prime the coach for feedback on selection of subjective and objective data. This allows the learner to proactively support their initial assessment. Second, learners should be asked to explicitly create and state their problem representation for each patient. A thorough problem representation should answer three questions [30]:

(a) Who is the patient? Include pertinent demographics and risk factors
(b) What is the temporal pattern of illness? Length (acute, subacute, chronic) and tempo (stable, progressive, resolving, intermittent,

waxing and waning)
(c) What are the key signs and symptoms?

The learner should also be asked to refine their problem representation once new clinical data are collected or revealed in various case-based scenarios.

Hypothesis Refinement (Fig. 9.2, Green Gear)

> Dr. Williams: *Ethan, your presentations are greatly improved. But now you seem to be presenting expansive differential diagnosis lists even after the diagnosis is relatively certain.*
>
> Ethan: *Yes, now that you mention it, I feel that I am now commonly considering many more diagnoses than I did previously. I thought that was a good thing.*
>
> Dr. Williams: *It is, but the next step is to focus in on a few most likely diagnoses.*

Learners sometimes assign diagnoses to individual pieces of data, but fail to consider the pattern in the data. This behavior emphasizes how knowledge is necessary but not sufficient for strong clinical reasoning, because this behavior can lead to over-testing and overtreatment when the clinician has a low tolerance for risk and uncertainty. An effective targeted exercise to address this phenomenon is known as "identify findings that matter" [23–25, 29], which asks the learner to identify findings that have the biggest impact on increasing or decreasing the probability of certain diagnoses. This helps them build more robust illness scripts.

Another exercise is to have the learner assume the role of a patient [23–25, 29]. The learner then describes how they would convince the coach (role playing a clinician) of a specific diagnosis in order to force prioritization of clinical details.

Working Diagnosis (Fig. 9.2, Blue Gear)

Ethan: *After all of the negative feedback that I have received, I guess I am afraid getting it wrong.*

Dr. Williams: *Ethan, this a common response. But you have worked hard, and your skills are improving. Now we need to work on building your confidence in your approach.*

Ethan: *Are there any exercises that I can use to check myself once I select a diagnosis so that I am less prone to bias and cognitive error?*

The coach can have the learner practice visual diagnosis using images, video, or bedside findings to enhance pattern recognition [23]. In addition, common cognitive biases include anchoring, confirmation, availability, and premature closure. Structured reflection on each step of a clinical case and engaging their metacognitive awareness may help learners prevent reasoning errors. More specifically, structured assessment of fit, a systematic procedure of reflective reasoning, can counteract bias [31, 32]. In this exercise, the coach asks the learner to list findings in support of the diagnosis (which also may result in confirmation bias), findings against the diagnosis, and findings expected for the given diagnosis, but not present.

Management Reasoning

Dr. Williams: Let's *spend some time on management reasoning so that you select the correct tests and treatments for your patients. This should enhance confidence.*

Table 9.2 Management script template worksheet

	All management options for diagnosis/syndrome	Patient-specific management selection
Laboratory studies		
Imaging studies		
Procedures		
Consults		
Medications		
Monitoring		

Creating management plans can be difficult, especially for early learners who lack context or significant clinical experience. Use of a management script template provides a scaffold, forcing the learner to consider all of the potential management options for a given diagnosis [22]. A sample management script template is given below (Table 9.2).

Next, the coach should ask the learner to select which interventions to perform (i.e., management option selection) based on patient-specific characteristics.

The management script template can be particularly effective for coaching learners who struggle with urgent clinical encounters where the clinician is typically required to make management decisions prior to having a refined differential diagnosis. In these cases, the patient's clinical response to management interventions, specifically testing and treatment, may iteratively guide prioritization of the differential diagnosis. Use of the management script template allows learners to practice delineating a broad list of potential management options from which to select interventions. Coaches can discuss with the learner the benefits and risks of each management option specific to a given patient. Improving management reasoning using this exercise can both improve the efficiency of decision-making in urgent clinical encounters and guide hypothesis generation.

Continuing Observation and Reassessment

Lessons learned through direct coaching are ideally fed forward, with the learner's permission, by the clinical reasoning coach to faculty evaluators for use during subsequent direct observation on scheduled clinical rotations. Equipped with data from the global and targeted appraisal, a coach can gather real-time feedback from these clinical rotations, creating a dynamic process of coaching and feedback (Fig. 9.3) [4].

In most cases, learners benefit from ongoing practice with the skills developed with the coach. All of the exercises summarized earlier can be used in the clinical learning environment, under the supervision of peer evaluators (i.e., supervising residents or fellows) or the attending evaluator of record. This practice tends to promote more frequent direct observation of the learner and provide structure and impetus for more regular, higher quality, formative feedback. In the authors' experience, summative evaluations in which the evaluator has participated in these exercises are generally more substantive and, often, more positive.

Introduction:

As you know, I currently serve as a clinical reasoning coach for ***, a role that necessitates obtaining as much feedback as possible about his/her function in the clinical environment. Please provide me as much feedback as you can, both positive and constructive, based on your direct observation of ***. All feedback is confidential.

Is the learner able to generate a broad differential when provided a chief complaint? (Hypothesis Generation)

Is the learner able to elicit key clinical information specific to a working differential? (Hypothesis driven data gathering)

Is the learner able to reprioritize their differential diagnosis as new information is provided? (Manipulate and reprioritize the differential)

Is the learner able to generate an accurate one or two sentence summary of the case and modify this statement as new information is revealed? (Problem Representation)

Is the learner able to effectively recall illness scripts for a given clinical presentation? (Illness scripts)

    Is knowledge triggered by a clinical case?

Please comment on the learner's clinical communication:

        Are their oral presentations/consults/handoffs easy to follow and well organized?

        Is the learner able to present a brief and highly synthesized oral presentation/consult/handoff?

        Do their oral presentations/consults show evidence that the learner has a developed understanding of the problem and is searching for missing elements?

Is the learner able to accurately differentiate "sick" versus "not sick"?

Is the learner able to formulate an appropriate, patient-specific management plan?

Thank you.

Fig. 9.3 A tool for obtaining feedback from direct observation. Use this communication tool to obtain informed feedback from continuing direct observation of the learner who has undergone targeted coaching

Conclusion

The approach and tools described here are derived from the latest research on the teaching and coaching of clinical reasoning. The reasoning process is inherently complex, and we recognize that many educators were never explicitly taught a process for clinical reasoning. For both educators who are undertaking remediation efforts and learners in need of additional coaching, we have designed a relatively linear approach that we have found to be highly effective. This coaching process works best when the learner takes ownership of their own educational development, and the learning becomes more self-directed (see Chap. 4). One of the main tenets of adult learning theory is that adults learn best when they are actively engaged in the learning process and self-direct their own learning goals and activities [33]. In the authors' experience, learners who learn to gain comfort in feeding forward, soliciting feedback, bringing this feedback back to the coach, and continuing to self-reflect and identify areas for continued work, are most likely to succeed.

References

1. Norman GR, van der Vleuten CPM, Newble DI, Dolmans DHJM, Mann KV, Rothman A, et al., editors. International handbook of research in medical education. Dordrecht: Springer Netherlands; 2002. https://doi.org/10.1007/978-94-010-0462-6.
2. Cook DA, Sherbino J, Durning SJ. Management reasoning: beyond the diagnosis. JAMA. 2018;319(22):2267–8.
3. Committee on Diagnostic Error in Health Care, Board on Health Care Services, Institute of Medicine, The National Academies of Sciences, Engineering, and Medicine. Improving diagnosis in health care. Balogh EP, Miller BT, Ball JR, editors. Washington, DC: National Academies Press (US); 2015. http://www.ncbi.nlm.nih.gov/books/NBK338596/.
4. Parsons A, Warburton K. A novel clinical reasoning coaching program for the medicine learner in need. MedEdPublish; 2019. p. 8. https://www.mededpublish.org/manuscripts/2112.
5. Guerrasio J, Aagaard EM. Methods and outcomes for the remediation of clinical reasoning. J Gen Intern Med. 2014;29(12):1607–14.
6. Guerrasio J, Garrity MJ, Aagaard EM. Learner deficits and academic outcomes of medical students, residents, fellows, and attending physicians referred to a remediation program, 2006–2012. Acad Med. 2014;89(2):352–8.
7. Warburton KM, Goren E, Dine CJ. Comprehensive assessment of struggling learners referred to a graduate medical education remediation program. J Grad Med Educ. 2017;9(6):763–7.
8. Dupras DM, Edson RS, Halvorsen AJ, Hopkins RH, McDonald FS. "Problem residents": prevalence, problems and remediation in the era of Core competencies. Am J Med. 2012;125(4):421–5.
9. Riebschleger MP, Haftel HM. Remediation in the context of the competencies: a survey of pediatrics residency program directors. J Grad Med Educ. 2013;5(1):60–3.
10. Tabby DS, Majeed MH, Schwartzman RJ. Problem neurology residents: a national survey. Neurology. 2011;76(24):2119–23.
11. Warburton KM, Shahane AA. Mental health conditions among struggling GME learners: results from a single center remediation program. J Grad Med Educ. 2020;12(6):773–7.
12. Croskerry P. A universal model of diagnostic reasoning. Acad Med. 2009;84(8):1022–8.
13. Elstein AS, Schwarz A. Clinical problem solving and diagnostic decision making: selective review of the cognitive literature. BMJ. 2002;324(7339):729–32.
14. Custers EJFM. Thirty years of illness scripts: theoretical origins and practical applications. Med Teach. 2015;37(5):457–62.
15. Eva KW. What every teacher needs to know about clinical reasoning. Med Educ. 2005;39(1):98–106.
16. Kostopoulou O, Lionis C, Angelaki A, Ayis S, Durbaba S, Delaney BC. Early diagnostic suggestions improve accuracy of family physicians: a randomized controlled trial in Greece. Fam Pract. 2015;32(3):323–8.
17. Bowen JL. Educational strategies to promote clinical diagnostic reasoning. N Engl J Med. 2006;355(21):2217–25.
18. Chang RW, Bordage G, Connell KJ. COGNITION, CONFIDENCE, AND CLINICAL SKILLS: the importance of early problem representation during case presentations. Acad Med. 1998;73(10):S109.
19. Nendaz MR, Bordage G. Promoting diagnostic problem representation. Med Educ. 2002;36(8):760–6.
20. Gavinski K, Covin YN, Longo PJ. Learning how to build illness scripts. Acad Med. 2019; 94(2):293.
21. Jones B, Brzezinski WA, Estrada CA, Rodriguez M, Kraemer RR. A 22-year-old woman with abdominal pain. J Gen Intern Med. 2014;29(7):1074–8.
22. Parsons AS, Wijesekera TP, Rencic JJ. The management script: a practical tool for teaching management reasoning. Acad Med. 2020;95(8):1179–85.
23. Parsons AS, Clancy CB, Rencic JJ, Warburton KM. Targeted strategies to remediate diagnostic reasoning deficits. Acad Med. 2022;97:616.

24. Audétat MC, Laurin S, Sanche G, Béïque C, Fon NC, Blais JG, Charlin B. Clinical reasoning difficulties: a taxonomy for clinical teachers. Med Teach. 2013;35(3):e984–9.

25. Stuart E, Blankenburg B, Butani L, Johnstone N, Long M, Marsico N. Thinking about thinking: coaching strategies to promote clinical reasoning. COMSEP Workshop. 2011.

26. Exercises in Clinical Reasoning | sgim. org. 2021. https://www.sgim.org/web-only/clinical-reasoning-exercises.

27. Stern SDC, Cifu AS, Altkorn D. Symptom to diagnosis: an evidence-based guide. 2015.

28. Wheeler DJ, Cascino T, Sharpe BA, Connor DM. When the script Doesn't fit: an exercise in clinical reasoning. J Gen Intern Med. 2017;32(7):836–40.

29. Stuart E, Blankenburg B, Butani L, Johnstone N, Long M, Marsico N. Thinking about Thinking: 2011;28.

30. Problem Representation Overview | sgim.org. 2021. https://www.sgim.org/web-only/clinical-reasoning-exercises/problem-representation-overview.

31. Mamede S, Schmidt H. Reflection in diagnostic reasoning: what really matters? Acad Med. 2014;89(7):959–60.

32. Walker M, Warburton KM, Rencic J, Parsons AS. Lessons in clinical reasoning—pitfalls, myths, and pearls: a case of chest pain and shortness of breath. Diagnosi. 2019;6(4):387–92.

33. Knowles MS, Holton EF, Swanson RA. The adult learner: the definitive classic in adult education and human resourced development. 7th ed. Burlington, MA: Elsevier, Inc; 2011.

Remediation for Technical Skills

10

Shareef Syed, Riley Brian, and Sanziana Roman

Introduction

During a surgery education and competency committee meeting, concern arises regarding the technical skills of Ralph (he/him), a third-year resident. Ralph will be rotating on your service next month, and the committee has asked you to "address" the resident's technical skills and update them at a subsequent meeting.

Though struggles with technical skills can be identified at different times during training, learning experiences in most procedural specialties follow a temporal sequence. Earlier periods in training typically emphasize the cognitive aspects of a procedural specialty: learning history-gathering and specialized physical examination skills; diagnostic and management reasoning; caring for the critically ill; and mastering diagnostic and therapeutic algorithms to identify indications for invasive interventions and detecting complications after such interventions. Early trainees often have exposure to simple proce-

dures or small parts of complex procedures but do not independently perform technical skills until later in the training process. This means that a trainee may be at an advanced stage in training before concerns regarding their technical skills are identified. A learner's advanced non-technical skill competence and accomplishments may potentially influence or delay reporting of struggles with technical skills.

This chapter will follow the remediation framework outlined in Chap. 6. We will begin with the domains that affect technical proficiency and then review cognitive load theory as it underpins and helps to structure the clarification and intervention phases of procedural skills remediation. Finally, we will describe methods of ongoing assessment.

Identification: Defining Technical Skills Domains

Assessment of technical skills can be conducted in and out of the operating/procedure room. Expert proceduralists observing a novice usually can discern when something does not look right but may be unable to specify how or why it is going wrong. This makes it especially difficult to provide the coaching that learners desire.

Objective tools force evaluators to rate learner behaviors on specific criteria. Many simulation and intraoperative performance scales are avail-

S. Syed (✉) · R. Brian · S. Roman
Department of Surgery, University of California, San Francisco, CA, USA
e-mail: shareef.syed@ucsf.edu; riley.brian@ucsf.edu; sanziana.roman@ucsf.edu

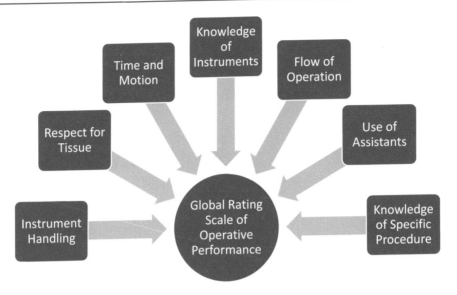

Fig. 10.1 Domains comprising technical skills performance [3]

able and are helpful for providing global assessment of trainees' technical skills. Objective structured assessment of technical skills (OSATS) is the most studied and validated in a lab setting [1]. Many of these tools have not been widely adopted into general educational practice, due to lack of expertise, infrastructure, time, and cost. Promising novel smartphone-based workplace assessment tools are also becoming available [2].

Even though these technical skills assessments only identify general deficiencies, they are useful in ascertaining individuals who might benefit from remediation. Figure 10.1 delineates the seven domains that comprise technical skills performance. We note that two of these domains overlap with the Accreditation Council for Graduate Medical Education (ACGME) core competency areas: underlying knowledge of the procedure, and use of assistants (a combination of interpersonal communication and systems-based practice).

Once the learner is identified, instructors must devote significant time and effort to remediating the learner's technical skills. An individual or a small group of instructors must commit to create relationship and optimize the learning environment (see below) for remediation success.

Because any combination of psychomotor, cognitive/knowledge, or affective issues may

influence a learner's technical skills, it is imperative that there is a high degree of trust between the coach and learner. Trust in this relationship increases the likelihood that a learner will be motivated to actively engage in the remediation process [4]. While trust is built over time, it is important to ensure that the learner-remediation coach relationship begins collaboratively by engaging the learner in co-creating the remediation plan to the extent possible. This includes discussing the learner's perceptions of their performance in a private and safe place (Chap. 6) prior to working in a "high stakes" environment, such as the operating room or simulation center. These discussions allow the trainee to understand the coach's motives, enthusiasm, and sincerity to help; ideally, they also allow the learner to speak freely, especially about potential meta-cognitive and affective struggles that may influence technical skills.

Refinement of technical skills is a lifelong journey for all proceduralists. Therefore, it may be appropriate to share the instructor's personal experiences and challenges in psychomotor skill acquisition. When done selectively and skillfully, sharing stories helps build rapport between the coach and the learner.

Clarification and Intervention: Cognitive Load Theory in Procedural Skill Learning

A body of literature has emerged around the contributions of cognitive load theory (CLT) to the clarification and intervention phases of remediating technical skills. CLT is an instructional design theory based on our knowledge of human cognitive architecture, in particular, the limitations of working memory [5] that can be used to understand workplace psychomotor learning. CLT proposes that at any one moment, humans have finite working memory resources or cognitive capacity for learning. "Cognitive load" refers to the relative proportion of working memory required to manage the information needed to do the task has been described in three types: extraneous, intrinsic, and germane.

Extraneous load (EL) is the portion of the learner's working memory that must processes information that is **not essential** to the task [6]. Practically, it encompasses methods by which learning tasks are presented as well as external distractions. In the surgical learning context, EL in operative settings includes operating room noise (communication in room not essential to the task, such as music, sounds of life support, and anesthetic machines), self-induced and instructor-influenced performance pressures, time limitations, and concerns for patients on the surgical floor.

Intrinsic load (IL) arises from the information-processing demands associated with the performance of the task itself. IL includes the effort needed to develop and organize knowledge essential to the task (e.g., sequence of the surgical procedure). Both task complexity and learner expertise determine the IL [7].

Germane load (GL) is the use of working memory to construct ways of organizing information into long-lasting schemas, for example, into flowcharts or algorithms. Therefore, it helps manage IL and contributes to long-term memory [7]. In procedural settings, learners can increase GL through thoughtful repetitive practice (see Simulation Training and Deliberate Practice sections below).

Reducing Extraneous Load

Learning Environment

Historically, surgical training followed an apprenticeship model. Early surgeon-barbers in the United Kingdom learned professional technical skills from a single mentor rather than through formal university or medical school training. This mentorship model still exists but is uncommon in most academic institutions for logistical reasons. In the modern context, trainees are expected to learn from many instructors and are exposed to significant diversity in techniques, communication, and entrustment. Although a diversity of approaches confers some learning advantages, it can also create uncertainty and instability for early learners or those who struggle. A coach can help such learners develop an approach for learning procedural skills in the face of conflicting models.

As noted above, the learning environment is crucial for effective procedural remediation. Technical procedures carry significant risk to patients. Adverse events during procedures make up a significant proportion of all adverse events, many of which are caused by technical faults [8]. The procedure/operating room is an intolerant environment due to patient safety issues, time pressure, and the stress of being observed, not only by supervisors but also by nursing staff and anesthesia providers. These all add to the learner's EL [9]. Learning environments outside of the procedure room, such as simulation and anatomy labs (see below) will reduce EL and may help increase GL for learners who struggle.

Affective Difficulties

During a procedure, you note that Ralph has a significant hand tremor which worsens during a difficult phase. During the case, he was very quiet and only was answering in very short sentences, and at times was incomprehensible. After the case, you note that Ralph's scrubs are drenched with sweat, and he appears visibly fatigued.

Learners may possess the cognitive and psychomotor skills to be successful, but they may lack confidence and/or suffer significant anxiety which may be exacerbated by a deep sense of responsibility to their patients and the stress of being observed. A trustworthy relationship with a coach can provide important support.

Performance anxiety is a significant issue in the execution of technical skills. As an adaptive mechanism that sharpens attention, anxiety can be helpful to a certain degree but if excessive can lead to impaired function. Unresolved performance anxiety in athletes and musicians may ultimately lead to personal and professional struggles; while less is known about performance anxiety in procedural specialists, early evidence suggests it is common and associated with burnout [10].

It is essential that the remediation coach empathize with the learner's affective issues. In addition, the learner can develop resilience mechanisms to reframe perceived stress through the development of specific cognitive habits [11]. These intra-procedural coping mechanisms, in conjunction with robust pre-procedural knowledge and technical preparation help, are critical for trainees to learn to manage inevitable deviations from the norm. Exposing the learner to high stress environments is uncomfortable. However, it is vital for the learner to develop skills to detect, control, and overcome stress.

Mindfulness-based interventions, such as focus on the breath, have been shown to enhance resilience and improve affect, executive function, and performance in other high-stress populations such as the Marines, police, special forces, and elite athletes. Mindfulness-based interventions can also serve as stress resilience training for physicians. Trainees completed procedural skills faster when they had completed mindfulness-based stress reduction training, compared with control participants. This may be explained by the influence of mindfulness-based interventions on attention, emotional regulation, and cognitive skills, which are increasingly recognized as critical for motor skill performance [11].

Addressing Intrinsic Load

Prior to your meeting with Ralph, you take time to review some of the prior rotation evaluations. You note that Ralph has scored well on his in-training knowledge exam and shows an outstanding level of responsibility to patient care. A few operative evaluations have been completed and reveal comments such as "apprehensive," "slow movement," "awkward technique," and "unable to modify with 'in the moment' feedback."

Learning psychomotor skills is separated into three graduated stages [12]: cognition (intellectualizing and executing the task); integration (refining the technique for efficiency and effectiveness); and automation (performing the task with minimal cognitive input).

Trainees are required to gather a large amount of sensory data when learning any psychomotor task, which can be overwhelming. Occasionally, simple medical interventions can optimize the learner's sight and hearing with appropriate prescription glasses or hearing aids. Haptics must also be addressed, to be sure learners understand how differently things feel with gloves on or how a particular suture feels, how an instrument unlocks, or how much pressure needs to be placed on a certain blade. Though these **sensory issues** are intuitive to some learners, they are not to others and can lead to challenges in learning psychomotor skills. Many of these very basic aspects can be easily discussed and practiced in an office setting.

Handedness is often a significant issue which is commonly overlooked and can affect around 10% of trainees. Procedural instructions, instrumentation, and exposure are frequently set up for a right-handed trainee. Many left-handed trainees voluntarily try to convert to a right-handed technique, but this adds additional complexity and IL, which can be perceived by observers as a struggle. Instructing a left-handed trainee requires significant adjustment to the exposure and approach. Making adjustments in the midst of a procedure usually results in a suboptimal experience for the trainee. This can be overcome by a discussion prior to the procedure to facilitate the left-hander's approach. Introducing the trainee to a left-handed proceduralist can be additionally important for them to discuss issues that a right-handed instructor may not appreciate, such as instrument and body positioning.

Ergonomics are also an important consideration, as most instruments (syringes, needle holders, and stapler devices) are designed for a "medium" sized hand, disadvantaging people with smaller hands. Again, a proceduralist and a learner who have similar hand sizes can discuss methods to overcome instrument design biases. Another example is ensuring that trainees with height differences adjust the height of the procedure table to optimize their body position and thereby their technical skills.

Once the baseline sensory, handedness, and ergonomic barriers are addressed, the instructor can subjectively and objectively evaluate the learner to identify any additional areas needing improvement, which can necessitate further intervention.

Addressing Intrinsic Load and Creating Germane Load

To an expert, foundational tasks, such as tying a knot or driving a needle, is a one-step process: they have automated a series of steps into a single task through use of GL. Novices, however, perceive the task as individual steps they must master. The instructor may have difficulty deconstructing these automatic tasks at first; however, the thoughtful coach can reduce IL and create GL with time and patience, clear instructions, careful observation and analysis, and actionable feedback to the learner.

Additional ways to address IL and create GL are through simulation training, facilitating deliberate practice, video coaching, and structuring learning opportunities.

Simulation Training

During your meeting, Ralph reports a growing sense of worry regarding his technical skills. He admits to struggling since coming back from his research year. You arrange to meet with him at the skills lab to review some foundational techniques.

Simulation provides a low-stakes, risk-free environment for learners to make and learn from errors. As Charles Mayo stated, "experience can mean making the same mistake over and over again" [13], which is not acceptable in the procedure room. Simulation provides a "safe" training ground for cognitive, metacognitive, and technical skill training, ideally focuses on and reduces IL [9], reduces learner EL, and aids GL development. In the simulation lab, learners can experiment with techniques and ask questions that they would not disclose in a real-life situation. They also have an opportunity to observe and discuss issues with any peers present in a facilitated and informal setting. This peer discussion and evaluation can help to reduce anxieties regarding their own skill level, further reducing EL.

Simulation of basic procedures (e.g., central lines, intubation) and laparoscopic/open surgery is widely available and practiced. Low-cost simulators can advance learners' skill level in a low-risk environment. Higher fidelity simulators may be largely unnecessary and are associated with greater and possibly prohibitive cost [14].

Cadaveric labs allow learners to revisit essential gross anatomy, which they may not have focused on since their earliest years of training. A fresh procedural context is powerful, reinforcing understanding of anatomic relationships and surgical planes, and enhancing interest and retention. Fresh frozen cadaveric models, although expensive, simulate the lifelike feel of tissue better than preserved models.

Animal models, are used sparsely but do enable practice with critically important scenarios such as intraoperative bleeding, which require technical (ability to expose and address); cognitive (understanding of anatomy and appropriate maneuvers for each situation); and metacognitive (understanding and creating overall strategies) skills. This experience is seldom obtained until the learner is advanced or independently performing tasks and can be an extremely valuable part of the remediation process.

Simulation is valuable in not only teaching core technical foundations but also maintaining technical skills between procedural experiences. Deliberate practice is a core principle in technical education and remediation (see below), and simulation provides a venue for the learner to integrate and automate movements.

Deliberate Practice

During the simulation session, you note some issues with Ralph's techniques and offer guidance, to which he responds readily. However, he shares that he feels unable to maintain the skills between procedures during low volume procedural months and that he finds real-life procedures very different from his experiences in simulation.

Deliberate practice (DP) is based on the theory that expert performance results from intentionally engaging in and choosing activities that improve and maintain high performance. It involves repeated practice on tasks and immediate feedback on performance that allows individuals to focus on improving where they struggle, while also refining other aspects of performance [8].

DP applies very successfully to procedural learning. In the setting of remediation, DP is critical to help learners overcome the technical issues they face. DP simulation studies show improvement in dexterity and global quality of performing procedural skills [15]. Creating simulators for the learner to practice and for instructors to provide feedback on a regular basis will improve procedural performance and reduce degradation of skills during low volume periods of training, ultimately leading to an increase in the learner's GL.

Video-Based Coaching

Prior to your first inguinal hernia case with Ralph, you ask to meet with him to review the operative steps. He displays appropriate knowledge of the operative steps and pertinent anatomy. You review a video of the procedure being performed by an expert and some of the subtle differences in your operative steps and technique.

Laparoscopic and endoscopic procedures are easily recorded; logistical challenges unfortunately interfere with effective recording of open procedures. Video-based coaching has been broadly studied and used successfully in technical education and remediation in both simulation and real-life procedural settings. Prerecorded video review of experts can also highlight specific techniques, anatomic landmarks, and planes. No significant difference between pre-procedure and post-procedure coaching has been noted; however, video-based coaching within a structured framework can increase GL and significantly improve technical performance [16]. A careful review of recordings of the learner performing the procedure, when available, can greatly help identify specific technical struggles.

Structuring Learning Opportunities

After the video review, you note that you have three inguinal hernia procedures today. You set expectations, informing Ralph that he will assist you in the first case; in the second case, he will perform the exposure and dissection, and you will implant the mesh; and in the final case, you will expose and dissect, and he will focus on mesh implantation. You arrange to have him assist in 2 other procedures that day, to try and remove some of the time pressure from the day and so that he can focus only on inguinal hernias.

By explicitly naming expectations with graded levels of responsibility throughout the day, learners can further develop GL.

Assessment: Intraoperative Remediation

The highest fidelity "model" of technical skills, and the locus of ultimate ongoing assessment of all the above elements, is in the operating/procedure room. As mentioned, the high-stakes nature of procedures creates a suboptimal learning environment for the initial phases of remediation. That said, intraoperative remediation is imperative to allow learners to understand errors in decision-making, identification of anatomic landmarks and surgical planes, and techniques.

Explicit discussion prior to the procedure will help set expectations and clarify the instructor's investment in their growth. It aids the trainee's focus, reduces uncertainty, and reduces the sense of failure if the instructor assumes the primary role. Trainees can thereby anticipate their participation level, reducing EL. Complex procedures, such as cardiac, vascular, and transplant surgery, can have thousands of steps and resultant high IL. Separating these complex procedures into smaller parts is helpful to reduce the learner's IL and increase GL.

The Instructor can give graduated responsibility and autonomy over time [17]. These steps (Table 10.1) provide a guide, with the instructor correcting behaviors that will lead to errors, and if an error has already occurred, to "take over" and correct the error.

Table 10.1 Sequenced stages of supervision [17]

Zwisch stage of supervision	Attending behaviors	Resident behaviors commensurate with this level of supervision
Show and tell	Does majority of key portions as the surgeon Narrates the case (i.e., thinks out loud) Demonstrates key concepts, anatomy, and skills	Opens and closes First assist and observes
Cues to advancement		When first assisting, begins to actively assist (i.e., anticipates surgeons' needs)
"Smart" help	Shifts between surgeon and first assist roles When first assisting, leads the resident in surgeon role (active assist) Optimizes the field/exposure Demonstrates the plane or structure Coaches for specific technical skills Coaches regarding the next steps Continues to identify anatomical landmarks for the resident	The above, plus: Shifts between surgeon and first assist roles Knows all the component technical skills Demonstrates an increasing ability to perform different key parts of the operation with attending assistance
Cues to advancement		Can execute the majority steps of procedure with active assistance
"Dumb" help	Assists and follows the lead of the resident (passive assist) Coaching regarding polishing and refinement of skills Follows the resident's lead throughout the operation	The above, plus: Can "set up" and accomplish the next step for the entire case with increasing efficiency Recognizes critical transition point issues
Cues to advancement		Can transition between all steps with passive assist from faculty
No help	Largely provides no unsolicited advice Assisted by a junior resident or an attending acting like a junior resident Monitors progress and patient safety	The above plus: Can work with inexperienced first assistant Can safely complete a caste without faculty Can recover from most errors Recognizes when to seek help/advice

Active coaching throughout the more advanced stages of autonomy is critical. Coaching should be offered supportively (see Chap. 6), and if possible, in the context of a longitudinal relationship. In addition to feedback and coaching in the moment, it is often useful to allow time for learners to reflect on and share their thoughts about the complete procedure, in writing, prior to an additional discussion regarding overall performance. This will importantly establish the habit of thoughtful and honest self-assessment. The resultant clarity of insight will enable trainees to grow into self-directed learners with strong self-regulation skills (see Chap. 4) for the remainder of their careers.

Once a clear mental model has been created, these conversations ultimately will mature into collegial discussions on the finer points of procedures and technical skills, including prior planning, anticipating technical challenges in specific anatomic or pathologic settings, and understanding adverse events and complications. Together with improved observed technical skill, this would serve as evidence that the trainee is developing into a competent proceduralist.

Conclusion

Remediation of technical skills is a time-consuming endeavor that requires significant commitment from both instructor and learner and can be guided by addressing and optimizing the three elements of cognitive load: extrinsic, intrinsic, and germane. Through creating an educational relationship, gathering specific information to understand a learner's technical issues, hearing the learner's perspective, supervising simulated tasks, and conducting effective feedback conversations, instructors can optimize GL to maximize learning [9]. The cornerstone of remediation is the formation of a trusting, bidirectional relationship, developed though empathy and clear communication that allows the transmission of honest reflections without fear of any retribution. Having a holistic yet focused theory-based perspective will allow the instructor to offer actionable advice and create opportunities for the learner to overcome many of the common obstacles they face in technical skill acquisition.

References

1. Martin JA, Regehr G, Reznick R, MacRae H, Murnaghan J, Hutchison C, Brown M. Objective structured assessment of technical skill (OSATS) for surgical residents. Br J Surg. 1997;84: 273–8.
2. George BC, Bohnen JD, Schuller MC, Fryer JP. Using smartphones for trainee performance assessment: a SIMPL case study. Surgery. 2020;167:903–6.
3. Niitsu H, Hirabayashi N, Yoshimitsu M, Mimura T, Taomoto J, Sugiyama Y, Murakami S, Saeki S, Mukaida H, Takiyama W. Using the objective structured assessment of technical skills (OSATS) global rating scale to evaluate the skills of surgical trainees in the operating room. Surg Today. 2013;43: 271–5.
4. Sandhu G, Thompson-Burdine J, Nikolian VC, Sutzko DC, Prabhu KA, Matusko N, Minter RM. Association of faculty entrustment with resident autonomy in the operating poom. JAMA Surg. 2018;153: 518–24.
5. Sweller J. Cognitive load theory. In: Mestre JP, Ross BH, editors. The psychology of learning and motivation: cognition in education. Cambridge, MA: Elsevier Academic Press; 2011.
6. Choi HH, van Merriënboer JJG, Paas F. Effects of the physical environment on cognitive load and learning: towards a new model of cognitive load. Educ Psychol Rev. 2014;26:225–44.
7. Young JQ, John M, Thakker K, Friedman K, Sugarman R, Sewell JL, O'Sullivan PS. Evidence for validity for the cognitive load inventory for handoffs. Med Educ. 2021;55:222–32.
8. Hashimoto DA, Sirimanna P, Gomez ED, Beyer-Berjot L, Ericsson KA, Williams NN, Darzi A, Aggarwal R. Deliberate practice enhances quality of laparoscopic surgical performance in a randomized controlled trial: from arrested development to expert performance. Surg Endosc. 2015;29: 3154–62.
9. Sewell JL, Boscardin CK, Young JQ, ten Cate O, O'Sullivan PS. Measuring cognitive load during procedural skills training with colonoscopy as an exemplar. Med Educ. 2016;50:682–92.
10. Dupley L, Hossain S, Ghosh S. Performance anxiety amongst trauma and orthopaedic surgical trainees. Surgeon. 2020;18:e33–8.
11. Lebares CC, Guvva EV, Olaru M, Sugrue LP, Staffaroni AM, Delucchi KL, Kramer JH, Ascher NL, Harris HW. Efficacy of mindfulness-based cognitive training in surgery: additional analysis of the mindful surgeon pilot randomized controlled trial. JAMA Netw Open. 2019;2:e194108.
12. Hamdorf JM, Hall JC. Acquiring surgical skills. Brit J Surg. 2000;87:28–37.
13. Thomas W. Teaching and assessing surgical competence. Ann Royal Coll Surg Engl. 2006;88: 429–32.

14. Massoth C, Röder H, Ohlenburg H. High-fidelity is not superior to low-fidelity simulation but leads to overconfidence in medical students. BMC Med Educ. 2019;19:29. https://doi.org/10.1186/s12909-019-1464-7.

15. Crochet P, Aggarwal R, Dubb SS, Ziprin P, Rajaretnam N, Grantcharov T, Ericsson KA, Darzi A. Deliberate practice on a virtual reality laparoscopic simulator enhances the quality of surgical technical skills. Ann Surg. 2011;253:1216–22.

16. Augestad KM, Butt K, Ignjatovic D, Keller DS, Kiran R. Video-based coaching in surgical education: a systematic review and meta-analysis. Surg Endosc. 2020;34:521–35.

17. DaRosa DA, Zwischenberger JB, Meyerson SL, George BC, Teitelbaum EN, Soper NJ, Fryer JP. A theory-based model for teaching and assessing residents in the operating room. J Surg Educ. 2013;70:24–30.

Evaluation and Remediation of Organization, Efficiency, and Time Management

11

Karen M. Warburton, Andrew S. Parsons, Peter Yen, and Eric Goren

Case 1

Ray (they/them) is a categorical internal medicine intern who is several months into their internship. Ray has already completed several inpatient rotations. Evaluations consistently comment that "Ray could benefit from improving their efficiency" and that "Ray has trouble getting their work done on time." Some evaluations are marked 'for concern' and detail that Ray always stays late on call days and comes in far earlier than anyone else on the team the next day. Ray undergoes a comprehensive assessment that does not reveal any concerns related to mental well-being and determines that organization and efficiency seems to be the most likely primary deficit. The coach, Dr. Suárez, reaches out to Ray to introduce her role and sets up a time to meet privately with Ray.

K. M. Warburton (✉)
Department of Medicine, University of Virginia School of Medicine, Charlottesville, VA, USA
e-mail: Kmw2g@virginia.edu

A. S. Parsons
Departments of Medicine and Public Health, University of Virginia School of Medicine, Charlottesville, VA, USA
e-mail: Asp5c@virginia.edu

P. Yen · E. Goren
Department of Medicine, Perelman School of Medicine, University of Pennsylvania, Philadelphia, PA, USA
e-mail: peter.yen@pennmedicine.upenn.edu; eric.goren@uphs.upenn.edu

Introduction

For many trainees, learning to perform and properly prioritize patient care tasks efficiently and completely comes naturally through observation and practice. These learners need little directed teaching, using the tricks, tips, and frameworks modeled by their supervisors and peers. Efficient management of daily clinical tasks, such as being prepared for clinic or team rounds by "pre-rounding" or admitting patents to the hospital, are typically minimum expectations of learners, yet many struggle in these fundamental areas. Deficiencies in time management and organization have been reported in specialty-specific surveys of program directors as well as retrospective reviews from single-center remediation programs. These deficits may become apparent when learners are late or unprepared for rounds, deliver disorganized presentations, produce poor quality documentation, or are unable to reliably complete their daily task lists. Such behaviors can be frustrating and disruptive to clinical care teams. Furthermore, a disorganized learner can make it more difficult for clinical educators to assess medical knowledge, clinical reasoning, and global achievement of clinical milestones. This chapter presents a systematic approach to the assessment and coaching of the learner struggling with organization and efficiency. The authors have developed and tested these interventions on medical students, residents, and fellows in the in- and outpatient settings. All these tools can be adapted for use with learners on interprofessional teams, including nursing and pharmacy trainees. As with other chapters in this section, we will follow the general framework and recommendations outlined in Chap. 6.

Identification: A Learner Appears "Disorganized"

"Disorganized" and "inefficient" are terms commonly used to describe learners who struggle at all stages of training. These descriptors map to a few overlapping domains and at least four of the six Accreditation Council for Graduate Medical Education (ACGME) competencies (patient care, interpersonal and communication skills, professionalism, and systems-based practice). Common behavioral patterns include the learner who is consistently late or unprepared for rounds, perpetually behind schedule in clinic, whose notes are completed very late in the day, and who cannot keep track of their materials and deadlines. These learners typically require a great deal of supervision, and thus their struggles may negatively impact the dynamics of the clinical care team.

Learners' struggles with organizational skills manifest in all clinical settings and include:

- New patient evaluations (admissions or new patient intake clinic visits)
- Pre-encounter preparation (pre-rounds, pre-clinic charting)
- Note-writing
- Managing a to-do list, triaging tasks

Organizational skills, referred to by neuroscientists and cognitive psychologists as executive functions, develop gradually and can change over the lifespan, peaking when the prefrontal cortex becomes fully myelinated, typically between the ages of 20 and 29. Probably due to the requirements of qualifying for entry into school, health professions trainees tend, as a group, to have relatively strong executive functions compared with age-matched peers; however, there is a range of abilities in all groups. Higher-order executive functions include planning, reasoning, and problem-solving. The set of cognitive processes underlying these functions have been delineated as attentional control, cognitive inhibitory control, working memory, and cognitive flexibility, all necessary for selecting and monitoring behaviors that facilitate goal attainment. In the authors' experience, it is not uncommon for even high performing learners to struggle with higher-order executive functions. Often these struggles go unnoticed until these learners enter clinical training, where the demands exceed their previous ability to compensate using other elements of their intelligence. Viewed through this lens, young adults can be expected to continue to develop stronger executive functions and benefit from coaching, practice, and use of adaptive tools.

There is limited literature to guide our approach to the learner who struggles with organization and efficiency, because we have not yet classified this as a unique competency. A survey of United States (US) Internal Medicine (IM) program directors performed in 2008 reported that, among trainees having performance difficulty, 41% had trouble with organization and prioritization [1]. Single-center reports from institutions with centralized remediation programs suggest that time management and organization are common problems, particularly among resident learners undergoing remediation [2–5]. A national survey of nephrology fellowship program leaders cited organization and efficiency as the second most common struggle requiring remediation among nephrology fellows over the preceding five years [6].

The Merriam-Webster dictionary defines "disorganized" as not having parts arranged in a neat and effective way or lacking coherence, system, or central guiding agency [7]. Simply put, some learners struggle to maintain many aspects of their life in an orderly fashion. Their problems lie on a continuum of global struggles in many aspects of their life to very specific issues particular to the context they are in. Learners with global deficits may arrive late to events because they have forgotten to record the meeting time, or failed to leave enough time to park, or realized too late that they do not have directions to their destination. They may appear flustered on rounds, shuffling papers and struggling to locate information or their belongings. Their patient presentations are often disorganized because they are unable to collect and record information in an effective manner. These learners may have inadequate systems for completing their work-related tasks or, more commonly, lack systems altogether. This chapter provides an approach to specific challenges related to clinical work. Global deficits require broader behavioral coaching not covered here.

Clarification: Delineating Underlying Causes of Executive Function Struggles

Specific organizational challenges are often predictable when one considers the learner's prior educational training and experience with the electronic health record. For instance, a learner who did not complete a sub-internship in which they functioned in the full capacity of an intern may have difficulties with organization and efficiency when they transition to the role of an intern. Similarly, someone who completed residency at a small community program may struggle as a subspecialty fellow in a busy academic

Table 11.1 Differential diagnosis of the learner who appears disorganized

Type of struggle	Behavioral clues
I. Struggles with organization, efficiency, or time management	– Lacks effective habits, approaches, or systems for completing daily work
A. Global	– Struggles in multiple aspects of life Difficulty meeting deadlines, bills unpaid, cluttered home or desk – Arrives late to meetings or rounds
B. Specific	– Lack of familiarity with specific information systems (e.g.. electronic medical record) – Prior educational/training program did not prepare learner for current program (e.g., size, complexity of patients, different expectations) – Unable to describe systems for evaluating new patients, preparation for rounds
II. Struggles with clinical reasoning	– Has not seen all patients prior to clinical rounds, unprepared for rounds in general – Spends an atypically long time evaluating new patients – Struggles to triage tasks in all clinical settings, may lack appreciation of urgency of tasks – Perpetually behind on all work – Scattered history-taking or physical exam

III. Mental well-being concern
  A. Medical impairment (e.g., metabolic disease, neurologic disease, side effect of prescribed medication)
  B. Fatigue
  C. Substance use
  D. Depression
  E. Anxiety
  F. Cognitive issue (e.g., ADHD, learning disorder)
	– Other signs of impairment (e.g., unsteady gait, slurred speech, lethargic, agitated, withdrawn, fidgety, inappropriate or uninhibited behavior, memory loss or confusion, disheveled appearance, loud, rapid, or nonsensical speech)
	– Known history of mental health condition(s)
	– Other issues with performance

hospital with a large and complex consult service.

Alternatively, learners who appear to be disorganized or inefficient may struggle primarily with clinical reasoning. Clinical reasoning, also not an ACGME competency, describes a complex, patient-centered process that involves the gathering, integration, and interpretation of information to form a working diagnosis and treatment plan [8]. A challenge at any point along the diagnostic [9] and management [10] reasoning pathway may present as a primary problem with organization. Learners with these struggles often lack training and experience in hypothesis-driven data gathering, triaging of large amounts of information, generation of an effective problem representation, development and selection of appropriate illness scripts, and generation of the differential diagnosis with reprioritization as new data are presented (see Chap. 9; [8, 11]).

Finally, disorganization and inefficiency at work may be the presenting symptoms of impairment or other mental well-being concern. Impairment may be the result of a medical condition, mental health diagnosis, fatigue, or substance use (see Chap. 6).

In some cases, these learners' struggles can be attributed to the overlap of more than one of these conditions. As much as possible, appropriately distinguishing between struggles related to organizational systems, clinical reasoning, and mental well-being is crucial, as each of these issues necessitates a unique remediation approach. Coaching to improve organization and efficiency is best accomplished through a structured process that deconstructs complex tasks into precise steps, with direct observation and feedback by a coach [5, 6]. In the authors' experience at two different institutions, peer coaching can be an effective component of this work.

Success in any remediation program requires systematic and accurate information-gathering of specific clinical performance struggles (Table 11.2; [3]). This clarification process includes a comprehensive review of the learner's performance in the current program and, when available, prior programs. Understanding the learner's trajectory can be very informative. An

Table 11.2 Comprehensive clarification phase: the learner needing help with organization and efficiency

I. Reconnaissance
  A. Written file[a]
     Here is an example of information to compile for Internal Medicine residency

Undergraduate Medical Education	Graduate Medical Education
[] Preclinical performance	[] Inpatient evaluations for residency and/or fellowship rotations
[] Clinical performance, including course evaluations from clerkships, subinternships	[] Outpatient evaluations for residency and/or fellowship rotations
[] Standardized test scores, including United States Medical Licensing Examinations (USMLE)	[] In-training, USMLE scores
[] Medical Student Performance Evaluation (MSPE) letter	[] Program director file from residency and/or fellowship, letters of recommendation

  B. Direct observation
  C. Direct communication with evaluators
II. Interview
  A. Build rapport with the learner, assess the learner's insight and perspective
  B. Assess for underlying issues
  C. "Review of systems" for specific deficits
     i. Medical knowledge
     ii. Clinical reasoning
     iii. Organization/efficiency
     iv. Professionalism and communication

[a] The written file is most relevant to the assessment of a US graduate medical learner. The approach can be adapted for international learners and learners in other professions such that the reconnaissance phase includes a review of the comprehensive written file in both the current (and prior, when available) programs, including objective and subjective data

abrupt change in trajectory may signal a challenging external circumstance, or acute or chronic issues with mental well-being. When possible, additional direct observation of the learner and direct communication with evaluators is recommended. An interview with the learner should assess for underlying issues such as stressors, mental well-being diagnoses such as depression, anxiety, history of learning differences (see Chap. 17), burnout (see Chap. 18), and impairment, including substance use. Specifically, the interview can distinguish between needs to support organization and efficiency as opposed to clinical reasoning. This can be accomplished by asking the learner to describe in detail their strategies for completing their daily work. It is also useful to review clinical cases to pinpoint specific challenges along the diagnostic or management clinical reasoning pathways (see Chap. 9).

It is often helpful, if possible, to designate someone other than the learner's direct supervisor, or program director, to conduct this clarification phase, as learners may be more willing to confide in a faculty member who is not part of their ultimate assessment process (see Chap. 2).

Intervention

An effective coaching plan must be individualized to the needs of and developed in collaboration with the learner. The plan should explicitly summarize the area(s) of struggle, outline specific goals and objectives, provide a timeline, and provide a method of reassessment. Detailed documentation throughout the process is key. Again, when possible, reassessment should be performed by someone independent of the coaching process.

> At the initial meeting, Dr. Suárez alerts Ray to the emerging pattern of concerns about inefficiency and time management on the written evaluations from inpatient rotations.
>
> *Dr. Suárez: Ray, do these comments resonate with your experience?*
>
> *Ray: It's definitely not the first time I've been given feedback that I don't get my work done quickly enough. I'll admit that I've consistently found myself needing to stay late and arrive early to get my work done. That does make me a little worried because it's wearing me down and taking a toll on my personal life.*
>
> *Dr. Suárez: I also worry that you feel residency is having an overwhelming impact on your personal life. I think if we figure out where exactly you're struggling, we can tackle these problems together. Tell me, what part of your workday seems to slow you down the most?*
>
> *Ray: Well, call days are particularly hard for me because it takes me a long time to work through a new admission. It feels like as soon as I finally have a grasp on one admission, the next one comes, and all my tasks are just suddenly piled up and I'm so far behind.*

With some targeted questioning, Dr. Suárez has identified inefficiency with new patient admissions as a notable weakness that Ray recognizes needs improvement. It will be important for her to observe Ray to pinpoint the specific issues.

Inefficiency with New Admissions

> **Identifying the Area of Struggle**
>
> *Dr. Suárez: Ray, let's have you walk me through your approach on a new admission.*
>
> Ray has a hard time verbally describing these steps, so the coach asks Ray to demonstrate the work on a hospital workstation. During the demonstration, Ray flips through multiple tabs in the patient chart, first reviewing the patient's most recent outpatient note, then acute Emergency Department (ED) vitals, and then reviewing the ED physician's assessment and plan. Ray's inefficiency becomes clear: Ray does not have a system for approaching new admissions.

Dr. Suárez works with Ray to identify key components of the task, emphasizing the importance of naming the steps of the process, and creating explicit steps for something many of us do subconsciously. She introduces and simulates how to use the "TRIAGE An H&P" tool (Fig. 11.1).

Dr. Suárez then outlines specific goals, providing a timeline and method of reassessment.

Setting a Goal and Timeline

Dr. Suárez: Okay, Ray. I want you to practice implementing the "TRIAGE An H&P" tool on five mock patient cases, then actively using this tool on all your admissions this week. Your goal will be to complete an admission from start to finish in 1.5 hours. Let's meet again next week after your next call cycle to review the call day.

"TRIAGE An H&P": Guide to Admitting a Patient

T	**Triage** Key Patient Data	**Obtain current objective data** • Vital Signs / CC / ED TRIAGE Notes • Quick review of Labs/Micro Data • Quick review of Current Imaging
R	**Review** Clinical Overview	**Chart Biopsy / "Clinical Overview" Medview** • Trend vitals • Trend labs (find out baseline Hgb, Cr, etc.) • Review PMH/Meds/Allergies • Review last EPIC outpatient progress note • Review last discharge summary / signout • Review pertinent prior imaging • Review last EKG / echo
I	**Investigate/Inquire**	**Review current ED MD or Clinic Note** • In-depth review of Vital Signs/ CC • Medications Given (abx, IVF, etc.) • U-dip, pregnancy tests, other ED work-up • ED MD/Clinician HPI and assessment **Doc-2-Doc from ER/Clinic Provider**
A	**Admit Orders /** Organize Thoughts	**Place General Admissions Orders in SCM** **Compose a draft problem list in signout document** • Acute (i.e. Neutropenic fever, SOB, etc.) • Chronic Problems (ie AML, HTN, DM, etc.)
G	**Go see** the Patient	**See the patient (problem-based, focused H/P)**
E	**Evaluate** Orders	**Place detailed orders in SCM** • Interventions (abx, IVF, heparin gtt, etc.) • Medication Reconciliation • Diagnostic tests (echo, CT, other labs, etc.)
An	**Assess**, Formulate Plan	**Formulate Assessment & Plan (complete signout)** • Prioritize acute problem list • Each problem should include 3 Ws: o What, Why, What next • What else? Chronic Problem List
H&P	*Write it / Put it in Chart*	**Complete H&P and place in chart**

Fig. 11.1 The "TRIAGE An H&P" tool is a comprehensive ordered list of tasks to accomplish during initial hospital admissions [5]

Inefficiency in Pre-rounding

> Over time, Ray's efficiency with new admissions improves, but they still come in very early to ensure readiness for rounds.
>
> Dr. Suárez: It seems your efficiency on admissions has improved. But you still seem to have to come in very early to be ready for rounds.
> Ray: Yes. If I don't come very early, I struggle to see everyone before rounds start. I don't feel like I have any organization or system. Each day I do things a bit differently.

Learners commonly struggle to efficiently review records and check-in with their hospitalized patients before the scheduled work begins. This "pre-rounding" time is rarely observed or explicitly directed. The "PRePPING" tool (Fig. 11.2) walks the learner through each pre-rounding step, starting with mentally preparing while traveling to the hospital, maximizing time with patients, and efficiently using any additional downtime before formal rounds begin. It also provides faculty areas for focused, direct observation of pre-rounding skills.

A similar approach applies to learners struggling with efficiency in the outpatient setting. The learner is encouraged to briefly review the charts of patients scheduled for the following day and estimate the amount of time they expect to

Fig. 11.2 The "PRePPING the Patient" tool is a comprehensive ordered list of tasks that help learners organize their preparation for hospital work and develop a plan for evaluating patients prior to hospital rounds [5]

"PRePPING" the Patients: Guide to Pre-Rounding

P	**Plan** the day	**On your way to work, think about:** • Planned discharges vs ongoing care plans • Current patient plans for the day *(CT scan, OR plan)*
Re	**Review** signout	**Obtain written and verbal signout, review overnight events**
P	**Prioritize**	**Make game plan:** • Assess need for urgent/emergent interventions based on signout – do you need to contact supervising resident? • Decide on rounding order based on acuity, geography, and discharge planning
P	**Prepare**	**Scan vitals, talk to RN, review individual overnight events**
I	**Inside** the room	**Perform focused ROS and physical exam, to answer these key questions (at least):** • Is the primary reason for hospitalization/primary complaint better, worse, or same? • Are the relevant physical exam findings better, worse or same? • Is the patient ready for discharge: Have you achieved all medical goals and they are eating, drinking, walking, and have a place to go?
N	**Note** your findings	**Complete S and O sections of note**
G	re**Group**	**After you have seen all your patients, you should:** • Check labs • Replete electrolytes, transfuse blood • Put in other routine orders • ***Reassess, Rename and Reprioritize*** each problem • Within each problem, **compose *the What, the Why, and the What Next*?**

spend in the room with each patient to address a limited number (e.g., 2–3) of key issues and tasks that must be addressed.

Inefficiency and Disorganization in Note Writing

Case 2
You are working with an intern, Arthur (he/ him), who is on his second inpatient rotation of the year. You have served as his ward attending for 1 week and are about to meet to provide feedback. He is enthusiastic and frequently shows a good fund of knowledge and clinical reasoning when asked questions during rounds. His new patient presentations are thorough with well-developed differentials, assessments, and therapeutic plans.

He does not yet have a large patient panel, but he consistently struggles with his daily work. You have noticed he rarely completes his notes before midday and never has notes ready for rounds, despite the expectation that notes be completed shortly after rounds. When he does finally submit the notes, they are often copied and pasted from prior days and lack pertinent, new information.

In the era of the electronic health record, many learners fall into the 'copy forward' note writing habit. Besides negatively affecting the quality of the written patient chart, this practice also represents a missed opportunity for learners to better understand a patient's clinical progression. We developed the inpatient "3R/3W" tool (Fig. 11.3), which provides the learner with a framework for updating notes. It reminds the learner to ask three questions aimed at *reassessing* a patient's trajectory based on information gathered in pre-rounds—"Is the patient better?" "Is the current diagnosis still the most likely?" "Is your current therapeutic plan still effective?" After reassess-

ing, it encourages the learner to rename the patient's diagnoses more precisely based on additional information (e.g., "Is the patient's fever now more aptly described as a symptom of newly diagnosed endocarditis?"). Finally, and most importantly, this tool encourages the learner to reprioritize issues on the problem list as issues resolve and others develop. This tool can be easily modified for coaching longitudinal care in the outpatient setting.

Inefficiency in Daily Tasks

With your help, Arthur becomes more accurate in his note-writing. However, he still struggles to complete his clinical duties. He often does not complete high-priority tasks until well after rounds and frequently requires reminders from you and the senior resident.

Arthur needs specific tools to help him better manage his "to do" list with proper triaging of tasks.

Too often, the feedback given to learners like Arthur is nonspecific: they need to be "more efficient." To provide specific and actionable feedback while also allowing for direct observation of the learner, start by asking the learner to share their "to do" list with you. While no single approach to organizing a task list is superior, having one is critical. An effective system should allow the learner to see all of their tasks in a concise and comprehensive way. Frequently, learners who struggle with task organization either have no system or have developed a system that is cumbersome.

After reviewing the learner's task management system, we resist the urge to completely overhaul it, but instead ask the learner to review their task list with us at the end of rounds. With this "fresh" task list, we ask the learner about their priorities. Then if need be, we work with the learner to prioritize tasks as

3Rs/3Ws: Guide to Composing Daily Notes

You've finished PRePPING your patient!   Before you start your note or give your oral presentation on rounds, think broadly about your patient:

R	**Reassess**	Is the patient better, worse, or the same? Is the current diagnosis still the most likely? Is your current therapeutic plan still effective?
R	**Rename**	Are the problem names as specific as possible, based on TODAY's data? • *Gram-negative rod UTI → Klebsiella UTI* • *SOB → Pneumonia*
R	**Reprioritize**	Is the most active problem listed first? Can you move resolved or chronic problems lower?
W	**What**	Name the problem, with current clinical status (eg Improved, Stable, Worse, New) • *Community Acquired PNA: Improved....*
W	**Why**	Describe the differential diagnosis and discuss how the current clinical exam, vitals, labs, and studies support your likely diagnosis.
W	**What Next**	What is the plan for the day? Will you be ready to discharge soon? What do we need to do in order to get the patient to move towards discharge?

Fig. 11.3 The "3Rs/3Ws" framework provides guidance for learners to update inpatient progress notes (see text for details) [5]

follows: (1) high priority for completion immediately following rounds; (2) intermediate priority (can be completed later in the day as time allows); (3) low priority for completion only by day's end; and (4) very low priority (can be delayed until the following day or later).

Using this approach, we can explore learners' reasoning around prioritizing tasks and give them very specific feedback about where their approach to prioritization could improve. Ideally, this requires only a brief discussion at the end of rounds and provides a topic for deeper exploration and reflection at a subsequent time. We often review task lists more than one day in a row to identify how changing contexts impact the learner's efficiency.

Assessment and Continuing Observation

Continuing direct observation with structured feedback is critical to solidifying new organizational and task management habits [3]. Optimally, supervisors would directly observe learners in their usual clinical environment, recording the timing of each step in accomplishing a task, eliciting structured reflection, and providing immediate feedback. Lessons learned through direct coaching should be documented by the coach and relayed to faculty and peer evaluators for use during subsequent direct observation on scheduled clinical rotations.

In addition, because effective organization, efficiency, and time management typically rely on appropriate decision-making at nuanced pivot points throughout the day, near-peer coaches can be particularly effective observers. Peer coaches should be familiar with the day-to-day tasks of the struggling learner, making them excellent at observing specifics and providing practical, real-time feedback. Peer coaches should also be at similar stages of training as the struggling learner to promote buy-in and limit stigmatization.

Conclusion

Proactively defining success in remediation coaching is essential. There is no standard definition of "success"; many remediation programs only report short-term outcomes without ongoing observation and reassessment after directed coaching [12]. Definitions of success should be individualized to the needs and developmental stage of the learner and the educational or training program. Demands of training frequently shift, and therefore what constitutes success will also evolve. Proactively defining success means looking forward to anticipating both short-term and long-term demands for a given learner. All stakeholders, including the learner, should have a common understanding of what defines successful remediation and when the learner can transition back into normal, full-time activities.

It is important to acknowledge that remediation is not always successful. In the authors' experience, remediation success is most closely tied to the type of struggle, the accuracy of the "diagnosis," and the level of learner insight and buy-in. Provided that the learner is motivated to change, struggles with organization and effi-

ciency are typically remediated promptly and successfully with effective coaching. If there is a failure to improve, the coach should return to the clarification phase and reconsider whether the learner has a clinical reasoning deficit or a mental well-being challenge, including cognitive dysfunction.

References

1. Dupras DM, Edson RS, Halvorsen AJ, Hopkins RH, McDonald FS. "Problem residents": prevalence, problems and remediation in the era of core competencies. Am J Med. 2012;125(4):421–5.
2. Guerrasio J, Garrity MJ, Aagaard EM. Learners deficits and academic outcomes of medical students, residents, fellows, and attending physicians referred to a remediation program, 2006-2012. Acad Med. 2014;89:352–8.
3. Warburton KM, Goren E, Dine CJ. Comprehensive assessment of struggling learners referred to a graduate medical education remediation program. J Grad Med Educ. 2017;9:763–7.
4. Warburton KM, Shahane AA. Mental health conditions among struggling graduate medical learners: results from a single-center remediation program. J Grad Med Educ. 2020;12:773–7.
5. DeKosky AS, Sedrak MS, Goren E, Dine CJ, Warburton KM. Simple frameworks for daily work: innovative strategies to coach residents struggling with time management, organization, and efficiency. J Grad Med Educ. 2018;10:325–30.
6. Warburton KM, Mahan JM. Coaching nephrology trainees who struggle with clinical performance. Clin J Am Soc Nephrol. 2018;13:172–4.
7. https://learnersdictionary.com/.
8. Bowen JL. Educational strategies to promote clinical diagnostic reasoning. N Engl J Med. 2006;355:2217–25.
9. Parsons AS, Clancy CB, Rencic JJ, Warburton KM. Targeted strategies to remediate diagnostic reasoning deficits. Acad Med. 2022;97:616.
10. Parsons AS, Wijesekera TH, Rencic JJ. The management script: a practical tool for teaching management reasoning. Acad Med. 2020;95:1179–85.
11. Parsons AS, Warburton KM. A novel clinical reasoning coaching program for the medicine learner in need. MedEdPublish. 2018;8(1):9. https://doi.org/10.15694/med.2018.000009.1.
12. Chou CL, Kalet A, Costa MJ, Cleland J, Winston K. Guidelines: the dos, don'ts and don't knows of remediation in medical education. Perspect Med Educ. 2019;8:322–38.

Remediation of Interpersonal and Communication Skills

12

Carol M. Chou, James Bell, Anna Chang, and Calvin L. Chou

Introduction

A colleague pulls you aside to tell you about Quinn (he/him), a student with whom she is working and about whom she has concerns. She has noted that Quinn's interactions with patients are awkward, and he appears to make patients uneasy. Your colleague knows that you will be working with this student in his next rotation and hopes that you can help.

The challenges in identifying and then remediating trainees who have difficulty in interpersonal communication are many. Occasionally,

C. M. Chou (✉)
Department of Medicine, Perelman School of Medicine, University of Pennsylvania, Philadelphia, PA, USA
e-mail: carol.chou@pennmedicine.upenn.edu

J. Bell
Daemen College, Amherst, NY, USA

Institute for Healthcare Communication, Buffalo, NY, USA
e-mail: jbell2@daemen.edu; jbell@healthcarecomm.org

A. Chang · C. L. Chou
Department of Medicine, University of California, San Francisco, CA, USA

Veterans Affairs Healthcare System, San Francisco, CA, USA
e-mail: anna.chang@ucsf.edu; calvin.chou@ucsf.edu

trainees are identified on clinical skills examinations, but often the need for remediation becomes evident while observing them in everyday clinical situations. Despite what we may observe in their outward behaviors, many of these learners wish desperately to connect effectively with others; most do not have a single identifiable, easily correctable area of struggle. We will first enumerate the most likely obstacles that learners encounter in achieving excellent patient-clinician interactions, and then the remediation strategies that we have used successfully. As with other chapters in this section, we will use the general approach to remediation outlined in Chap. 6.

Identification

Learners often face several obstacles to effective communication simultaneously. To identify specific focus areas for remediation, the faculty member should begin by observing the learner in real-time clinical situations using the mini-clinical evaluation exercise ("mini-CEX"; [1]) or a Brief Structured Clinical Observation [2], and/or with simulation case scenarios. It is critical to base the next clarification step of remediation on accurate low-inference observations of trainee behaviors, because struggles in other areas of medical knowledge or patient care may masquerade as communication skills struggles (see below); implicit bias may also influence judgment of the observer or examiner [3, 4].

Clarification

Suboptimal communication skills may be due to gaps in knowledge, attitude, or skills. It is important to note that struggles with clinical reasoning (see Chap. 9) and issues such as culturally-influenced interaction styles (see Chap. 3), as well as psychological and psychiatric factors, can manifest as struggles with communication skills.

1. Knowledge gap: The learner may not have a systematic approach to the patient-centered interview (Table 12.1). Alternatively, since clinical fund of knowledge informs the content and organization of the interview, a poor knowledge base will negatively affect interviewing skills. Students early in their clinical immersion experiences (e.g., medical students on their first clinical clerkship) often struggle to balance listening and empathy skills with clinical reasoning and the diagnostic process.
2. Attitude gap: Once they have learned basic communication skills principles, a learner may determine that further honing their patient-clinician interaction skills is less important than focusing on other areas of clinical competence.
3. Skills gap: The learner may lack skills in any of the fundamental relationship-centered communication skills known to enhance the trust between patient and clinician [5]. These include building rapport, demonstrating empathy, showing respect, actively listening for both content and emotion, reflective listening and summarizing, and identifying and interpreting nonverbal cues.
4. Psychological and psychiatric factors: Learners suffering from clinical depression or excessive anxiety (either generalized or specific to performance) may find these conditions to be barriers to effective patient interactions. In these instances, educators can help by empathically eliciting the learner's perspective and then encouraging follow up with a mental health professional.
5. Interactional diversity: Learners from minoritized cultural or language groups may not fully understand communication norms implicitly assumed by indigenous groups or native language speakers. Highly introverted individuals may appear to have communication struggles when in fact they simply require extra time for internal information and emotional processing.

Learners referred for communication skills remediation may have a higher incidence of a global communication condition, which the Diagnostic Statistical Manual of Mental Disorders fifth edition (DSM-5) divides into social communication disorder (SCD) and autism spectrum disorder (ASD), sometimes referred to as a neuroatypical interaction style. Often, trainees with SCD or ASD (diagnosed or undiagnosed) have adequate coping skills for and/or are socially accepted for their differences earlier in training, but stressors may outstrip internal resources in demanding academic or clinical training settings [6, 7]. Such learners are espe-

Table 12.1 Fundamental relationship-centered communication skills [5]

Skill Set 1
Establish rapport quickly
Elicit the list of all items
Negotiate the agenda
Skill Set 2
Open the conversation
Explore perspectives and name emotions
Respond with empathy
Skill Set 3
Share information incrementally
Assess understanding
Summarize and clarify with teach-back

cially challenged by and can experience frustration functioning within the healthcare systems where implicit interpersonal interactions rules continually change. These settings challenge the learner's ability to achieve clinical competence.

Two main features of autism spectrum conditions include 1) persistent challenges with social communication and interaction, and 2) restricted and repetitive behaviors, activities, and interests [8]. We strongly recommend that educators ensure that a diagnosis of ASD be made by professionals with specific training because inaccurate use of this diagnostic term risks stigmatizing the learner. We have witnessed the value in making a diagnosis of autism spectrum condition during health professions training, as it can also be revelatory for the learner, providing an explanation for and demystifying years of unexplained negative feedback, and enhancing self-compassion [7].

Potential Causes of Challenges in Communication and Interpersonal Skills
- Knowledge Gap
  - Approach to relationship-centered interviewing
  - Clinical fund of knowledge
  - Inability to balance communication skills with clinical reasoning
- Attitude Gap
- Skills Gap
  - Active and reflective listening
  - Identification of nonverbal or emotional cues
  - Development of rapport
  - Demonstration of empathy
- Psychological/Psychiatric Factors
- Differences in culture, language, or ways of communicating, including neuroatypical interaction style
- Diversity Issues

Intervention and Assessment

When Quinn arrives on your rotation, you observe his interactions with patients and indeed find his mannerisms to be distracting and awkward. Specifically, you observe that Quinn makes poor eye contact and often stammers when speaking. After a patient completes a series of statements and awaits the student's responses, there is often an uncomfortable pause. When a patient says something with emotional valence, Quinn moves forward with clinical questions without acknowledging what the patient has said.

Review of previous coursework showed that there had been no prior concerns about Quinn's knowledge base; he had performed at the class mean on most written exams before beginning clinical rotations. Comments from faculty observers in his interviewing skills course showed no glaring issues. However, standardized patients in an Observed Structured Clinical Examination commented that they detected a general awkwardness, without specifically describing ineffective behaviors.

You say to Quinn, "I'd like to have a discussion with you about your interactions with patients. Can we meet tomorrow afternoon to talk about this further?"

We model our strategy for remediating learners on Relationship-Centered Communication (RCC) skills [5]; the same communication skills that we use to establish meaningful relationships with patients are also used to develop meaningful relationships with learners. (There are many other frameworks of healthcare communication skills to choose from [9–16]; coaches may opt for a framework used at their institution.)

The first meeting with Quinn should address these concrete goals:

1. Set the stage and establish rapport.
2. Model the desired communication skills.
3. Elicit the learner's perspective.
4. Encourage reflection on strengths.
5. Focus on small successes.
6. Assist the learner to develop their own learning plan.
7. Revisit the learning plan and modify future goals.

Step 1: Set the Stage and Establish Rapport

Conversations about remediation should begin with the equivalent of taking a patient's social history. Showing genuine interest in the learner maximizes the possibility of establishing a strong partnership founded on trust and unconditional positive regard [17]. In addition, stating an explicit commitment to work with the learner and to be as nonjudgmental as possible can enhance the learning climate.

Sample statements: *"As we begin our work together, it is important to me to get to know you as a person. Tell me about yourself. What influenced you to choose the health professions as a career? If you were not in a health profession, what would you be doing?"*

These questions are not idle cocktail party conversation. Sought with genuine interest and gentle prompting, answers to these questions can reveal the learner's underlying passions, motivations, and strengths. Eliciting learner strengths in this appreciative manner helps coaches link personal attributes to potential goals.

Step 2: Model the Desired Communication Skills

It is essential that coaches of communication skills exhibit fluency and flexibility in one or more models of communication (see example, Table 12.1) and use those same principles when

interacting with learners who struggle. The process of remediating communication skills depends as much on modeling exemplary behaviors as it does on teaching and facilitating learner behaviors. Too often, trainees undergo passive learning practices, where coaches merely share their perspective without first eliciting the learner's thoughts. This approach may result in the learner becoming passive about their learning. To explicitly apply principles of relationship-centered communication skills to the remediation process, we favor an iterative process of interactional "AART" (see box).

Iterative, Interactional "AART"

Ask and frequently elicit the learner's thoughts

Actively listen and reflect the content of the learner's words

Respond with empathy

and only then:

Tell new insights from the coach's perspective

Step 3: Elicit the Learner's Perspective

You learn that Quinn felt great shame about his poor performance. He knew something was not working but could not identify exactly what he was doing wrong. He felt anxious whenever interacting with patients, and this anxiety was heightened when he was being observed. He felt that all his classmates were "superstars" that he could never compete with.

Learners who struggle with patient-clinician interaction skills often feel a range of emotions, including embarrassment, frustration, sadness, awkwardness, and defensiveness. Many equate poor communication performance with not being a "nice" person, or worse yet, being devoid of compassion. This becomes a condemning self-judgment. Often learners will say, in self-defense, "when I'm in a *real* clinical situation [as opposed to a standardized or observed encounter], my patients like me."

Therefore, it is helpful to uncover the emotions behind the learner's reactions. Connecting emotionally with a learner undergoing remediation helps to build trust in the relationship. By expressing empathy and forming a personal connection, the work of remediation becomes a collaborative partnership. Rather than reacting only with statements like, '*Well, you need to perform on this exam,*' or, '*I can only evaluate you on what I observe,*' authentic relationship building statements such as those patterned after the mnemonic PEARLS © [5] can be very helpful in addressing learner resistance:

- **P**artnership: "*I want you to know that I am committing to working with you on this.*"
- **E**motions: "*I imagine it is frustrating to feel that you are being judged on situations that may feel inauthentic to you.*"
- **A**pology/Appreciation: "*I'm sorry you're having to go through this process.*"
- **R**espect: "*You have done a lot of work; I'm glad to hear that your patients work well with you.*"
- **L**egitimization: "*These exercises can feel contrived. Anyone might feel awkward about having to go through this learning experience.*"
- **S**upport: "*We can use your strengths to build skills and help lessen your frustration.*"

Empathizing with the learner is highly powerful: from an empathic stance, a coach can more easily explore additional topics, such as:

"I'd like to hear your ideas about how you might succeed on this exam, given that it doesn't feel completely real to you."

A word of caution: just because you may acknowledge the learner's emotions initially doesn't mean they will remain dormant for the remainder of the remediation process. The emotions arise again and again. Continued attention to emotional connection with the learner will reap continued rewards.

Step 4: Encourage Reflection on Strengths

Once the emotional connection develops, supporting the learner's strengths and passions can restore some of their confidence. Often in remediation, the tendency is for both coach and learner to focus on deficit detection—what the learner is not doing well, behaviors that the learner most wishes to change—and elimination. An alternative approach is appreciative inquiry [18], a process for learning through building on success rather than focusing on deficits. The premise underlying the appreciative inquiry model is that learners should have successes upon which they can build. Focusing on behaviors that encourage positive outcomes allows the learner to start from a place of known strength and comfort, which enhances the likelihood of further success. Additionally, having the student identify and reflect on good examples they have seen may also be helpful, because it serves as a point of inspiration for learners with challenges identifying anything laudatory in their own performances.

"Based on the video of your interaction with this patient, I'd like to hear from you about areas that you believe you are doing effectively."

"I agree that you use steady eye contact when introducing yourself to the patient."

One caveat, is that low-performing learners may overestimate their abilities; deft handling of these situations, without reinforcing ineffective behaviors is key.

(In discussing an area of possible disagreement): *"I am hearing that you think your eye contact with the patient effectively communicated caring."*

Quinn desperately wished to connect with patients and was highly motivated to learn specific techniques to accomplish this connection. He reports he has been an excellent test-taker because he just buckles down and forces the information into his head.

Communication Remediation Coach: *"It sounds like one of your strengths is not only to take tests but also to assimilate information in a way that makes sense to you. I'm glad to hear that connecting with patients is very important to you, and I'm excited to work with you to develop those skills. This work will probably require new ways of learning since "forcing" is not usually successful in communication. What ideas do you have about how you will best learn in this domain?"*

Step 5: Focus on Small Successes

Direct observation—whether in real time or via review of video recorded encounters, whether using role-play or with a real or standardized patient—provides primary data for analysis. We recommend following the same "AART" process used to get to know the learner: begin with **A**sking the learner for their own assessment of performance, **A**ctively listen to the learner's responses and compare their self-assessment with your own impressions, and begin to determine if the learner's strengths can be drawn on to effect needed changes. Then, continue by **R**esponding with empathy, affirming those things they did effectively and demonstrating your understanding of the learner's self-assessment, and conclude by **T**elling your own impressions of the learner's areas of strengths as well as areas that need work, and discussing next steps for practice and improvement. Learners who struggle tend to perceive their own skills as better than they objectively are [19, 20]; therefore, to ensure continual improvement of skills, it is key to help the learner increase the accuracy of their self assessments. Using the "AART" pro-

cess of eliciting self-assessment and providing reinforcing feedback early, often, and iteratively in the relationship can help the learner to gain that accuracy and achieve sustained success.

Initially, Quinn wished to work on skills using role play, with the coach playing a range of patient presentations, as this approach felt manageable. The coach understanding Quinn's goals, designed practice exercises specifically to meet his needs.

Deliberate practice with structured feedback is a fundamental strategy in developing expertise [21]. It is important to provide the learner opportunities for small successes that build on each other. For example, one can start with a controlled or simulated scenario that allows the learner to employ strategies highlighting one of their own strengths. Focusing feedback on the learner's effective behaviors prepares them with the confidence to face incrementally more challenging practice sessions. The educator can then deliver specific feedback, homing in on the desired skills.

Remediation can be anxiety-provoking. Frequent, planned feedback sessions initially focused on reinforcing strengths, rather than providing corrective behavior modifications, reduce the anxiety for the learner and the faculty member. One simple format for feedback, using the AART framework noted above, is to follow these steps:

1. Create an environment that allows for privacy and comfort.
2. Take an emotional reading of the learner: *"How do you feel that went?"*
3. Elicit the learner's perception of successful aspects of the interaction.
4. Confirm the learner's view of specific successful actions, and add any not noted by the learner.
5. Elicit the learner's self-critique.

6. Confirm or refute this critique, and add any specifics not noted by the learner, limiting these to the few most important and modifiable issues to avoid negative impact on learning.
7. Ask the learner for their "take-home" points to be practiced.
8. Summarize and plan next steps.

Using a structure for feedback reduces the potential negative emotional impact and enhances collaboration.

Step 6: Assist the Learner to Develop Their Own Learning Plan

> Upon initiating feedback after a simulated patient encounter involving a disengaged teenager, Quinn is frustrated with the lack of progress toward understanding the patient's motivation and the amount of time he "wasted" during the interview. The coach acknowledges the frustration, indicates that teenage patients are often challenging to engage, and points out that Quinn's frustration is an indication that he is perceiving communication barriers, an important step toward addressing such barriers.

Effective learning plans are written documents with specific goals and strategies to address these goals. Learners often struggle at first to develop personal learning plans because they may not have had prior experience generating learning goals and strategies. Work by Knowles in adult learning theory suggests that learner-generated interventions and goals result in increased frequency of application of interventions and increased success toward goals [22]. Coaches should develop an approach to eliciting a learner's goals. Some starting prompts include:

> "Tell me an area where you would like to improve."

> "When you watch the video of that interaction, where did you feel that you struggled?"

Often, learners name many goals that coaches have not considered. After identifying several of the learner's own goals, the coach can take the opportunity to ask for permission to add another goal or two.

> "Are you open to a suggestion or two from my perspective?"

> "You mentioned earlier that your eye contact helped your communication with patients. I have a different perspective and would like to analyze those phases of these encounters with you more closely. Can we agree to put that on your learning plan?"

Goals as part of learning plans are most effective when they are "SMART": specific, measurable, attainable, relevant, and time-bound [23]. While the learner can be challenged to draft a learning plan based on the discussion, it is important for the faculty coach to revise the learning plan with the student to improve the plan's utility. Some sample learning plans for this student might be:

> "The next time I need to prepare a patient for hearing bad news in an encounter, I will change my tone of voice to be serious, not lighthearted, and I will make a statement that gives them a warning that the news is serious. I will say…"

> "When the patient starts to cry, I will allow silence in the room instead of continuing to speak. After I count to 10 or when the sobbing has subsided, I will gently ask them to share their experience by saying…"

Step 7: Revisit the Learning Plan

> *Because Quinn's strengths were about test-taking and desire to connect, goals developed with his coach included: using a structured, standardized approach to each encounter; making certain to use at least one empathic statement during each encounter; remembering to ask about the patient's explanatory model of illness; and using the teach-back technique to check his understanding of the patient's illness.*

A learning plan is best used as a guide for continued intervention. Frequent review of the learning plan during remediation serves to verify intervention strategies and monitor and celebrate progress. As the student works through the goals, new goals may emerge, updating the learning plan.

Common Remediation Scenarios

We have applied the seven-step approach successfully to most of our remediation work in communication skills. We now describe adaptations of the approach to three common scenarios.

Learners Who Lack Verbal Rapport-Building Skills

It is common for learners to claim to feel compassion and empathy, but not verbalize these feelings in ways that patients can appreciate.

> Coach: [after eliciting effective behaviors from the learner and other areas to improve] *I wonder if I could bring up an observation.*
> Learner: *OK.*
> Coach: *I noticed that while your eye contact and vocal tone showed caring, I didn't hear a specific empathic statement.*
> Learner: *But I was empathetic.*

> Coach: *I saw your intention, but I'm not certain that the patient did. I was guessing that you were feeling the patient's frustration, but to make sure the patient experiences that, verbal empathy is helpful.*
> Learner: *That sounds too touchy-feely.*
> Coach: *I'm hearing you feel uncomfortable saying words that communicate emotion. At the same time, did you know that studies have shown that for both surgeons and internists, using a verbal empathic statement actually shortens their office visits?*
> Learner: *No, I didn't.*
> Coach: *It's hard for patients to read our minds. I wonder if you could find expressions that would allow you to connect verbally with a patient without sounding too hokey.*

Learners Exhibiting Resistance to Learning This Material

Understanding of the learner's ultimate professional goals provides the opportunity to connect these goals with the importance of mastering communication skills. For instance, succeeding in fields based on interactions between colleagues of different disciplines and professions invariably requires excellence in interpersonal skills.

> Learner: *I don't need to learn this stuff. My patients will like me because I can save their lives.*
> Coach: *I'm glad to hear that you plan on establishing such important and satisfying medical expertise. I would like to support you to be clinically masterful in a sustainable way. What do you know about relationship development and the effect on patients and clinicians?*
> Learner: *I'm not sure I know much about that.*
> Coach: *It turns out that clinicians have better long-term career satisfaction, and patients recover faster with less pain and psychological distress. Communication skills distinguish masterful from merely good clinicians. I want to get you to that masterful level.*

Another approach uses appreciative inquiry (see above) to challenge the learner to define characteristics of exemplary clinicians.

> Coach: *Tell me of a time when you saw one of your role models do something admirable.*

Coach: *What are some examples you've seen of expert clinicians who effectively used communication skills to achieve desired clinical outcomes?*

After establishing the learner's perspective, use the opportunity to share knowledge about outcomes and pitfalls of ineffective communication skills for any practicing clinician, including inefficiency, increased malpractice risk, poor patient outcomes and experiences of care, and poor well-being (see Chap. 18).

I'm curious if you know data on the relationship between the quality of interactions of exemplary clinicians in your field and malpractice risk.

Learners with an Autism Spectrum Condition

There is reason to be optimistic about remediation for learners with an autism spectrum conditions as long as they are otherwise motivated to address their challenges. A highly structured approach such as the one we have outlined above will help many learners. Two other widely available resources can particularly support learners and remediation teams. First, highly analytical trainees may find the Facial Action Coding System (FACS) helpful [24]. Popularized by Paul Ekman, who famously has consulted for Pixar films to humanize faces of animated cartoons, FACS systematically details facial expressions, provides approaches to decode them, and gives insight into what one intends to convey and what others perceive. Second, having trainees read poignant narratives written by people reflecting on their ability to function with autism can inspire them with motivational techniques to address unintended interactional challenges due to their communication styles [25–27]. An additional potential resource for remediation team members specializing in working with trainees on the autism spectrum is Social Cognition and Interaction Training, to help learners define emotions, link facial expressions to these emo-

tions, help detect and interpret social cues, and address multiple explanations for ambiguous social situations [28].

Through these resources, and patience and compassion on the part of learner and remediation team, a trainee's fear of needing a "personality transplant" will gradually dissipate, along with the recognition of the value that the trainee brings to individual encounters and to healthcare in general.

Other Coaching Considerations

Methods to ascertain the learner's communication skill level include: observation by qualified faculty arbiters in real-time clinical settings, assessment in an Observed Structured Clinical Examination or similar simulation by trained standardized patients, and/or video review of either real-time or simulated encounters.

To enhance the success of these and future coaching interactions, faculty coaches must also self-reflect, investigate their own blind spots or issues of countertransference with learners, and be open to consultation with trusted colleagues and experts in these skills. Courses such as those held by the Academy of Communication in Healthcare (www.achonline.org) can also deepen fundamental skills, expand coaching tools, and provide connections and feedback from colleagues and experts.

Finally, curricular elements at programmatic and institutional levels must undergo review. Opportunities to improve explicit teaching of communication skills may be identified. In addition, it is important to examine the hidden curriculum that might de-emphasize communication skills ("soft skills") in favor of "hard" science; hierarchical or other cultural influences that interfere with effective role-modeling of effective communication; or toxic work environments necessitating resilience interventions (see Chap. 18).

Conclusion

Remediation can be a challenging endeavor for the learner as well as for the coach.

We presented an effective seven-step approach to support learners with communication skills struggles. Though the examples in this chapter have focused on patient-clinician interactions, this approach to coaching communication skills applies to many different settings, including interactions between colleagues (with tips from the professionalism literature (see Chap. 14)); faculty members struggling to connect with learners; and leadership interactions with team members. This broad application makes coaching interpersonal communication skills a versatile practice that we have found repeatedly helpful for learners at all levels.

Acknowledgment The authors thank Stephen Bent for his helpful review.

References

1. Norcini JJ, Blank LL, Duffy FD, Fortna GS. The mini-CEX: a method for assessing clinical skills. Ann Intern Med. 2003;138:476–81.
2. Kuo AK, Irby DI, Loeser H. Does direct observation improve medical students' clerkship experiences? Med Educ. 2005;39:518.
3. Stroud L, Herold J, Tomlinson G, Cavalcanti RB. Who you know or what you know? Effect of examiner familiarity with residents on OSCE scores. Acad Med. 2011;86:S8–11.
4. Yeates P, Moreau M, Eva K. Are examiners' judgments in OSCE-style assessments influenced by contrast effects? Acad Med. 2015;90:975–80.
5. Chou CL, Cooley L, editors. Communication Rx: transforming healthcare with relationship-centered communication. New York: McGraw Hill Education; 2017.
6. Moore S, Kinnear M, Freeman L. Autistic doctors: overlooked assets to medicine. Lancet Psychiatry. 2020;7:306–7.
7. Price S, Lusznat R, Mann R, Locke R. Doctors with Asperger's: the impact of a diagnosis. Clin Teach. 2019;16:19–22.
8. American Psychiatric Association. Diagnostic and statistical manual of mental disorders. 5th ed. Washington, DC: American Psychiatric Publishing, Inc.; 2013.
9. Cole S, Bird J. The medical interview: the three function approach. St. Louis: Mosby, Inc.; 2000.
10. Frankel RM, Stein T. Getting the most out of the clinical encounter: the four habits model. Perm J. 1999;3:79–88.
11. Makoul G. The SEGUE framework for teaching and assessing communication skills. Patient Educ Couns. 2001;45:23–34.
12. Kurtz SM, Silverman JD. The Calgary-Cambridge referenced observation guides: an aid to defining the curriculum and organizing the teaching in communication training programmes. Med Educ. 1996;30:83–9.
13. Makoul G. Essential elements of communication in medical encounters: the Kalamazoo consensus statement. Acad Med. 2001;76:390–3.
14. Kalet A, Pugnaire MP, Cole-Kelly K, Janicik R, Ferrara E, Schwartz MD, Lipkin M Jr, Lazare A. Teaching communication in clinical clerkships: models from the Macy initiative in health communications. Acad Med. 2004;79:511–20.
15. Fortin AHVI, Dwamena FC, Frankel RM, Smith RC. Smith's patient-centered interviewing: an evidence-based method. 4th ed. New York: McGraw Hill; 2019.
16. Windover AK, Boissy A, Rice TW, Gilligan T, Velez VJ, Merlino J. The REDE model of healthcare communication: optimizing relationship as a therapeutic agent. J Patient Exp. 2014;1:8–13.
17. Rogers C. On becoming a person. Boston: Houghton Mifflin; 1961.
18. Cooperrider DL, Whitney D. Appreciative inquiry: a positive revolution in change. San Francisco: Berrett-Koehler Publishers, Inc.; 2005.
19. Langendyk V. Not knowing that they do not know: self-assessment accuracy of third-year medical students. Med Educ. 2006;40:173–9.
20. Srinivasan M, Hauer KE, Der-Martirosian C, Wilkes M, Gesundheit N. Does feedback matter? Practice-based learning for medical students after a multi-institutional clinical performance examination. Med Educ. 2007;41:857–65.
21. Ericsson KA. Deliberate practice and the acquisition and maintenance of expert performance in medicine and related fields. Acad Med. 2004;79:S70–81.
22. Knowles M. Adult learning. In: Craig RL, editor. The ASTD training and development handbook. New York: McGraw Hill; 1996.
23. Chang A, Chou CL, Teherani A, Hauer KE. Clinical skills-related learning goals of senior medical students after performance feedback. Med Educ. 2011;45:878–85.
24. Ekman P. Emotions revealed: recognizing faces and feelings to improve communication and emotional life. New York: Holt Paperbacks; 2007.
25. Finch P. Somewhere inside: a path to empathy. New York Times. https://www.nytimes.com/2009/05/17/style/modern-love-somewhere-

inside-a-path-to-empathy.html; read on podcast by Daniel Radcliffe at https://www.nytimes.com/2020/04/08/style/modern-love-podcast-daniel-radcliffe.html?searchResultPosition=1.

26. Finch P. The journal of best practices: a memoir of marriage, Asperger syndrome, and one man's quest to be a better husband. New York: Scribner; 2012.

27. Grandin T. Thinking in pictures: my life with autism. New York: Vintage Books; 2008.

28. Turner-Brown LM, Perry TD, Dichter GS, Bodfish JW, Penn DL. Brief report: feasibility of social cognition and interaction training for adults with high functioning autism. J Autism Dev Disord. 2008;38:1777–84.

Professionalism Lapses as Professional Identity Formation Challenges

13

Verna Monson, Muriel J. Bebeau, Kathy Faber-Langendoen, and Adina Kalet

Introduction

Most trainees begin their journey toward becoming health professionals with the best of intentions. However, it is common that actions do not always align with intentions. Our recommendations for remediating lapses in professionalism are guided by Rest's Four-Component Model (FCM) of Morality, an evidence-based psychological theory whose central premise is that specific psycho–social–emotional capacities are essential to consistent moral behavior [1]. Initial use of this model was supported by data from 20 cohorts of professional school students who completed an ethics curriculum designed to promote the capacities defined by the theory. We have since refined measures based on the FCM for use in remediation coaching of medical students and residents.

The phrase "lapses in professionalism" is now preferred to the term *unprofessionalism* in the literature [2–4]. This phrase adjusts for the tendency to over-generalize from behavior to person, i.e., avoiding the tendency to deem a person as being of poor character based on a single episode or a pattern of behaviors [5]. In our view, professionalism is neither solely constituted of behaviors nor of character, but instead is a capacity for actions and decisions that are consistent with the requirements and expectations of the profession. We assert that consistent professional behavior is a function of (1) the individual's level of identity development, or professional identity formation (PIF) [5–9] and (2) the organizational or institutional culture [2, 5, 10]. Accordingly, with a combination of coaching methods guided by principles of adult developmental theory, supportive mentors and instructors, and an environment conducive to growth, the individual can improve in order to meet the expectations and requirements of the institution and the profession [2, 5, 9, 11]. We consciously use both "lapses in professionalism" and "unprofessional behavior" synonymously throughout the chapter to remain consistent with the literature and to emphasize that professionalism is more than either the sum

V. Monson (✉) · A. Kalet
Kern Institute for the Transformation of Medical Education, Medical College of Wisconsin, Milwaukee, WI, USA
e-mail: akalet@mcw.edu

M. J. Bebeau
School of Dentistry, University of Minnesota Twin Cities, Minneapolis, MN, USA
e-mail: bebea001@umn.edu

K. Faber-Langendoen
Center for Bioethics and Humanities, State University of New York Upstate Medical Center, Syracuse, NY, USA
e-mail: faberlak@upstate.edu

of a checklist of behaviors or solely attributable to the developmental level of the individual, but a complex integration of both [12].

Papadakis et al. demonstrated that unprofessional behaviors in medical students predicted disciplinary actions taken by medical boards against those individuals when they were in practice [13]. Since then, there has been growing commitment to understanding root causes of unprofessional behaviors, intervening early, and remediating effectively. Educators now have more sophisticated tools for these processes to enhance individuals' capacity for lifelong professional behavior. However, continued reluctance to report identified lapses in professionalism limits the impact of remediation. While one-fifth of clinician–educators observe unprofessional behaviors, only 3–5% report them to someone with the responsibility and skills to remediate [2]. Barriers to reporting lapses in professionalism include a lack of clarity about or trust in our ability to effectively intervene [14]. In this chapter, we hope to provide the health professions educator community and our trainees with an optimistic view of the need to routinely identify and effectively address lapses in professional behavior.

The Evolving Definition of Unprofessional Behaviors

Of course, context matters in how individuals enact their professionalism. While aspects of the ethical codes of many professions have remained fundamentally unchanged over very long time periods, significant shifts, reinterpretations, and updates have occurred with cultural, economic, and political movements. War and natural disasters such as pandemics present new professionalism challenges [15]. With increasing scrutiny regarding what constitutes professional behavior [16], health professions faculty must exercise considerable wisdom, diligence, curiosity, and compassion when investigating lapses in professionalism [11].

Research has identified four patterns of unprofessionalism behaviors (see Chap. 14), including involvement (e.g., tardiness submitting assignments, unexcused absences, interpersonal conflicts), integrity (e.g., plagiarism, false reporting of data), interaction (e.g., disruptive behavior, harassment, inappropriate use of social media, breaches of confidentiality), and introspection (e.g., avoiding/resisting feedback, blaming others for lapses, being insensitive to others' needs, lacking insight) [2]. Mak-van der Vossen and colleagues identified wide-ranging factors associated with these four dimensions [2, 3]. Individual factors include lack of awareness about competencies, neuro-atypical conditions (see Chap. 12), coping with physical and mental health or substance misuse/abuse, lack of motivation to become a health professional, and language limitations. Broader factors include lack of clarity about expectations of professionalism behaviors, lack of role models, "unwarranted evaluations," prevalence of racially discriminatory microaggressions in learning environments (see Chap. 3), cultural differences, difficulties in adapting to a hierarchical culture, or "feeling overwhelmed by stressful circumstances" [16].

Of the unprofessional behaviors, issues of integrity may be the most high-profile, challenging, and likely to lead to dismissal. Fargen and colleagues [17] found that plagiarism, cheating on examinations, and listing fraudulent publications were reported in 5% to 15% of student and resident populations. Self-reported cheating ranges from 0 to 58% [18].

When educational activities abruptly shifted to remote formats due to the COVID-19 pandemic, issues of academic integrity and changes in how to address unprofessional acts became highly publicized. At West Point Military Academy, at the height of the first wave of the pandemic in May 2020, 73 cadets were accused of cheating on a remotely administered calculus exam [19]. Fifty-nine admitted to cheating and voluntarily entered a rehabilitation process that allowed them to continue in the academy, a departure from previous policies of automatic suspension [20]. Similarly, at Dartmouth Medical School in May 2021, 17 students were accused of cheating on an exam administered through the learning management system, based on digital activity data [21]. After much debate and investigation, deliberate student cheating was not proven, all allegations were dropped, and apologies were issued [22]. Health professions educators have recently moved significantly from punitive toward developmental approaches, although not without controversy. Strategies employed vary from providing additional mentoring or coaching to requiring mental health counseling [23].

In addition, remediation can reinforce stigma and shame among learners, particularly in those with preexisting mental health challenges, because of the fear of being labelled unfit for practice. The negative effects of remediation may occur at a disproportionately higher rate among learners who have experienced adverse childhood events (ACEs). Researchers found that ACEs that most strongly predicted referrals for lapses in professionalism were those categorized as "boundary violations," including "feeling unwanted or unloved or caretaker substance use" [24]. Therefore, educators involved in remediation must use trauma-informed approaches [24–26].

How, then, should health professions schools develop a coherent approach to remediation that maintains learning environments where ongoing formative assessment is the norm [27]? We propose a theoretically and empirically grounded approach that considers the full complexity of factors involved in remediating cases of unprofessionalism [6]. We introduce a conceptual model that has been well-validated in health professions education [5], followed by a discussion of potential assessments that are shown to be useful in remediation of lapses in professionalism.

A Theoretical Approach to Professionalism Remediation

Beginning in the early 1980s, Bebeau and colleagues designed and validated theoretically grounded performance measures used to both identify the need for an ethics educational intervention and demonstrate long- and short-term program effectiveness (see [5] for a summary of the various measures). In addition to designing ethics educational programs for dentistry stu-

dents [1], MJB designed individualized ethics remediation programs for over 50 professionals disciplined by a licensing board [28, 29]. VM and AK built on this foundational work, applying it to extensive professionalism remediation efforts with medical students, residents, and colleagues. Utilizing two of four components of morality—moral judgment and moral motivation, they designed remediation programs that effectively promote professional identity formation (PIF). This approach empowers professionals and students to recognize and reflect on developmental challenges as a path toward understanding and guarding against lapses in professional behavior. Below, we briefly review the theoretical framework and share our experience with dental and medical students highlighting assessments and coaching strategies that help with commonly encountered lapses in professionalism [30].

The Components of Morality

In the early 1980s, Rest reviewed morality research from multiple theoretical perspectives to illuminate the internal processes—in addition to moral reasoning and judgment—that might explain lapses in moral behavior. He suggested four independent reasons for moral failure: moral blindness, defective reasoning, lack of commitment to moral ideals, and deficiencies of character and competence [31]. Rest proposed that for consistency in moral action, especially in the context of challenging professional practice, individuals must have four core social–emotional and cognitive capacities that lead to conscious and effective, rather than accidental or unreflective, ethical decision-making (Table 13.1).

Wide-ranging evidence supports that each of Rest's capacities develops throughout life [28, 29]. Thus, at any given time point, for example, one's inadequately developed competence in any of the four capacities could result in behavior that others judge as evidence of a moral failing that requires remediation. For example, a patient might report a professional to the licensing board, initiating investigation and, eventually, a judgment. If the judgment suggests someone has

Table 13.1 Rest's four-component model of ethical decision-making and moral action

Capacity	Assessment	Mental capacities of morality: growth trajectory
Moral sensitivity	Dental Ethical Sensitivity Test	From moral or ethical blindness to full awareness of ethical issues that encompass multiple, diverse perspectives
Moral judgment	Defining Issues Test	From justifications centered on self-interest to ones that are humanistic and advocate for justice and the greater good
Moral implementation	Observed structured clinical examinations Multiple mini interviews	From communication that is ineffective, self-interested, or paternalistic to communication that enacts principles of respect, autonomy, do no harm, justice
Moral motivation *(or professional identity)*	Professional Role Orientation Inventory or the Professional Identity Essay	From a professional identity that seeks external guidance and direction and prioritizes self-interest to PIF that is internalized ("I am a physician, therefore I..."), committed to aligning personal values to the profession's, managing competing values, and contributing to well-being and the common good

been harmed or wronged, questions emerge about that professional's competence and intentions. MLB has used this framework, and assessments associated with each component, to determine the professional's relative strengths and weaknesses in each of the capacities. Then, the professional engages, with coaching, in self-reflection, goal-setting, and development and implementation of a learning plan with the goal of enhancing ethical competence and reducing the chances of unprofessional behaviors in the future.

We describe two practical measures that relate to PIF, their scoring, and interpretation of the results. Though trainees are often referred for remediation based on unacceptable behaviors (e.g., [30]), the specifics of those behaviors may not translate directly into remediation strategies. We have shown that remediation, guided by two measures of the individual's capacities and understandings that drive the behavior, can be effective because they enhance self-awareness and identify targets for educational intervention [29]. The Defining Issues Test (DIT-2) provides a general assessment of the moral arguments that the individual finds persuasive when confronted with a moral problem. The Professional Identity Essay (PIE) elicits the individual's concept of a professional's role in contemporary society.

Measuring Moral Judgment: The Defining Issues Test

The DIT-2 [32] is an extensively validated and widely used measure of moral judgment development and, unlike many preference measures, is highly resistant to social desirability bias, particularly to "faking" high scores [33]. It asks respondents to choose among alternative actions when confronted with a series of moral dilemmas presented as brief written cases. Each dilemma is followed by 12 statements that reflect each of three general moral schemas (a Personal Interests Schema, a Maintaining Norms Schema, and a Postconventional Schema) that adults tend to use to justify their action preferences as well as a few irrelevant phrases that serve as a reliability check (see Table 13.2; see [5] for details of scoring). The DIT-2 takes 25–30 min to complete, on average.

To gauge the development of moral judgment, respondents are asked to rate each statement, select four of the 12 deemed most important to their decision-making about the case, and further rank-order the selected statements. Scoring responses across cases reveals (1) whether the individual has a preferred moral schema; (2) whether the individual tends to use the preferred schema in decision-making; and (3) whether the individual responded with reasonable consistency across cases and distinguished between coherent and irrelevant statements. Recall that a

Table 13.2 Descriptions of DIT-2 domains

Index	Index abbreviation	Reflects arguments that appeal to…
Personal interests	PI index	Personal interest and/or maintaining one's loyalty to family/friends
Maintaining norms	MN index	Maintaining existing laws, rules, and/or societal norms (also called "conventional arguments")
Post-conventional	P index	Procedural justice and/or to moral principles and ideals upon which conventions, norms, rules, laws are based

moral dilemma isn't just a tough problem that is hard to resolve, but a situation that presents competing claims that thoughtful people can disagree with. Although there isn't one "right answer" to many difficult moral dilemmas, some answers are more defensible than others. (For information on the availability of the DIT-2, and an updated bibliography, see http://www.ethicaldevelopment.ua.edu/.)

Respondents' selections are reported as percentages across the three categories, and the patterns can then be interpreted and discussed. Overall, the DIT-2 does not indicate whether someone is a good person, but it does help them see what kinds of justifications they find most persuasive compared to others. It also does not discriminate among types of personal interest arguments or among the more complex theoretical approaches used by moral philosophers and ethicists; it simply shows whether the individual prefers arguments that appeal either to procedural fairness or to ideals.

Higher education, especially a liberal arts education, has a powerful effect on moral judgment development. A preference for post-conventional thinking (or principle-based thinking) on the DIT-2 tends to increase with higher educational attainment, such as with additional health professions training, and is necessary for effective moral reasoning in highly complex situations. Conversely, a DIT-2 score distribution which shows a relatively low preference for post-conventional thinking (and therefore higher personal interest or maintaining norms scores) have been

associated with malpractice claims in practicing orthopedic surgeons [34]. Our experience in remediation aligns with DIT-2 research showing that individuals use all three arguments to some degree in their moral thinking. Under some circumstances, DIT-2 scores are useful in helping those undergoing remediation understand why they are perceived as unprofessional and suggests effective remediation strategies.

A formal curriculum in professional ethics has been shown to enhance moral reasoning development during professional school [32]. We have found that while most students undergoing professionalism remediation have DIT-2 patterns like their peers (high post-conventional scores), suggesting they are exceptionally capable of principle-based moral reasoning, for the relatively unusual health professions student with "immature" DIT-2 scores (Personal Interest scores >10%), a structured, cognitively intensive individualized curriculum does help them gain insight.

Elwin (he/him) was referred for remediation by the school's Honor Council because he was episodically reported to be disrespectful to peers, supervisors, and staff. His DIT-2 revealed a high Personal Interest score compared with peers (~30% compared with ~5%). Through reflection on his behavior both in writing and through dialogue with his coach, he gained insight into how his occasional tendency to justify his actions based on his own needs (e.g., "I left rounds because I wasn't learning anything," "The nurse was wasting my time") was perceived by those around him as arrogant and unprofessional. He also underwent a focused curriculum, including selected readings reviewing basic professional ethics and principles, analytic and reflective essays, and discussions with a faculty member with advanced medical ethics training. These activities motivated him to strengthen his capacity to consistently apply the principles of professionalism, in particular the expectation of interpersonal respect, in work relationships.

Professional Identity Formation (PIF) and the Professional Identity Essay (PIE)

Unlike the general population, persons granted a license for professional practice are expected to adhere to codes of professional responsibility and engage in actions that benefit others [32, 35–38]. Certainly, professionals vary in how reflective, deliberate, and resistant to self-interest they are in their daily work. However, health professionals are expected to reflect on the moral basis of their actions and to place a patient's interests before their own. We see PIF as a developmental process by which professionals internalize values, aspirations, and actions into their identity and develop increasingly complex understandings of what it means to be a professional. This process begins prior to entry into professional education programs and continues across the professional lifetime. Figure 13.1 describes a staged professional developmental theory [33, 39].

Ideally, as one achieves competence in reasoning and an understanding and commitment to professional values and expectations, idiosyncratic factors influencing action are reduced, and individuals are more likely to behave consistently with professional norms.

The Professional Identity Essay (PIE) consists of a series of open-ended questions designed to elicit the individual's conception of a profession-

al's role in contemporary society [5]. Responses are scored based on criteria adapted from Kegan's life-span model of self-development [7]. Kegan's approach to the study of identity formation is based on constructivist notions that individuals are by nature engaged in making sense of the world and thereby form conceptions of various social categories such as the self, the self as a member of society, a professional, a parent, etc. Kegan and colleagues propose a lifelong developmental model in which individuals can be located in terms of prototypic identity formation.

We reworked Kegan's model to focus on how one comes to understand their specific professional role and incorporated Blasi's [40] view that individuals differ in which moral considerations penetrate the conception of self. In this view, *seeing oneself as responsible is at least part of the bridge between knowing what one ought to do and doing it.* Because students in health professions programs can often express themselves well in writing, we use a series of open-ended questions to elicit understanding of a professional identity consistent with Kegan's descriptions of development stages. Questions prompt learners to reflect on how they construct meaning about becoming a professional, what they expect of the profession, what is expected of them, and what they anticipate being the most salient con-

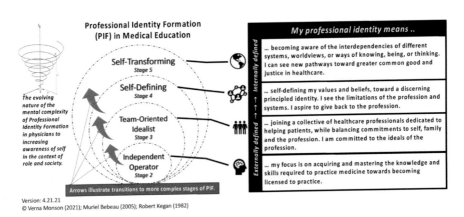

Fig. 13.1 Professional identity formation as a developmental construct in medical education

flicts or failures that could result from taking on their professional role.

A PIE stage scoring guide offers descriptions followed by prototypic statements that characterize stages and transition phases of professional identity [41]. In validation studies, trained raters have achieved high levels of intra- and inter-rater reliability in judging levels of development [42], including in medical students, law students, and counseling students.

Although we initially used these assessments only in professionalism remediation, we began assigning the PIE as a formative assessment to engage all students in self-assessment and reflection as to their location on a developmental continuum typical of professional life, and to develop a reasonable plan for self-development. Assigned during orientation to medical school, orientation to clinical clerkships, and after completing their advanced clerkships, students engage in a debriefing and reflective writing exercise as a component of a professional development curriculum. PIE stage scores are positively correlated with DIT-2 scores [33], increase through medical school, and predict small but significant increases in clinical communication skills [43]. In addition, these measures of PIF may have utility as part of a panel of "non-cognitive" measures in holistic medical school admission processes [44].

Trainees undergoing professionalism remediation complete both DIT-2 and PIE. DIT-2 is scored for a small fee by the Center for the Study of Ethical Development (https://ethicaldevelopment.ua.edu). The PIE is stage scored by an expert (VM), and an individually tailored, detailed report is generated (see Table 13.3 for excerpts from a coding rubric). Each report includes DIT-2 scores, the PIE stage score, and feedback in the form of "questions for ongoing reflection." These questions are designed to facilitate both self-assessment and coaching which can begin with the questions or the learner's felt needs or goals to engage in deeper and ongoing reflection, both verbally and in reflective writing.

Coaching Using the Professional Identity Essay (PIE)

Establishing the Relationship and Expectation of Active Self-Reflection

Coaching has rapidly gained recognition as an important and effective approach to facilitating PIF and conducting professionalism remediation [9, 45, 46]. In addition, the Accreditation Council of Graduate Medical Education [47] has established the expectation that residents demonstrate the skill of "coach[ing] others when their behavior fails to meet professional expectations" as a competency milestone.

We have found that having a trainee begin a professionalism remediation by completing a PIE provides a strong learner-centered basis for PIF coaching. Discussing feedback from the PIE helps identify the trainee's perspectives of their needs and challenges and facilitates action on their self-defined values as goals for remediation work. Deepening the trainee's ability to reflect on their thoughts and emotions, rather than providing a socially desirable response, is a prerequisite for tapping into their implicit assumptions, values, and sources of tension or anxiety that surface deeper identity structures [41, 48]. Based on close reading of thousands of PIE reflective writing assessments, we note that trainees in professionalism remediation benefit from coaching to strengthen their reflectiveness and develop a more nuanced understanding of their professional role. These tools help students understand how reflection on one's assumptions and beliefs can enhance their self-awareness, rather than attain more knowledge or display surface conformity with textbook definitions of professionalism.

Given the sometimes sensitive nature of trainees' written responses to the PIE questions, we advise that programs strongly respect confidentiality, to reassure learners that their responses will not become part of their academic record, and that the assignment is, while perhaps required, purely

Table 13.3 Professional Identity Formation (PIF). Major criteria for analysis of developmental level from reflective writing or interview data. © Verna Monson, Ph.D., 4.9.2020

Cumulative levels of increasing complexity of professional identity formation (PIF)

Criteria related to stage	Independent operator (stage 2) Externally defined	Team—oriented (stage 3)	Self—defined (stage 4) Internally defined	Self—transformed (stage 5)
	2a. Professional identity is subject to (inseparable from) external authorities, institutions, achieving specific concrete goals and rewards	3a. Professional identity subject to (inseparable) others' views—family, peers, physician mentors or supervisors, and the profession as an institution	4a. Professional identity of team-orientation is now object (seen as separate) from one's self-definition, forged through experiences (real or vicarious) that demand greater complexity	5a. Self-defined professional identity is now object (seen as separate), and its limitations are recognized
	2b. May struggle with emotions, showing empathy toward others, lack sensitivity to ethical issues	3b. Can empathize with patients, but may over-prioritize meeting their expectations, failing to see the limitations of patients' understanding or their own biases, barriers to understanding, or access to resources	4b. Can step back and identify one's emotions, and self-regulates within the professional role	5b. Draws upon different disciplines, ideologies, or worldviews to revise or refine one's self-defined professional identity
	2c. May present as confident, but hold fears and doubts privately	3c. May struggle with accepting constructive criticism and be dependent on others to validate and soothe one's self	4c. Can self-assess one's limitations and biases, accept constructive criticism, strive to improve, self-validate, and self-soothe	5c. Revising or refining one's professional identity is seen as an iterative process of self-transformation and incorporates increasing complexity
	2d. Prioritizes performance on objective tests that demonstrate knowledge and skills	3d. Embraces the core principles of the profession, but may not see their limitations	4d. Views problems and conflicts as opportunities to problem solve with others, improve, and/or take leadership	5d. Limitations of existing systems or principles are acknowledged
	2e. Prone to oversimplifications or false dichotomies, e.g., issues that are black/white, all/nothing, friend/foe, or win/lose when facing setbacks and failures	3e. Avoids disclosing views that could destabilize peer, working group, or support system cohesion. May avoid questioning the norms of groups. Views conflicts and disruption as dysfunctional	4e. Retains core principles of the profession, but can acknowledge the limitations of the profession is meeting the social contract with society	5e. May understand failure or setbacks as symptomatic of systems that are dysfunctional or broken
	2f. May catastrophize when considering a hypothetical failure or the "worst that could happen"	3f. May view out-group peers, supervisors, or patients as the "other"	4f. Understand failure or setbacks as a part of the learning process, and not personalize or catastrophize failure	5f. Is motivated to find deeper purpose and meaning related to the social contract between medicine and society
	2g. Self-interest predominates, but may reflect motivation toward self-preservation, rather than character or personality	3g. Views the "worst that could happen" as being judged, shamed, or rejected by peers, patients, or authorities in the profession	4g. May view the "worst that could happen" as a failure to meet one's self-defined goals	
			4h. Prone to becoming entrenched in one's self-defined worldview	

formative. Once the coach establishes their trust-worthiness and commitment to being facilitative and respectful of privacy, trainees may disclose personal experiences such as encountering bias or microaggressions, which then become meaning-ful opportunities for empathic coaching. When coaches identify clinically significant symptoms of depression or anxiety, early referral to a mental health professional may proactively address soci-etal stigma regarding mental illness [49]. Coaches can emphasize that the lifelong process of self-discovery requires a level of openness and curios-ity that cannot be attained merely by excelling in coursework or exams. Coaching involves "nurtur-ing continuous reflection and embracing failure as an opportunity for learning" and "provides a model that aligns assessment and professional identity formation" [45].

Working with the "Alienated Idealist"

We have found that some trainees become openly cynical or jaded early in training. These "alien-ated idealists" come to the profession with high expectations that members of the profession will *all* exhibit great skill, unbridled altruism, and devotion to the profession. When the trainee observes that many clinicians fail to meet these expectations, they may disengage or become aggressively disrespectful, believing that only a select few truly understand professional values. These attitudes can thus lead to lapses in profes-sionalism, such as expressing active disregard for teachers and peers, bringing them to the attention of educational leaders and signaling a need for remediation. Coaching such a trainee an be chal-lenging, but also rewarding. We have found that it is critical to engage the learner by identifying, acknowledging, and expressing respect for the high standards the trainee has set for themselves and others. Encouraging them to articulate a spe-cific interest or problem in society that requires putting one's ideals into action may help them engage in self-directed reflection on their inten-tions and actions, thereby guiding them to explore ways to refine and act upon their idealized goals, refrain from blaming or criticizing others, and act on their own ideals. Coaching can then focus on the learner's experience of putting their ideals

into practice, reflecting on the nuances inherent in the "real world," engaging in pragmatic activi-ties, and enhancing their ability to take the per-spective of and therefore develop empathy toward colleagues and peers. Role playing the communi-cation skills and emotional self-management needed to engage in respectful disagreement and debate can provide these trainees with strategies that enhance their capacity to navigate complex environments. An important assumption of the exercise is that it is normal to adjust one's goals, narrowing the scope to a realistic level. For example, a student who has expressed interest in contributing to the problem of access to health-care or disparities of healthcare outcomes could seek out opportunities to volunteer in a free clinic doing outreach to raise awareness about the importance of routine health screenings. Once the coach has reviewed the proposal, we ask the student to complete a professional development plan utilizing SMART goals [Chap. 6; 50] that relate to an overarching general expectation of the self, the profession, or society, and can build upon their responses to the PIE [41]. Students who feel alienated from their ideals benefit from guidance from potential mentors who can sup-port those ideals and serve as role models for individualized, meaningful career planning.

With an Eye Toward the "I" in Professional Identity

"… it becomes more apparent that there is an I who coordinates the facets of personality, who 'owns' the house of self and is comfortable in all of its rooms" [51]

Coaches should become comfortable discuss-ing PIF as a nonlinear process of setting goals and reaching them. It is also important to acknowledge that trainees, who are usually highly goal-driven, may need a moratorium on committing to specific goals. Movement toward self-definition (the fourth PIF stage) involves questioning one's assumptions and then making refinements or major changes to how they define their professional identity. Contemporary student identity theorists emphasize the importance of integrating specific aspects of one's personal identity (e.g., gender, race, or ethnicity) into one's professional identity, a topic of interest to health professions education as we consider the need for an intersectional view of professional identity [52]. The process of identity development must also consider the context of "historical events and social and cultural conditions emanating from family and ethnic heritage" [53], from which a stable sense of self can grow.

Remediation of Professionalism Lapses: Coaching Principles and Process

As noted, health professions learners are often in the throes of a highly pressured personal and professional maturation process. Internal motivations may conflict with other aspects of one's identity. Health or wellness routines are difficult to reconcile with the demands of health professions school. Making sense of how the hidden curriculum or social milieu of the learning environment conflicts with the stated higher standards of professionalism is personally challenging. Coaches must strive to incorporate into their practice well-established developmental psychology approaches that embrace a growth mindset and the identification of underlying assumptions and beliefs that interfere with acting upon one's intentions [9, 54].

The PIF coach must balance two needs: to guide the learner supportively throughout the remediation process, and to require accountability, engagement in the process, and evidence of improved performance. This process takes time. *A professionalism remediation should not be viewed as a short-term process.* Coaches and trainees need time to establish a growth promoting relationship in which they can co-create and negotiate a variety of strategies. Therefore, while the coach might need to report regularly on progress, time pressure should be resisted. Steinberg cautions medical educators of the need to "be aware of our power and the ability to injure as much as to influence, yet to positively modify and help co-construct and co-create professional (and yes, personal) identity" [55].

We provide two case vignettes to illustrate coaching approaches (consistent with those proposed in Chap. 6) to support trainees who have been identified as having lapses in professionalism.

Two Cases Illustrating Coaching Principles, Processes, and Approaches

Coaches should be sensitive to the difference between technical and adaptive challenges facing professional learners [54]. Initially, coaches should focus on relationship development and actively resist the desire to give technical advice. For instance, if a learner's issues include tardiness or failure to respond promptly to emails, coaches may feel tempted to suggest setting up one's smart phone for calendar alerts. However, most health professions students do not attain admission by being disorganized or unresponsive to requests from administrators or faculty. Something else is often going on.

> **Case 1: DB (He/Him)**
> **Identification Phase**
> *DB recently missed two required learning sessions. When asked by the Associate Dean to explain what happened, he stated that he thought he had informed the program director that he had a conflict, but the email did not go through. On three other occasions, he arrived late to small group sessions. A classmate reported that DB was unprepared to discuss a group project. Another faculty member noted he seemed unwilling to accept feedback during a clinical simulation assessment.*

Table 13.4 illustrates the explanations or hypotheses that coaches can generate to help learners meet behavioral expectations: one that is more technical, and another that relies on a more complex, adaptive approach, resulting in more sustained behavior [54]. Both approaches may be needed at different times.

Clarification Phase

To help DB, rather than rushing to develop a specific plan of action, the PIF coach should initially focus on establishing the relationship with attentive listening and observation for signs of depres-

Table 13.4 Two approaches to helping DB

Technical change: *may help short-term; suggests a "quick-fix"*

- DB is disorganized and/or distracted by personal problems.
- He needs to develop a system of organizing his email inbox.
- He needs to use the calendar on his phone and set up reminders.
- He needs to communicate more responsively and frequently with faculty and peers.

Adaptive change: *more effective in the long run; requires high trust relationship with coach*

- DB explains that his purpose and motivation to become a health professional is getting lost amidst the dense workload.
- He sees little value in some small group activities and believes that what really matters is passing his exams.
- He states that he feels isolated from his family and friends.
- DB confides to you that he has observed racial microaggressions recently, and is questioning whether to say anything or just let it go.

sion, clinical anxiety, or indicators of potential self-harm or abuse. One of the coach's key roles is to help normalize talking about feelings and if needed consulting with a mental health professional. Making this referral may precipitate an emotional reaction in which DB's beliefs about seeking help to cope with difficult emotions might be revealed, e.g., with shame, anger, or denial. The coach also must ascertain if DB might be at risk for self-harm or suicide. Given the prevalence of depression, burnout, and suicide in the health professions, it is vital to maintain communication and trust throughout this process.

Secondly, it is important to assess whether DB has an adequate and accessible support system. Coaches can and should determine if the student has at least one mentor. Depending on the situation, ideally, each student would have access to mentors who share important aspects of their background or identity (e.g., race/ethnicity, gender, immigrant status, etc.) without being prescriptive (see Chap. 3, section on Location of Self).

Intervention Phase

Following the supportive clarification phase with DB, formulating a remediation plan can begin

with assigning and then reviewing a PIE. This can guide further brief reflective writing assignments (Table 13.5). The coach can tailor self-assessment exercises based on elements of the PIF rubric (Table 13.3) or related to health and wellness to issues identified during the remediation. The coach can also assess DB's organizational and time management strategies (see Chap. 11) with attention to how these capacities might have changed over time.

Table 13.5 Question prompts for interviewing or reflective writing

Facilitating the shift from an external to internal definition

- What does it mean to you to become a professional, personally? What motivates you to want to care for people who are ill or suffering?
- What does the profession expect of you?
- What was a time when you experienced being "the other?" Felt excluded or invisible?
- How do you make sense of the benefits of reaching out to your peers who are different from you, forming friendships, and learning about their lived experiences?
- How do you make sense of the privilege(s) you were born with?
- What kind of experiences could you engage in that would be enriching (e.g., clinical rotations abroad or in the community, volunteering)?
- How can you build a bridge for understanding and empathy that goes beyond dichotomies of "right/wrong," "left/right," or "good/bad"?

Facilitating a more fully self-defined professional identity

- How does the social contract between the health professions and society shape what our role and responsibilities are in becoming a professional?
- How could you cultivate leadership capacities in helping your peers, patients, or others grow to see greater complexity and the humanistic implications of divisive issues?
- How can you build your support system and find mentors who "get you?"
- In what ways can you be fully present as a professional while claiming your identity as someone who is, e.g., female, Black, Asian-American, Latinx, IMG, indigenous, LGBTQ, living with a disability, a first-generation physician during residency and your fellowship?
- How can people from backgrounds of privilege interrupt patterns/incidents of unprofessionalism that threaten well-being and patient safety? How can they support peers who are recipients of microaggressions, racism, bullying, or other acts of unprofessionalism?

Case 2: Selina (She/Her)

Identification Phase

Selina is a PGY-2 pathology resident [56]. *She shows up for work at 6 AM and leaves after 6 PM. Her peers say she spends her evenings studying pathology, and she comes in on weekends to review unknowns and work on projects. She has limited social interactions and no known outside interests. Within the last month, laboratory personnel have commented that she has become more indifferent in her work and in her relationships with them. Faculty comments suggest she is "cutting corners" during gross specimens and not taking the required sections. A patient's complaint about Selina's lack of respectful communication was lodged during her last transfusion medicine rotation.*

Table 13.6 Selina's differing assumptions by professional identity formation level

Version A: Externally defined PIF	Version B: Internally defined PIF
I'm worried that peers will never accept me as one of them—I think they even look down on me. I'm ashamed to even tell my parents that I've been isolating myself because of this. They want the best for me.	I can't afford to do a lot of activities with my peers right now, and I'm OK with that. But I think it makes me kind of an outsider to them.
Some patients just don't care about their health and think I'm being rude when I'm trying hard to get them to take their health seriously.	Some patients will always see me as "not a real physician," but I've learned to not take it personally.
When Dr. H asked me about the specimens for Patient X, I thought he was trying to get me in trouble. I'm terrified to do work for him now.	When Dr. H asked if I had taken enough sections of the specimen for Patient X, I realized I had made a mistake, and I will be more careful in the future.

Clarification Phase

In facilitating Selina's remediation process, the professional identity coach should first assess her current state of health and wellness considering the possibility that she may be in a state of burnout, experiencing clinical level of anxiety or depression, or utilizing unhealthy coping mechanisms. Referring to a primary care physician or a mental health professional should be considered as an additional step in ensuring the trainee's safety and ruling out conditions requiring urgent medically guided treatment. In parallel, reflective writing assignments, such as the PIE, may help to uncover Selina's current adaptive PIF challenges by revealing assumptions and beliefs that are related to the lapse. The overarching goal of coaching is to facilitate self-directed growth towards an internally defined PIF along with the capacity to develop strategies to prevent future lapses (Table 13.6).

If Selina's responses are more like Version A, an externally defined PIF in Table 13.6, then she appears to struggle with the two developmental challenges: separating the self from important others and managing emotions resulting from balancing learning with her need for autonomy as she moves from an external to an internally defined professional identity. These challenges can be explored in either written reflection or through discussion to encourage her to aspire to a more internally defined PIF.

Intervention Phase

To facilitate the shift from an externally defined to an internally defined professional identity, the coach can first create the space and psychological safety for Selina to examine those emotions and thoughts and to recognize patterns leading to states of mind that precede lapses in professionalism (e.g., discomfort or anger with peers resulting in self-isolation). Subsequent options include assigning readings or self-assessments that introduce concepts related to PIF growth, or reflective writing prompts to explore emotions and thoughts related to the lapse [48]. Additionally, the SMART Goals framework can also be useful; however, it is important to be cognizant of the fact that remediation of professionalism lapses is not a "quick fix" but comprises an ongoing need to balance providing additional support and setting appropriate challenges [57].

Last, coaching for remediation of PIF can benefit from tools such as the Immunity to Change process [54].

Assessment for Coaching Effectiveness

There is little research to guide professionalism remediation coaching. One key outcome is to prevent future professionalism lapses; another is to promote the learner to develop a mature internalized professional identity, where they are capable of complex reasoning and actions consistent with good intentions. Scholarship from other fields supports the importance of attention to the psychosocial capacities that enable consistent moral sensitivity, judgment and reasoning, implementation, and motivation, as well as the centrality of wellness or well-being to consistent professional behavior. We encourage collecting and sharing best practices and narrative outcomes from individual remediation coaching cases to build on any one coach's experiences, thereby contributing to the overall community of practice. We also urge health professions schools to make explicit that remediation interventions are aimed at both changing behaviors to meet the expected standards set by the profession and preserving or even enhancing the trainee's holistic well-being. We acknowledge that with some egregious lapses or in cases of persistent inability to reach a minimum level of competency, remediation coaching might conclude with dismissal from training. More often, however, a learner may choose to leave health professions training, accepting that they are on the wrong path and need to pursue another. While difficult in the short run, this is likely a best outcome for all involved.

Summary and Conclusions

We agree with Shulman [58] that professional education will always need to address the formation of professional identity "with a moral core of service and responsibility around which the hab-its of mind and practice should be organized." As educators, we do not fulfill our responsibility if we assume that trainees will always intuit professional values and expectations from the general socialization process. Instead, early in professional education, we must assess capacities that are known to be necessary conditions for behavior, and then engage trainees in self-assessment and reflection regarding attainment of these capacities. Just as curricula provide for the development of technical knowledge and its application to clinical care, we advocate assessment, instruction, reflection, and further assessment of PIF for all students, not just those who "hit the radar" when they lapse. In the end, of course, each trainee is responsible for their own learning and is expected to maintain competence throughout a lifetime of professional practice. Coaching for PIF centers on the learner's goals and understanding, leading to reliable consistency between their intentions and actions. Coaches must consider that developmental growth is not linear. While ideally all learners will grow toward a fully self-defined professional identity, expectations should be realistic. Developmental growth can best occur when learners are sufficiently supported to identify a specific goal related to the lapse in professionalism, and to formulate a sufficiently challenging plan of action. Steinberg describes this as reframing professionalism "as a verb," describing the role of coaching as follows:

"…We nurture, mature, grow, and transform by multimodal communication in every venue in which we do communicate, and by professionalism—not only as rigid laws and commandments, but professionalism as a verb: the hidden acculturation, socialization, and action-ethics that are yet ill-defined and underacknowledged by our profession and that must be synonymous with trust and security" [55].

References

1. Bebeau MJ. Promoting ethical development and professionalism: insights from educational research in the professions. Univ St Thomas Law J. 2008;5(366):386.

2. Mak-van der Vossen M, van Mook W, van der Burgt S, Kors J, Ket JCF, Croiset G, Kusurkar RA. Descriptors for unprofessional behaviors of medical students: a systematic review and categorization. BMC Med Educ. 2017;17:164.

3. Mak-van der Vossen M, de la Croix A, Teherani A, van Mook W, Croiset G, Kusurkar RA. A road map for attending to medical students' professionalism lapses. Acad Med. 2019;94:570–8.

4. Mak-van der Vossen M, Teherani A, van Mook W, Croiset G, Kusurkar RA. How to identify, address and report students' unprofessional behavior in medical school. Med Teach. 2019;42:372–9.

5. Bebeau MJ, Faber-Langendoen K. Remediating lapses in professionalism. In: Kalet A, Chou CL, editors. Remediation in medical education. New York: Springer; 2014. p. 103–27.

6. Kalet A, Chou CL, Ellaway RH. To fail is human: remediating remediation in medical education. Perspect Med Educ. 2017;6:418–24.

7. Kegan R. The evolving self. Cambridge, MA: Harvard University Press; 1982.

8. Lewin LO, McManamon A, Stein MTO, Chen D. Minding the form that transforms: using Kegan's model of adult development to understand personal and professional identity formation. Acad Med. 2019;2019(94):1299–304.

9. Vipler B, McCall-Hosenfeld J, Haidet P. Remediation through transformation: applying educational theory to the struggling resident. J Gen Intern Med. 2019;35:3656–63.

10. ten Cate O, Snell L, Carraccio C. Medical competence: the interplay between individual ability and the health care environment. Med Teach. 2010;32:669–75.

11. Chou CL, Kalet A, Costa MJ, Cleland J, Winston K. The dos, don'ts, and don't knows of remediation in medical education. Perspect Med Educ. 2019;8:322–38.

12. Antiel RM, Kinghorn WA, Reed DA, Hafferty FW. Professionalism: etiquette or habitus? Mayo Clin Proc. 2013;88:651–2.

13. Papadakis MA, Teherani A, Banach MA, Knettler TR, Rattner SL, Stern DT, Veloski JJ, Hodgson CS. Disciplinary action by medical boards and prior behavior in medical school. N Engl J Med. 2005;353:2673–82.

14. Ziring D, Frankel RM, Danoff D, Isaacson JH, Lochnan H. Silent witnesses: faculty reluctance to report medical students' professionalism lapses. Acad Med. 2018;93:1700–6.

15. Wald HS. Optimizing resilience and wellbeing for healthcare professions trainees and healthcare professionals during public health crises: practical tips for an 'integrative resilience' approach. Med Teach. 2020;42:744–55.

16. Lee JH. The weaponization of medical professionalism. Acad Med. 2017;92:579–80.

17. Fargen KM, Drolet BC, Philibert I. Unprofessional behaviors among tomorrow's physicians: review of the literature with a focus on risk factors, temporal trends, and future directions. Acad Med. 2016;91:858–64.

18. Kusnoor AV, Falik R. Cheating in medical school: the unacknowledged ailment. South Med J. 2013;106:479–83.

19. Zaveri M, Phillipps D. Backlash over leniency at west point after 73 cadets are accused of cheating. New York Times https://www.nytimes.com/2020/12/23/nyregion/west-point-cheating-scandal.html. Accessed 22 Dec 2022.

20. United States Military Academy. Character program (gold book). New York: West Point; 2015.

21. Singer N, Krolik A. Online cheating charges upend Dartmouth medical school. The New York Times https://www.nytimes.com/2021/05/09/technology/dartmouth-geisel-medical-cheating.html. Accessed 22 Dec 2022.

22. Singer N. Dartmouth medical school drops online cheating cases against students. The New York Times. https://www.nytimes.com/2021/06/10/technology/dartmouth-cheating-charges.html. Accessed 22 Dec 2022.

23. Thaxton RE, Jones WS, Hafferty FW, April CW, April MD. Self vs. other focus: predicting professionalism remediation of emergency medicine residents. West J Emerg Med. 2018;19:35–40.

24. Williams BW, Welindt D, Hafferty FW, Stumps A, Flanders P, Williams MV. Adverse childhood experiences in trainees and physicians with professionalism lapses: implications for medical education and remediation. Acad Med. 2021;96:736–43.

25. Substance Abuse and Mental Health Services Administration. SAMHSA's concept of trauma and guidance for a trauma-informed approach. HHS Publication No. (SMA) 14–4884. Rockville, MD: Substance Abuse and Mental Health Services Administration; 2014. https://ncsacw.acf.hhs.gov/userfiles/files/SAMHSA_Trauma.pdf. Accessed 22 Dec 2022.

26. Rougas S, Gentilesco B, Green E, Flores L. Twelve tips for addressing medical student and resident physician lapses in professionalism. Med Teach. 2015;37:901–7.

27. Konopasek L, Norcini J, Krupat E. Focusing on the formative: building an assessment system aimed at student growth and development. Acad Med. 2016;2016(91):1492–7.

28. Bebeau MJ. Enhancing professionalism using ethics education as part of a dental licensure board's disciplinary action. Part 1. An evidence-based process. J Am Coll Dent. 2009;76:38–50.

29. Bebeau MJ. Enhancing professionalism using ethics education as part of a dental licensure board's disciplinary action. Part 2. Evidence of the process. J Am Coll Dent. 2009;76:32–45.

30. Ainsworth MA, Szauter KM. Student response to reports of unprofessional behavior: assessing risk of subsequent professional problems in medical school. Med Educ Online. 2018;23:1485432.

31. Rest JR, Narvaez D, Bebeau MJ, Thoma SJ. Post conventional moral thinking: a neo-Kohlbergian approach. Mahwah, NJ: Erlbaum; 1999. p. 229.
32. Bebeau MJ. The defining issues test and the four component model: contributions to professional education. J Moral Educ. 2002;31:271–95.
33. Kalet A, Buckvar-Keltz L, Harnik V, Monson V, Hubbard S, Crowe R, Song HS, Yingling S. Measuring professional identity formation early in medical school. Med Teach. 2017;39:255–61.
34. Baldwin DC Jr, Adamson TE, Self DJ, Sheehan TJ, Oppenberg AA. Moral reasoning and malpractice. A pilot study of orthopedic surgeons. Am J Orthop (Belle Mead NJ). 1996;25:481–4.
35. Gutmann A, Thompson D. Democracy and disagreement. Cambridge, MA: Belknap Press of Harvard University Press; 1996. p. 422.
36. Kegan R. The evolving self: problem and process in human development. Cambridge, MA: Harvard University Press; 1982. p. 318.
37. Welie JV. Is dentistry a profession? Part 3. Future challenges. J Can Dent Assoc. 2004;70:675–8.
38. Bebeau MJ. Professional responsibility curriculum report. American college fellows serve as expert assessors. Teaching ethics at the University of Minnesota. J Am Coll Dent. 1983;50:20–3.
39. Rule JT, Bebeau MJ. Dentists who care: inspiring stories of professional commitment. Chicago, IL: Quintessence Publishing Co.; 2005. p. 176.
40. Blasi A. Moral identity: its role in moral functioning. In: Kurtines WM, Gewirtz JL, editors. Morality, moral behavior, and moral development. New York: Wiley; 1984. p. 129–39.
41. Monson VE. Professional Identity Essay (PIE) assessment: a practical guide for educators in the professions. 2020.
42. Bebeau MJ, Monson VE. Professional identity formation and transformation across the life span. In: McKee A, Eraut M, editors. Professional learning over the life span: innovation and change. New York: Springer; 2012. p. 2012.
43. Kalet A, Ark TK, Monson V, Song HS, Buckvar-Keltz L, Harnik V, Yingling S, Rivera R Jr, Tewksbury L, Lusk P, Crowe R. Does a measure of medical professional identity formation predict communication skills performance? Patient Educ Couns. 2021;104:3045–52.
44. Yingling S, Park YS, Curry RH, Monson V, Girotti J. Beyond cognitive measures: empirical evidence supporting holistic medical school admissions practices and professional identity formation. MedEdPublish. 2018;7:274.
45. Sawatsky AP, Huffman B, Hafferty F. Coaching versus competency to facilitate professional identity formation. Acad Med. 2020;95:1511–4.
46. Wolff M, Hammoud M, Santen S, Delorio N, Fix M. Coaching in undergraduate medical education: a national survey. Med Educ Online. 2020;25(1):1699765.
47. Accreditation Council of Graduate Medical Education (ACGME). Internal Medicine Milestones, Internal Medicine, ACGME Report Worksheet. p. 21. https://www.acgme.org/globalassets/pdfs/milestones/internalmedicinemilestones.pdf. Accessed 22 Dec 2022.
48. Wald HS. Professional identity (trans)formation in medical education: reflection, relationship, resilience. Acad Med. 2015;90:701–6.
49. Schwenk TL, Davis L, Wimsatt LA. Depression, stigma, and suicidal ideation in medical students. JAMA. 2010;2010(304):1181–90.
50. David SA, Clutterbuck DA, Megginson D, editors. Beyond goals: effective strategies in coaching and mentoring. New York: Routledge; 2013.
51. Chickering AW, Reisser L. Education and identity. 2nd ed. San Francisco, CA: Jossey-Bass; 1993. p. 49.
52. Hardemann R, Perry S, Phelan SM, Przedworski JM, Burgess DJ, van Ryn M. Racial identity and mental Well-being: the experience of African American medical students. J Racial Ethn Health Disparities. 2016;2016(3):250–8.
53. Pascarella ET, Terenzini PT. Theories and models of student change in college. In how college affects students, volume 2, a third decade of research. San Francisco: Jossey-Bass; 2005.
54. Kegan R, Lahey L. Immunity to change: how to overcome it and unlock the potential in yourself and your organization. Cambridge, MA: Harvard Business Press; 2009.
55. Steinberg JJ. Residency as identity transformation: the life stages of the homo medicalis. J Grad Med Educ. 2010;2:646–8.
56. Conran RM, Powell SZ-E, Domen RE, McCloskey CB, et al. Development of professionalism in graduate medical education: a case-based educational approach from the College of American Pathologists' graduate medical education committee. Acad Pathol. 2018;2018(5):2374289518773493.
57. Kegan R, Congleton C, David SA. The goals behind the goals: pursuing adult development in the coaching enterprise. In: David SA, Clutterbuck DA, Megginson D, editors. Beyond goals: effective strategies in coaching and mentoring. New York: Routledge; 2013. p. 229–42.
58. Shulman L. Foreword. In: Cooke M, Irby DM, O'Brien BC, editors. Educating physicians: a call for reform of medical school and residency. San Francisco, CA: Jossey-Bass; 2010. p. 3–4.

Nuts and Bolts of Professionalism Remediation

14

Marianne Mak-van der Vossen, Sjoukje van den Broek, Walther van Mook, and Marian Wolters

Introduction

Professionalism is the basis for society's trust in healthcare professionals. In medicine, malpractice claims and healthcare complaints are often based on physicians' unprofessional behavior [1, 2]. Papadakis found that unprofessional behavior during medical training is predictive of unprofessional behavior as a physician, making it clear that having a permissive approach toward unprofessionalism during the early phases of medical education is not defensible [3].

M. Mak-van der Vossen (✉)
Department of General Practice, Amsterdam UMC,
University of Amsterdam,
Amsterdam, The Netherlands
e-mail: m.mak@amsterdamumc.nl

S. van den Broek
Education Center, Department of Clinical Skills
Training, University Medical Center,
Utrecht, The Netherlands
e-mail: w.e.s.vandenbroek@umcutrecht.nl

W. van Mook
Department of Intensive Care Medicine, Academy for
Postgraduate Training and School of Health
Professions Education, Maastricht University and
Maastricht University Medical Center,
Maastricht, The Netherlands
e-mail: w.van.mook@mumc.nl

M. Wolters
Center for Research and Development of Health
Professions Education, University Medical Center,
Utrecht, The Netherlands
e-mail: m.s.wolters@umcutrecht.nl

Professionalism should ultimately result in an optimal combination of individual performance (based on knowledge, skills, and reflective ability), self-care, collaboration with other health professionals, and provision of quality patient care. As clinical trainees progress in their educational careers, they will predictably encounter moments of conflicting interests in these dimensions. In learning how to handle such conflicts, they will sometimes fail. Evidence suggests that somewhere between 3 and 20% of all medical students show unprofessional behavior at some point in their training [4–11]. This wide range of percentages may be attributed to the differences in the definition of unprofessional behavior and methods of reporting and assessment.

In the experience of many educators, remediating professionalism is more complicated than remediating knowledge and skills. US internal medicine residency program directors report that remediation is most successful for medical knowledge (85.8%) and least successful for professionalism (41.2%) [12]. Although we agree that remediation trajectories can be complex, we assert that failings in professional behavior also provide learning opportunities. We believe that providing students support and opportunities to reflect on their struggles early in their training may enable sustained professional behavior through their entire career.

How to Teach Professionalism?

We recommend that schools formally teach theoretical content about professionalism at the onset of the undergraduate curriculum. Providing trainees with necessary knowledge about the history and nature of professionalism will set expectations and give clear rationale for these behaviors [13–16]. Additionally, students must formally learn and practice necessary skills associated with professionalism, such as communication and reflection.

Box 14.1: Knowledge Aspects of Professionalism

History [17]
  Virtues
  Professional behavior
  Professional identity
Definitions [18, 19]
Attributes [13, 20, 21]
  Interpersonal skills
  Understanding of roles
  Capacity for teamwork
  Cultural humility
  Collegiality
  Respect for patients and colleagues
  Ethical conduct
  Social contract [22]
  Rights and obligations of the profession
  Independence and self-regulation of the profession

As learners progress into graduate and postgraduate training, professionalism teaching and learning becomes largely informal and often *implicit* [13, 23, 24]. In fact, most of the teaching and learning of professionalism takes place through this 'hidden curriculum' [25], in which implicit beliefs, attitudes, and behaviors of educators and other role models, positive or negative, influence trainees' professional development.

These influences are frequently inconsistent with the formal curriculum. To enable trainees to grapple with the numerous nuances throughout their training, programs must provide formal opportunities to reflect on, explore, and unveil the hidden curriculum as a component of professionalism education [25].

How to Assess Professionalism?

In many educational settings, measuring professionalism takes place through scheduled evaluations [26]. Formative assessments of trainee performance drive individual learning, while only summative assessments are included in the final grade. Scheduled formative and summative evaluations can take place in both preclinical and clinical settings. Many institutions use locally developed versions of In-Training Evaluation Reports (ITERs) that describe directly observed behaviors in clinical or teaching settings, Objective Structured Clinical Examinations (OSCE's), and moral reasoning assessments [27]. In addition to regularly scheduled assessments, critical incident reports are a necessary part of documenting unprofessional behavior, particularly for egregious and unlawful behaviors, such as sexual harassment, intimidation, plagiarism, or falsifying official records [27]. Emerging issues, such as the possibility that trainees may post protected patient information on social media, must be addressed directly as a matter of curriculum [28].

In professionalism evaluations, trainees receive a subjective judgment from their teachers and supervisors. Subjectivity is most helpful when it is part of a programmatic assessment procedure [29]. Scheduled and incidental measurements of professionalism (Fig. 14.1) are ideally integrated in a program of assessments in which trainees' professionalism is evaluated early and frequently, using a variety of methods, in various settings, and ideally by a myriad of experienced and well-trained assessors [30, 31].

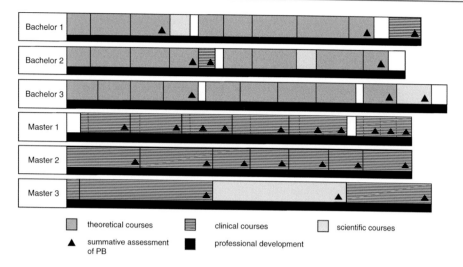

Fig. 14.1 Example of a scheme of training and assessment of professional behavior (PB) from the undergraduate medical curriculum of the Faculty of Medicine VU Amsterdam. This school has the typical European structure of a 3-year bachelor's, followed by a 3-year master's program. Theoretical courses are primarily aimed at knowledge acquisition, scientific courses are aimed at experiencing research practices, and clinical courses are aimed at gaining practical experience [32]

Box 14.2: Example of a Scheduled Summative Professional Behavior Assessment

At the undergraduate medical education program in Utrecht, all students receive scheduled assessments for professional behavior from frontline teachers at least twice during their rotations. The assessment form has eight items:

1. Decency and respect
2. Communication with patients
3. Managing emotions of patients
4. Collaboration with colleagues
5. Managing own emotions, values, and norms
6. Self-assessment, reflection, and handling feedback
7. Commitment
8. Responsibility, integrity, reliability, and knowing one's own boundaries

Students are rated on a scale from 4 to 10 (this is a regularly used scale in The Netherlands: 4–5 below expectation; 6–8 expected level; 9–10 above expectation) and there is a blank space to add open comments (strengths and aspects of improvement).

The assessment forms are reviewed at the administration office, and the Professionalism Remediation Supervisor (see below) is informed in following cases:

A score of 5 on any one item, or more than one score of 6, triggers an overall assessment of 'needs attention'. A school-wide Examination Committee (see Box 14.3) refers the student for professionalism coaching, while the student continues in their courses.

If a student receives a score of 4, or a score of 5 on any 2 items, this triggers an overall "unsatisfactory" assessment. The student is obliged to engage in professionalism coaching and not allowed to start rotations again until the Examination Committee has approved. Approval is based on the student's progress during coaching. Progress is assumed if the student demonstrates adequate self-awareness and can critically reflect on their functioning.

Assessment of professionalism is very challenging for educators. Educators and clinicians often *'fail to fail'* trainees even after they have directly observed unprofessional behavior [33, 34]. As a result, unprofessionalism goes undocumented, and the opportunity to identify and address the stagnation of a trainee's professional identity formation is lost [35, 36]. Educators would benefit from a better understanding about how to identify trainees who behave unprofessionally, how to help these trainees improve their behavior, and what steps to take if a trainee persists in displaying unprofessional behavior [33]. Failing a trainee would then become an opportunity to help them in the goal of optimally serving future patients and healthcare colleagues. We therefore assert that assessing performance and providing feedback on professionalism is the responsibility of all educators.

Four Phases of Professionalism Remediation

Below, we describe practical guidelines for identifying, evaluating, and intervening in medical trainees' unprofessional behaviors. We describe four phases of professionalism remediation (Fig. 14.2) that are congruent with the structure presented in Chap. 6 [37]. While *all* educators have a role to 'intervene' when they observe unprofessionalism, we use the term 'remediate' to describe specific teaching activities conducted with individual students alongside the regular curriculum by designated professionalism educators.

We list *do's and don'ts* for each phase and recommendations for educators' roles and activities when a trainee shows no improvement. Although the nature and consequences of professionalism issues may differ, the process of identifying,

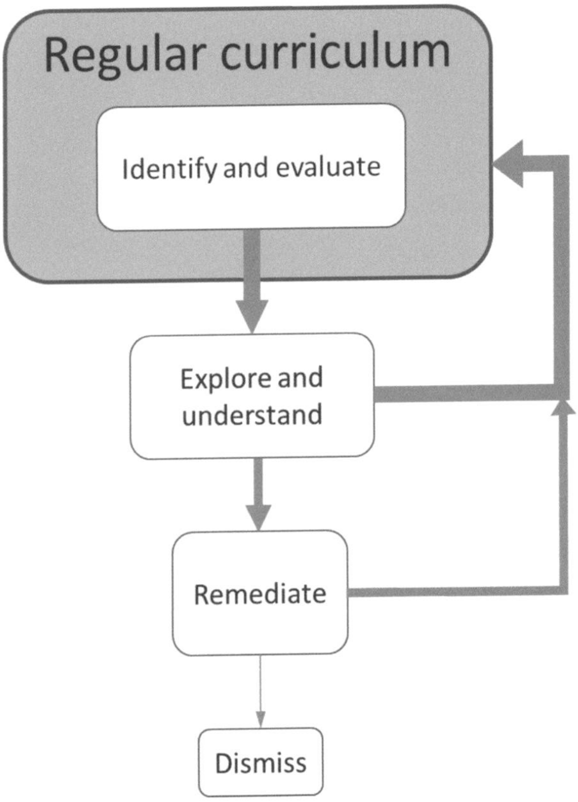

Fig. 14.2 Phases of professionalism remediation and their relation to the regular curriculum. Teachers in the regular curriculum identify and evaluate students showing unprofessionalism. They often start clarifying underlying causes, and if necessary refer their students to the next phase for further exploration. The thickness of the arrows represents the relative number of students. While most students can return to and proceed in the regular curriculum, some of them will need professionalism remediation support first. A small number of students will eventually be dismissed

exploring, and remediating is essentially comparable across undergraduate and postgraduate trainees and practicing professionals [38, 39]. We describe professionalism remediation strategies based on findings from both our research and our experiences in The Netherlands, with examples from our own institutions. While we try to provide a general and international perspective, local contexts and situations will differ, and cultural context will influence applicability of these guidelines.

Identify and Evaluate

Professionalism is generally not considered an innate trait, but a capacity to behave consistently and in alignment with expectations of the profession. Trainees in all health professions curricula should be taught these expectations as explicitly as possible [13, 14, 40, 41]. By teaching and evaluating trainees' professionalism, educators can identify trainees who need additional help to develop into clinicians who consistently demonstrate professional behavior.

4 I's Model of Unprofessional Behaviors

Unprofessional behaviors have been categorized in different ways [42–48]. Based on a systematic review of the literature of medical students' unprofessional behaviors as witnessed by educators or students, Mak-van der Vossen et al. proposed the 4 I's model of medical students' unprofessional behaviors (Fig. 14.3): lack of *Involvement*, a lack of *Integrity*, poor *Interaction*, and poor *Introspection* [49].

The 4 I's model provides a framework for frontline educators to identify, prioritize, discuss, and document concerns about unprofessional student behavior. The model, which originates from

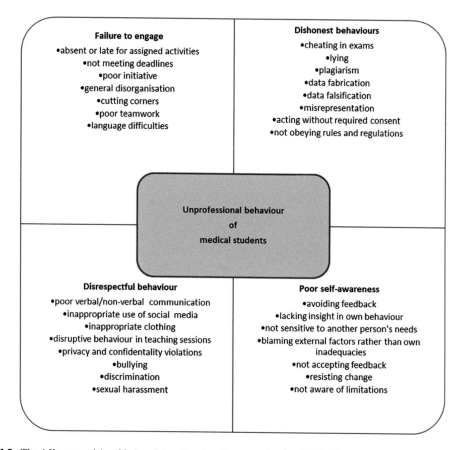

Fig. 14.3 The 4 I's, comprising 30 descriptors for signaling unprofessional behaviors among medical students [49]

undergraduate medical education, has been validated for graduate general practice specialist training [50]. The framework helps trainees and educators talk about unprofessionalism and explore how individual issues and the educational context may influence student behavior. We see frontline educators as members of the coaching trajectory team, who need to feel free to contact a designated professionalism educator if any questions around patient safety issues or other concerns should arise.

> *Andrea (she/her) is a resident in general practice. Her supervisor notices that she leaves at 5 PM sharp every day, sometimes leaving unfinished work behind for her colleagues. They discuss this during a routine formative evaluation. The supervisor and Andrea share their expectations of what it means to be a professional general practitioner. To the supervisor, this means that "you are always there for your patients." To Andrea, it is paramount that a practitioner attends to their own well-being and private life. Both agree that their goal is to serve patients best. They agree that to avoid misunderstandings and ensure that the patient's needs are attended to, Andrea will explicitly provide a written hand-off of patient care to her colleagues and inform her patients she is doing so. This improves the situation, and the summative evaluation is satisfactory.*

Roles and Responsibilities

In Dutch medical schools, frontline educators are responsible for teaching trainees how to behave professionally, identifying a trainee's unprofessional behavior, and including this in assessments. If needed, a Professionalism Remediation Supervisor (PRS) is often available for consultation. The PRS regularly chairs a small committee of educators, the Professionalism Progress Committee (PPC), to monitor trainees' remediation and progress.

Box 14.3: Terminology for Role Descriptions Used in This Chapter

- **Frontline teacher/frontline educator/ frontline supervisor:** teacher in standard course, clerkship, or regular part of postgraduate education
- **Professionalism Remediation Supervisor (PRS):** faculty member with a dedicated central role in remediation. In institutions with a formal remediation program, the PRS oversees the process of remediation, knows all trainees who are referred for remediation, and makes ultimate decisions. In some institutions, the Dean of Student Affairs is the PRS.
- **Professionalism Progress Committee (PPC):** a group of educators, often directed by the PRS, that supervises trainees' professional development by synthesizing and aggregating assessment data from frontline teachers in various contexts over time (51).
- **Remediation coach:** dedicated faculty member who is trained in the coaching of students during the process of remediation of unprofessional behaviors and who is involved in the remediation trajectories of individual students.
- **Examination Committee (EC):** A school-wide body that is responsible for the quality and validity of the examinations. The EC objectively and expertly determines whether a student meets the conditions laid down by education and examination regulations with regard to knowledge, insight, and skills necessary for obtaining a degree.

Do's and Don'ts for Frontline Educators in the Identify and Evaluate Phase

Do:

- Start a conversation about professionalism soon after observing any of the 4 I's.
- Provide feedback to the trainee within a for-

mative assessment to foster learning.

- Ask for help from the PRS if you doubt the trainee's reflectivity and/or ability to grow.
- Give the trainee an unsatisfactory grade if the performance does not improve despite your feedback.

Don't:

- Blame the trainee as an individual. Blame-free handling of underperformance means discussing both personal and institutional causes and supporting better adjustment to circumstances.
- Give a marginal grade out of convenience or a sense of mercy. This neither addresses the behavior nor ensures better behavior in the future.

After an unsatisfactory summative assessment, the trainee is generally referred to the PRS and their advisors, which marks the transition to the *Explore and Understand* phase [51].

Explore and Understand

This phase involves one or more conversations with the trainee in which the educator (or PRS) explores and clarifies underlying causes for unprofessional behaviors. Educators can help increase a trainee's awareness of the gap between their intentions and displayed behaviors, inducing reflection on the observed behavior and ideally motivating professional growth [52]. This phase both serves the individual trainee and promotes a culture that accepts failure in professionalism, once addressed, as a learning opportunity for both trainee and supervisor, fostering a learning environment in which failures are seen as growth opportunities [52–55]. The process of exploring and discussing the unprofessional behavior in regularly scheduled meetings with the trainee may in and of itself constitute an "intervention" [56].

Exploration of Unprofessional Behavior: Ten Questions

Unprofessional behavior can be attributed to personal circumstances, factors in the educational context, and cultural differences. A trainee's ultimate behavior is also influenced by the trainee's intentions and beliefs about the behavior and its outcomes, social norms, and perceived control [57]. Based on the literature and our experience, we propose ten questions which can help frontline teachers and/or PRS's understand what happened and why (Table 14.1). The order of these questions is flexible.

Four Patterns of Unprofessional Behavior

Based on observations and interactions (including the answers to the ten questions) with the trainee, and depending on the levels of reflectiveness and adaptability of the trainee, it might be useful for frontline teachers and/or PRS's to distinguish from among four different patterns of unprofessional behavior (Fig. 14.4) that suggest different remediation approaches [58].

Our experience is that most trainees who demonstrate accidental unprofessional behavior are aware of their lapse and experience feelings of shame and guilt [59]. While guilt helps the trainee identify and focus on the behavior, shame is a generalized bad feeling about who they are as a person and is more likely to have enduring negative consequences for the trainee. Such feelings may stand in the way of an effective coaching trajectory. Bynum and colleagues defined three ways in which teachers, supervisors, and remediation coaches may lead trainees to a 'shame-free' response to unprofessional behavior: by acknowledging the presence of shame and guilt in the learner, by avoiding humiliation, and by leveraging effective feedback [59].

During the coaching trajectories, remediation coaches and other supervisors may worry that

Table 14.1 Ten questions to explore a trainee's unprofessional behavior in a conversation [58]

	To be explored	Question	Examples of what educators are listening for in the trainee's answers
1.	Trainee's perspective about the facts	What happened?	• Are there any differences between the assessor's feedback and the trainee's narrative? • Does the trainee differentiate between facts and their opinion about the situation?
2.	Intentions	What did you intend to do?	• Behaviors could be well-intended yet be seen as unprofessional. What was the trainee's intention?
3.	Beliefs	What did you expect to happen?	• Does the trainee show insight into the consequences of the behavior?
4.	Context	What circumstances influenced your behavior?	• Are there any explanatory or modifiable circumstances, such as time pressure, poor relationships with peers or supervisors, personal tasks outside the learning environment, problems with health and well-being of the trainee or the trainee's relatives?
5.	Power	Were you able to influence the circumstances?	• Was the behavior complicated by power differences? • Did the trainee try to act differently?
6.	Effect on others	How do you think your behavior affected others?	• Is the trainee willing and able to reflect on consequences for peers, supervisors, patients?
7.	Emotions	How do you feel about the situation now?	• Does the trainee express feelings of shame, guilt, anger, or fear of consequences?
8.	Causes	Compared with your peers, are there any circumstances that make it more difficult for you to comply with the professionalism expectations?	• Does the trainee understand their own strengths and weaknesses?
9.	Plans	How will you act in a similar situation next time?	• What are trainee's plans and learning goals for subsequent similar challenges? • What does the trainee need to learn or rehearse? • Does the trainee see difficulties in learning alternative behavior?
10.	Alignment with teacher's perspective	Do you agree that what you did could be seen as unprofessional behavior?	• Does the trainee agree or disagree with the assessor's view? • Is the trainee willing and able to take the perspective of others/the assessor?

trainees are 'saying the things they want to hear' or displaying desirable behaviors without having internalized the underlying professionalism values. Clinical teachers need to become skillful in eliciting the trainee's values. Doing so helps distinguish between the awkwardness of a novice practicing a new behavior as their own professional identity matures and one who is simply trying to 'game the system', accelerating their progress through the coaching trajectory without sincerity [58]. It is therefore essential for a trainee to practice and demonstrate their intended revised behaviors in authentic (clinical) settings with the attendant complexities, where it will be more obvious if a trainee is struggling or simply 'faking' the new behavior.

Sometimes trainees lack awareness of the impact of their behavior or frankly disagree that their behavior is unprofessional, thus showing the pattern of *disavowing behavior* (see Table 14.2). These trainees will move to the *Remediate* phase.

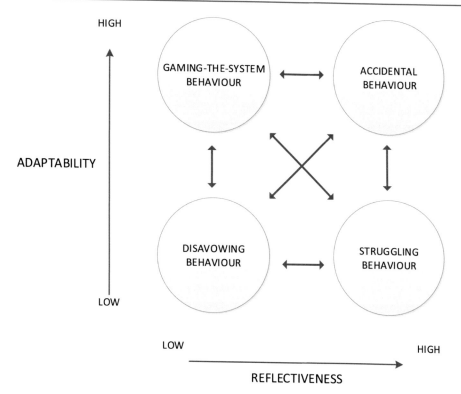

Fig. 14.4 Four patterns of unprofessional behavior. Reflectiveness is the ability and willingness to identify one's own strengths and relative weaknesses in detail. Adaptability is the ability and willingness to adjust to different conditions or circumstances. Each of the four behavioral patterns warrants a different remediation approach [58]

Table 14.2 Four behavioral patterns in professionalism remediation

	Description	Remediation	Goal
Accidental unprofessional behavior	Trainee seems to understand what happened and why it happened. Trainee can prevent future professionalism lapses with help from frontline teachers in the regular curriculum	Create awareness, offer help to deal with dilemmas	Learning from lapses
Struggling behavior	Trainee understands what went wrong and why but is not able to adapt to the professionalism expectations, often due to external constraints (for instance, personal problems)	Offer practical support to address deficiencies in competence and/or reflectiveness	Influencing causal factors
Gaming-the-system behavior	Trainee does not seem to reflect on professional values yet strategically follows the instructions, aiming to pass the exams or remain undetected by others	Show relevance of professionalism	Internalizing professional values (a more mature stage of medical professional identity—see Chap. 14)
Disavowing behavior	Trainee does not acknowledge their repetitive unprofessional behavior and/or blames others, despite remedial work	All of the above	Improving introspection

Roles and Responsibilities

Frontline teachers and the PRS work together in this phase to create a valid and reliable picture of a trainee's behavioral pattern over time. Allowing educators access to past assessments or providing them with education handovers is valuable in ensuring safety for patients and trainees [60, 61].

Do's and Don'ts for Teachers and Professionalism Remediation Supervisors in the Explore and Understand Phase

Do:

- Keep lines of communication open between the PRS and frontline teachers.
- Make organizational or contextual causes of professionalism lapses transparent to the institution.
- Recognize, appreciate, and follow up with frontline educators who have referred a trainee for remediation.

Don't:

- Underestimate gaming-the-system behavior.

If a trainee shows inadequate progress or a need for more support, the Professionalism Progress Committee can decide to refer the trainee for expert remediation, which initiates the *Remediate* phase.

Remediate

While most trainees with accidental unprofessional behavior will gain insight with support for change by frontline educators or the PRS, anyone with persistent, repetitive, or serious professionalism lapses will require help from dedicated *remediation coaches*.

Remediation coaches should be consulted early and made available to frontline teachers in the workplace for informal, confidential advice on how to approach a trainee. We recommend a structured and formal referral process, transparently shared with the trainee, where the PRS provides the remediation coach with information such as the name of the trainee, stage of training, description of the unprofessional behavior, and steps already taken. The remediation coach can then gather additional relevant subjective information, such as the trainee's emotional reactions during the process and their reactions to feedback, and feelings triggered in the supervisors or colleagues by the trainee's behaviors. At some point in the process, remediation coaches should also have access to the trainee's academic history and prior assessments to gain a complete and longitudinal overview of the trainee's situation.

Ideally, being identified for remediation would be a transformative experience for the trainee. If a coach can harness the trainee's self-awareness and the trainee engages in the remediation process with enthusiasm, the work can produce durable changes in understanding and behavior. Under these circumstances, we assert that punitive actions are counterproductive because they limit the trainee's emotional engagement with the process and attitude toward failures in the future. We view the professionalism remediation process as primarily educational and therefore best accomplished through supportive, optimistic, and growth-promoting strategies. However, unprofessional behaviors have consequences. Illegal acts should be referred to the proper authorities for adjudication. In relatively rare instances, for example, egregious cheating on high-stakes assessments, falsification of data, or harassment or threatening of others, a single episode may be an indication for serious institution-level academic consequences such as probation and dismissal (see Chaps. 20, 26, 29). Institutions should have and follow specific and transparent protocols for such punitive actions. This could be a reason to skip the Remediate phase and move directly to dismissal. However, most lapses in professionalism do not reach this threshold and can be addressed effectively through a pedagogically framed remediation process.

Remediation coaches should have freedom and creativity to refer trainees to others for help, for example, mental or physical health professionals, ethicists, drama coaches, communication experts, and courses on personal development. Specific resources should be easily available [62].

Ben (he/him) is a first-generation academic student from a minority background doing his first clerkship rotation. The supervising teacher notices that he stays in the back of the group during rounds and does not participate actively in group discussions. The supervisor identifies this behavior on the formative evaluation form and interprets it as a lack of engagement. The supervisor brings this issue up in discussion with Ben, who explains that he has always been shy and introverted. As a preclinical student, he worked diligently and never missed an exam. On this, his first clinical rotation, he enjoys speaking to and engaging with patients. He acknowledges that in this phase of his studies, he would learn more if he interacted more intensively with supervisors and peers. He asks for support to understand his introversion and improve his communication skills. The supervisor recognizes the student's struggling behavior, and to maximize the chances for success, refers him to the remediation coach. As a result of this voluntary professionalism remediation, where the coach and student engaged in a series of discussions guided by written reflections, selected readings, simulations that rehearsed engagement with supervisors and peers around case discussions and guidance around cultural norms, and social interactions outside of the learning setting, Ben thrived on subsequent clinical rotations.

Distinction Between Coaching and Assessment

When resources allow, the teams doing coaching and assessment should ideally be separate groups. For example, frontline teachers and supervisors in the workplace can initially assess and refer the trainee; a specific supervisor or another faculty member, such as a remediation coach, can support the trainee during remediation; and the PPC can assess ultimate remediation success. This structure provides a safe space for the trainee to express emotions with the remediation coach without being overly concerned about being assessed and judged. (See Chap. 2 for further information about the distinction between coaching and assessment.)

Elements of Coaching

The trajectory of professionalism coaching should be individualized. It will vary widely depending on the behavioral pattern of unprofessionalism, the institutional context, preferences of coaches, and the reflectiveness and adaptability of the trainee (Table 14.2).

The coach should ensure that the following elements are part of every coaching trajectory:

- Private, and if possible, confidential, conversations with the coach, which create a safe space for the trainee to speak freely, honestly, and vulnerably. When a student is obliged to undergo remediation by the Examination Committee, the coach reports regularly to the committee on whether the student is cooperating and making progress in their trajectory but does not include information on the content of conversations with the student. Assessment and feedback on professional behavior is done by frontline teachers during rotations.

- Clear explanations to the trainee of what will and will not be communicated to the medical school leadership about remediation progress [63].
- Regular reassessment and adaptation of goals, approach, frequency, and duration of the coaching.
- A requirement that the trainee routinely provides reflections in writing and through discussion on the progress of the coaching [64].
- When applicable, with the trainee's awareness, monitoring by the coach of feedback from others (supervisors, teachers, peers, other important persons in the trainees' environment) for evidence of progress.
- Plans for and rehearsals of how to best handle similar or related challenges in the future.
- Creation of space where the trainee will have productive failures in authentic situations and will receive feedback on what does and doesn't work for them. Support from the coach is critical to ensure adoption of effective strategies.
- A mutual understanding that the coaching trajectory will not be terminated until both the trainee and coach feel comfortable with the plan for new behavior, and the trainee has demonstrated the ability to be successful. This takes significant time.

Remediation Plan

Either the remediation coach or the PRS creates a *remediation plan* in collaboration with the trainee. They attend to the causal factors for unprofessional behaviors and to what extent they are of personal, contextual, or cultural origins [65]. Remediation might consist of measures to improve the trainees' knowledge of how professional values are important to health care, to foster reflectiveness, or support to overcome barriers that hinder growth. To determine the success of professionalism remediation, PRS's and remediation coaches should pay attention to the determinants of reflectiveness and adaptability [51].

The main goal of the remediation plan is to support the trainee in reaching shared learning objectives for professionalism. Several intervention options exist: individual coaching, relevant reading or reflective writing assignments ([66]; see Chap. 15), practice in simulated situations, or group remediation, e.g., including community work [67]. However, a recent literature review on the effectiveness of interventions to remediate professionalism lapses in medical trainees and doctors revealed a paucity of evidence to guide best practices [68]. We believe that a successful remediation plan is tailored to the underlying cause of the unprofessional behavior and results in growth of the trainee's reflective capacities, engagement in remediation activities, responsiveness to feedback, and ultimately, consistent exemplary professional behavior.

Although many trainees and educators may believe that *feeding forward* (educational handovers) will negatively bias future evaluations, we disagree and stress that feeding forward, done with respect for the learner's privacy, helps develop a remediation plan and is a necessary step in the process. See Chap. 2 for more information on this topic.

Documentation

Once a trainee has started remediation, the PRS or remediation coach monitors the trainee's progress. Careful documentation is necessary (see Chaps. 20, 26, 29), particularly because the training timeline may be extended, and because dismissal is a possible outcome of remediation [69].

The trainee's dossier should contain well-documented information on:

- The trainee's assessments over time and reflection assignments
- Information on procedures, including all the remediation steps, who made the relevant decisions, and when and by whom the trainee was informed about these decisions.

Roles and Responsibilities

The role of remediation coaches is to motivate and guide the trainee's change process. This includes spending more time with frontline educators who may provide assignments and give feedback.

Do's and Don'ts in the Remediate Phase

Do's

- Facilitate and encourage referrals from frontline educators to remediation coaches.
- Provide space for the trainee to practice their new intended behavior.
- Inform frontline teachers about a trainee's professionalism learning goals.
- Assemble a team of experts who can consult as necessary, and form a community of faculty involved in professionalism remediation to share experiences and support each other.

Don't

- Take a punitive approach unless necessary

Not every trainee develops a mature professional identity. If individual remediation does not lead to improvement in a reasonable amount of time and with a practical amount of effort, then the next phase should commence.

Gather Evidence for Dismissal

In this phase, the main goal shifts from helping the trainee enter the profession to guiding them out of it [51]. In the United States, where dismissal from medical school often leaves a trainee with significant debt and without credentials or obvious alternatives, there is an emerging recognition of the need for compassionate off-ramps from medical education [70, 71]. In the Netherlands, dismissing a trainee from medical school is only possible after carefully adhering to very strict legal procedures, and in cases where patients are at risk [72]. In all contexts, moving to this phase warrants the gathering of sound evidence (see Chap. 29). We generally believe that lack of progression in the overarching elements of reflectiveness, adaptability, and enthusiasm for remedial work will more likely result in dismissal than any specific unprofessional behavior.

Chris (she/her), an early pre-clerkship student, has been scheduled to do a 4-week outplacement in a nursing home. She submitted her signed and stamped evaluation form indicating having fulfilled the internship showing satisfactory professional behavior. Later, the examiner of the internship was surprised when asked by the nursing home supervisor how the school dealt with the student's 3-week absence.

In a meeting with the PRS to explore and understand the behavior, Chris denied her absence, stating that her presence was not noticed because she went to another ward. As this contradicted the local supervisor's information, the PRS referred the student to the Examination Committee (EC) to gather documentation about possible evaluation form falsification.

Only after the EC confronted Chris with evidence, she admitted having falsified the evaluation form. She explained that she was not able to attend the internship because she had to take care of her sick child, and she thought no one would notice her absence and wanted to avoid a delay in graduation. The EC suspended Chris from her studies for a year and referred her to a faculty member for professionalism remediation.

The coach asked Chris to reflect on her professional attitude. They discussed themes of balancing private and professional challenges, being aware of limitations, making difficult choices, and admitting failure. The coach supported Chris in writing a professional development plan including individual learning goals and encouraged her to discuss this with peers. After the suspension ended, Chris resumed her medical study and successfully repeated the nursing care internship. As a result of this case, the school recognized the need for improved guidance about attendance on placements for both external supervisors and students.

Gatekeeper of the Profession

Faculty must take their responsibility to society very seriously. Less than 2% of all learners referred for remediation continually disavow and show a persistent pattern of unprofessional behavior despite remediation [4, 46, 73, 74]. Early identification of this irremediable professional behavior is important since a trainee's time, energy, and financial resources can then better be directed elsewhere [38].

The decision to start on a path toward dismissal is challenging. We have found moral case deliberation, a framework borrowed from clinical decision-making, to be helpful in guiding these decisions [75], since legal requirements in most countries stipulate that trainee deserve due process (see Chap. 29), and the school must defend itself against possible legal actions.

Dismissal

Once it is determined that a trainee is unable to provide the ultimate standard of high quality and safe patient care, educators and PRS's hand off the trainee to those within the institution with the authority and responsibility to decide on dismissal, such as the director, dean, EC, or judicial board [51, 76]. Subsequent referral to nationally operating bodies or councils may be necessary or even demanded by the candidate. While in the Dutch context, dismissal can only take place through formal legal procedures, in the United States, a school may dismiss a trainee for cause. US trainees reserve the right to appeal a dismissal determination (see Chap. 29).

Denis (he/him) is in his final year of medical school. He has been studying medicine for more than ten years, during which he received multiple unsatisfactory professionalism evaluations, due to poor involvement. He remediated these by repeating the courses, doing additional assignments, and repeating exams. Once, he received a critical incident report about plagiarizing another student's work, for which he was suspended for three months. He underwent a professionalism remediation provided by expert faculty aiming to enhance his insight into his own behavior and the consequences of this behavior for others, which he completed successfully.

Then, a new critical incident report reached the PRS. The hospital received a complaint by a patient, in which the patient stated that the student invited her to engage in a relationship and after her refusal, had been stalking her for the subsequent half year.

Immediately, the dean suspended Denis for the duration of the investigation. After careful additional exploration of the facts by the Committee on Professionalism, Denis was asked to discontinue his studies. He refused. Considering the severity of the offense, the dean started a legal procedure to dismiss the student.

Roles and Responsibilities

The establishment of a PPC is pivotal in all phases of remediation because such a committee can, over time, accumulate expertise in making judgments about the common patterns of unprofessionalism, and develop policies and procedures that align. This becomes especially important when disciplinary intervention or dismissal is indicated. Ultimately, it is the responsibility of the director or dean to dismiss a student from the institution.

Do's and Don'ts in the Gather Evidence for Dismissal Phase

Do's:

- Acknowledge that not every trainee will be able to or should graduate as a physician.
- Gather strong evidence for dismissal from summative evaluations—especially evaluations from authentic, clinical, and other workplace contexts.

- Take concerns about patient safety very seriously.
- Treat trainees fairly through very clear processes that are specified in institutional policy documents.
- Offer the trainees compassionate off-ramps from medical training.

Don't:

- Limit indicated remediation out of fear of legal liability
- Forget to learn from these procedures

Concluding Thoughts

This chapter aims at providing the reader with an overview of the steps that can be taken in remediating a trainee's unprofessional behavior. We have proposed four consecutive phases in attending to professionalism lapses. Figure 14.5 shows an overview of the remediation process and its relation to the regular curriculum. The process

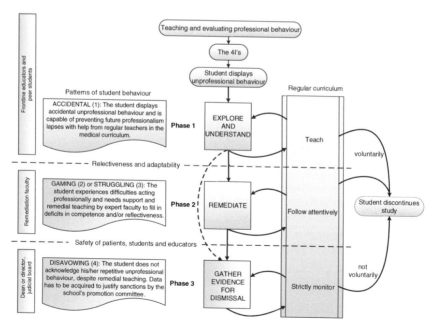

Fig. 14.5 Model for remediation of medical trainees' unprofessional behavior [51]

starts with teaching and evaluating professional behavior (Identify phase), and if there are lapses in professional behavior, trainees move to phase 1 (Explore and Understand), phase 2 (Remediate) and, if necessary, phase 3 (Gather Evidence for Dismissal).

Each of the phases for attending to professionalism lapses asks educators to assume a different role [51, 77]. Initially they have the role of a *concerned teacher*, then a *supportive coach*; finally, if ongoing behaviors threaten the safety of patients, fellow trainees, or educators, educators become *gatekeepers of the profession*. For the remediation coach, taking on the gatekeeper role conflicts with their former roles where they primarily acted to support the trainee. Thus, we strongly recommend distributing the guidance and assessment roles to different individuals, as we have described (see Chap. 2).

Professionalism remediation is a challenging task that generally consumes far more faculty time and effort than remediation of academic knowledge and skills struggles [46]. This is the case in all phases described in this chapter and calls for specific faculty development. All individuals involved in the remediation process ideally form a *community of practice* to share experiences and support each other [69].

Finally, every remediation trajectory is an opportunity for the institution to learn essential information on their curriculum and institutional culture. For example, a higher failure rate at a specific rotation site or by certain supervisors, or insufficient guidance to trainees about course or rotation expectations, should trigger a review of those curricular contexts/components or individual educators. As we expect trainees to learn and adapt, so must programs and institutions continually learn from remediation trajectories to avert future unintended consequences.

References

1. Van Mook WNKA, Gorter SL, Kieboom W, Castermans MG, de Feijter J, de Grave WS, et al. Poor professionalism identified through investigation of unsolicited healthcare complaints. Postgrad Med J. 2012;88(1042):443–50.
2. Morrison J, Wickersham P. Physicians disciplined by a state medical board. JAMA. 1998;279(23):1889–93.
3. Papadakis MA, Hodgson CS, Teherani A, Kohatsu ND. Unprofessional behavior in medical school is associated with subsequent disciplinary action by a state medical board. Acad Med. 2004;79(3):244–9.
4. Papadakis MA, Teherani A, Banach MA, Knettler TR, Rattner SL, Stern DT, et al. Disciplinary action by medical boards and prior behavior in medical school. N Engl J Med. 2005;353(25):2673–82.
5. Hickson GB, Pichert JW, Webb LE, Gabbe SG. A complementary approach to promoting professionalism: identifying, measuring, and addressing unprofessional behaviors. Acad Med. 2007;82(11):1040–8.
6. Parker M, Luke H, Zhang J, Wilkinson D, Peterson R, Ozolins I. The "pyramid of professionalism": seven years of experience with an integrated program of teaching, developing, and assessing professionalism among medical students. Acad Med. 2008;83(8):733–41.
7. Howe A, Miles S, Wright S, Leinster S. Putting theory into practice—a case study in one UK medical school of the nature and extent of unprofessional behaviour over a 6-year period. Med Teach. 2010;32(10): 837–44.
8. Van Mook WNKA, Gorter SL, De Grave WS, van Luijk SJ, Wass V, Zwaveling JH, et al. Bad apples spoil the barrel: addressing unprofessional behaviour. Med Teach. 2010;32(11):891–8.
9. Leape LL, Shore MF, Dienstag JL, Mayer RJ, Edgman-Levitan S, Meyer GS, et al. Perspective: a culture of respect, part 1: the nature and causes of disrespectful behavior by physicians. Acad Med. 2012;87(7):845–52.
10. Barnhoorn PC, Bolk JH, Ottenhoff-de Jonge MW, van Mook WNKA, de Beaufort AJ. Causes and characteristics of medical student referrals to a professional behaviour board. Int J Med Educ. 2017;8:19–24.
11. Burns CA, Lambros MA, Atkinson HH, Russell G, Fitch MT. Preclinical medical student observations associated with later professionalism concerns. Med Teach. 2017;39(1):38–43.
12. Dupras DM, Edson RS, Halvorsen AJ, Hopkins RH Jr, McDonald FS. "Problem residents": prevalence, problems and remediation in the era of core competencies. Am J Med. 2012;125(4):421–5.

13. Stern DT, Papadakis M. The developing physician—becoming a professional. N Engl J Med. 2006;355(17):1794–9.
14. Cruess SR, Cruess RL. Professionalism must be taught. BMJ. 1997;315(7123):1674.
15. O'Sullivan H. van MW, Fewtrell R, Wass V. integrating professionalism into the curriculum: AMEE Guide No. 61. Med Teach. 2012;34(2):e64–77.
16. Cruess RL, Cruess SR, Steinert Y. Teaching medical professionalism. Cambridge UK: Cambridge University Press; 2008.
17. Irby DM, Hamstra SJ. Parting the clouds: three professionalism frameworks in medical education. Acad Med. 2016;91(12):1606–11.
18. Holmboe E, Bernabeo E. The 'special obligations' of the modern Hippocratic oath for 21st century medicine. Med Educ. 2014;48(1):87–94.
19. Parsa-Parsi RW. The revised declaration of Geneva: a modern-day Physician's pledge. JAMA. 2017;318(20):1971–2.
20. Van Herwaarden CLA, Laan RFJM, Leunissen RRM. Blueprint 2009: common objectives of medical education in The Netherlands. Dutch Federation of University Medical Centres (NFU); 2009.
21. Frank, J. R. (2005). The CanMEDS 2005 physician competency framework. http://www.ub.edu/medicina_unitateducaciomedica/documentos/CanMeds.pdf.
22. Cruess R, Cruess S. Updating the Hippocratic oath to include medicine's social contract. Med Educ. 2014;48(1):95–100.
23. Cruess SR, Cruess RL, Steinert Y. Role modelling-making the most of a powerful teaching strategy. BMJ. 2008;336(7646):718–21.
24. Whitehead C, Selleger V, Van de Kreeke JJS, Hodges B. The 'missing person' in roles-based competency models: a historical, cross-national, contrastive case study. Med Educ. 2014;48(8):785–95.
25. Hafferty FW. Beyond curriculum reform: confronting medicine's hidden curriculum. Acad Med. 1998;73(4):403–7.
26. Arnold L. Assessing professional behavior: yesterday, today, and tomorrow. Acad Med. 2002;77(6):502–15.
27. Van Mook WNKA, van Luijk SJ, Fey-Schoenmakers MJ, Tans G, Rethans JJ, Schuwirth LW, et al. Combined formative and summative professional behaviour assessment approach in the bachelor phase of medical school: a Dutch perspective. Med Teach. 2010;32(12):e517–31.
28. Pronk SA, Gorter SL, Van Luijk SJ, Barnhoorn PC, Binkhorst B, Van Mook WNKA. Perception of social media behaviour among medical students, residents and medical specialists. Perspect Med Educ. 2021;10(4):215–21.
29. Ten Cate O, Regehr G. The power of subjectivity in the assessment of medical trainees. Acad Med. 2018;94(3):333–7.
30. Lynch DC, Surdyk PM, Eiser AR. Assessing professionalism: a review of the literature. Med Teach. 2004;26(4):366–73.
31. Schuwirth LW, Van der Vleuten CP. Programmatic assessment: from assessment of learning to assessment for learning. Med Teach. 2011;33(6):478–85.
32. Mak-van der Vossen MC, Peerdeman S, Kleinveld J, Kusurkar RA. How we designed and implemented teaching, training, and assessment of professional behaviour at VUmc School of Medical Sciences Amsterdam. Med Teach. 2013;35(9):709–14.
33. Ziring D, Frankel RM, Danoff D, Isaacson JH, Lochnan H. Silent witnesses: faculty reluctance to report medical students' professionalism lapses. Acad Med. 2018;93(11):1700–6.
34. Lankshear A. Failure to fail: the teacher's dilemma. Nurs Stand. 1990;4(20):35–7.
35. Byszewski A, Gill JS, Lochnan H. Socialization to professionalism in medical schools: a Canadian experience. BMC Med Educ. 2015;15(1):1–9.
36. Van den Goor M, Silkens M, Heineman MJ, Lombarts K. Investigating physicians' views on soft signals in the context of their peers' performance. J Healthc Qual. 2018;40(5):310–7.
37. Steinert Y. The "problem" learner: whose problem is it? AMEE guide no. 76. Med Teach. 2013;35(4):e1035–45.
38. Van Mook WNKA, van Luijk SJ, Zwietering PJ, Southgate L, Schuwirth LW, Scherpbier AJ, et al. The threat of the dyscompetent resident: a plea to make the implicit more explicit! Adv Health Sci Educ Theory Pract. 2014;20(2):559–74.
39. Seehusen DA. Understanding unprofessionalism in residents. J Grad Med Educ. 2020;12(3):243–6.
40. Swick HM. Toward a normative definition of medical professionalism. Acad Med. 2000;75(6):612–6.
41. Hochberg MS, Kalet A, Zabar S, Kachur E, Gillespie C, Berman RS. Can professionalism be taught? Encouraging evidence. Am J Surg. 2010;199(1):86–93.
42. Teherani A, Hodgson CS, Banach M, Papadakis MA. Domains of unprofessional behavior during medical school associated with future disciplinary action by a state medical board. Acad Med. 2005;80(10 Suppl):S17–20.
43. Cullen M. Not all behaviors are equal: the creation of a checklist of bad behaviors. Med Teach. 2017;39(1):85–91.
44. Ginsburg S, Regehr G, Stern D, Lingard L. The anatomy of the professional lapse: bridging the gap

between traditional frameworks and students' perceptions. Acad Med. 2002;77(6):516–22.

45. Hays RB, Lawson M, Gray C. Problems presented by medical students seeking support: a possible intervention framework. Med Teach. 2011;33(2):161–4.

46. Guerrasio J, Garrity MJ, Aagaard EM. Learner deficits and academic outcomes of medical students, residents, fellows, and attending physicians referred to a remediation program, 2006-2012. Acad Med. 2014;89(2):352–8.

47. Yates J, James D. Risk factors at medical school for subsequent professional misconduct: multicentre retrospective case-control study. BMJ. 2010;340:c2040.

48. Yates J. "Concerns" about medical students' adverse behaviour and attitude: an audit of practice at Nottingham, with mapping to GMC guidance. BMC Med Educ. 2014;14:196.

49. Mak-van der Vossen MC, van Mook W, van der Burgt S, Kors J, Ket JCF, Croiset G, et al. Descriptors for unprofessional behaviours of medical students: a systematic review and categorisation. BMC Med Educ. 2017;17(1):164.

50. Barnhoorn PC, Nierkens V, Mak-van der Vossen MC, Numans ME, van Mook WN, Kramer AW. Unprofessional behaviour of GP residents and its remediation: a qualitative study among supervisors and faculty. BMC Family Practice. 2021;22(1):1–1.

51. Mak-van der Vossen MC, Croix A, Teherani A, Mook WNKA, Croiset G, Kusurkar RA. A road map for attending to medical students' professionalism lapses. Acad Med. 2018;94(4):570–8.

52. Dweck CS, Yeager DS. Mindsets: a view from two eras. Perspect Psychol Sci. 2019;14(3):481–96.

53. Levinson W, Ginsburg S, Hafferty F, Lucey CR. Understanding medical professionalism. New York: McGraw Hill Professional; 2014.

54. Lucey C, Souba W. Perspective: the problem with the problem of professionalism. Acad Med. 2010;85(6):1018–24.

55. Mak-van der Vossen MC. Learning from lapses: how to identify, classify and respond to unprofessional behaviour in medical students. 2019. Doctoral thesis, VU University Amsterdam. ISBN 978-94-6323-526-6.

56. Barnhoorn PC, Houtlosser M, Ottenhoff-de Jonge MW, Essers GTJM, Numans ME, Kramer AWM. A practical framework for remediating unprofessional behavior and for developing professionalism competencies and a professional identity. Med Teach. 2018;41(3):303–8.

57. Jha V, Brockbank S, Roberts T. A framework for understanding lapses in professionalism among medical students: applying the theory of planned behavior to fitness to practice cases. Acad Med. 2016;91(12):1622–7.

58. Mak-van der Vossen MC, Teherani A, van Mook WNKA, Croiset G, Kusurkar RA. How to identify,

address and report students' unprofessional behaviour in medical school. Med Teach. 2020;42(4):372–9.

59. Bynum WE, Goodie JL. Shame, guilt, and the medical learner: ignored connections and why we should care. Med Educ. 2014;48(11):1045–54.

60. Morgan HK, Mejicano GC, Skochelak S, Lomis K, Hawkins R, Tunkel AR, et al. A responsible educational handover: improving communication to improve learning. Acad Med. 2020;95(2):194–9.

61. Humphrey-Murto S, LeBlanc A, Touchie C, Pugh D, Wood TJ, Cowley L, et al. The influence of prior performance information on ratings of current performance and implications for learner handover. Acad Med. 2019;94(7):1050–7.

62. Kalet A, Chou CL, Ellaway RH. To fail is human: remediating remediation in medical education. Perspect Med Educ. 2017;6(6):418–24.

63. Chou CL, Kalet A, Costa MJ, Cleland J, Winston K. Guidelines: the dos, don'ts and don't knows of remediation in medical education. Persp Med Educ. 2019;8(6):322–8.

64. De la Croix A, Veen M. The reflective zombie: problematizing the conceptual framework of reflection in medical education. Persp Med Educ. 2018;7(6):394–400.

65. Williams BW, Welindt D, Hafferty FW, Stumps A, Flanders P, Williams MV. Adverse childhood experiences in trainees and physicians with professionalism lapses: implications for medical education and remediation. Acad Med. 2021;96(5):736–43.

66. Ziring D, Danoff D, Grosseman S, Langer D, Esposito A, Jan MK, et al. How do medical schools identify and remediate professionalism lapses in medical students? A study of U.S. and Canadian Medical Schools. Acad Med. 2015;90(7):913–20.

67. Findyartini A, Sudarsono N, Sudarsono NC. Remediating lapses in professionalism among undergraduate pre-clinical medical students in an Asian Institution: a multimodal approach. BMC Med Educ. 2018;18(1):88.

68. Brennan N, Price T, Archer J, Brett J. Remediating professionalism lapses in medical students and doctors: a systematic review. Med Educ. 2020;54(3):196–204.

69. Kalet A, Guerrasio J, Chou CL. Twelve tips for developing and maintaining a remediation program in medical education. Med Teach. 2016;38(8):787–92.

70. Bellini LM, Kalet A, Englander R. Providing compassionate off-ramps for medical students is a moral imperative. Acad Med. 2019;94(5):656–8.

71. Santen SA, Christner J, Mejicano G, Hemphill RR. Kicking the can down the road—when medical schools fail to self-regulate. N Engl J Med. 2019;381(24):2287–9.

72. Bonke B, Luijk SJV. Protocol Iudicium Abeundi. 2010. https://www.nfu.nl/sites/default/files/2020-08/Protocol_Iudicium_Abeundi.pdf (in Dutch).

73. van Mook WNKA, Gorter SL, De Grave WS, van Luijk SJ, Wass V, Zwaveling JH, et al. Bad apples spoil the barrel: addressing unprofessional behaviour. Med Teach. 2010;32(11):891–8.

74. Bennett AJ, Roman B, Arnold LM, Kay J, Goldenhar LM. Professionalism deficits among medical students: models of identification and intervention. Acad Psych. 2005;29(5):426–32.

75. Widdershoven G, Stolper M, Molewijk B, Metselaar S. How to support patient and family in dealing with ethical issues? The relevance of moral case deliberation. Am J Bioeth. 2020;20(6):70–2.

76. Stringham RV, Whitlock J, Perez NA, Borges NJ, Levine RE. A snapshot of current US medical school off-ramp programs—a way to leave medical school with another degree. Med Sci Educ. 2021;31(2):341–3.

77. Bourgeois-Law G, Regehr G, Teunissen PW, Varpio L. Educator, judge, public defender: conflicting roles for remediators of practicing physicians. Med Educ. 2020;54(12):1171–9.

David Hatem

By three methods we may learn wisdom: first, by reflection, which is noblest; second, by imitation, which is easiest; and third, by experience, which is the most bitter.—Confucius

We don't see things as they are, we see things as we are.—Anais Nin

"All there is to thinking," he said, "is seeing something noticeable which makes you see something that you weren't noticing, which makes you see something that isn't even visible."—Norman MacLean, *A River Runs Through It*

Introduction

Health professions education historically has emphasized facts and the latest scientific knowledge. It has been oriented toward achievement, action, and outcomes, to the exclusion of other relevant domains of learning and ways of knowing. Nowhere else is this more manifest than in the prerequisite coursework for school applications. The set of admissions expectations has traditionally dissuaded students from exploring fields of study unless they are directly related to the goal of getting into professional school and therefore becoming a clinician [1, 2]. This emphasis, among many other powerful forces, has led to a culture of "unreflective doing" in health professions education, resulting in an underdeveloped capacity to learn by reflecting on practice.

As it has become clear that mastering foundational knowledge is necessary but not sufficient to being a competent health professional, there have been renewed calls for reform in education [3] and initiatives designed to facilitate that change [4]. Professional organizations such as the Accreditation Council for Graduate Medical Education (ACGME) have set expectations that reach beyond technical knowledge [5]. The behavioral and social sciences [6], an expanded understanding of social determinants of health [7], and health systems science competencies [8] are increasingly integrated into health professions school courses. Preprofessional course and testing requirements and admission processes are broadening for the first time in decades [9–14]. Beyond suggesting additional content, the landmark Carnegie Foundation report proposed that there be explicit focus on the processes of integration of knowledge and experience, habits of inquiry, and improvement to promote excellence, identity formation, and the process of developing and refining professional values [3]. All these efforts require individual clinicians to master a set of cognitive abilities that enable lifelong, self-directed learning. The capacity to reflect before, during, and after practice is foundational to this emerging area of competence [15]. Yet the literature suggests these skills are underdeveloped in learners and faculty [16].

D. Hatem (✉)
Department of Internal Medicine, University of Massachusetts TH Chan School of Medicine, Worcester, MA, USA
e-mail: david.hatem@umassmemorial.org

Reflection as a Competency

Reflection is particularly important in making a successful transition from a student-focused classroom setting to a patient-focused, experiential learning environment [17]. It is also foundational to efforts at continuous professional development and Maintenance of Certification initiatives [18, 19]; in professional practice, the "high hard ground," where problems are solved through the application of research-based theory, differs from the "messier" real world, where complex problems characterized by uncertainty and values conflicts defy clear technical solutions. In these indeterminate zones of practice, technically rational evidence-based solutions often do not emerge. Because experience alone is insufficient to guarantee learning, reflection—critically considering what one does before, during, and after doing it—is necessary [20]. Reflection is central to clinical problem-solving [21] and self-directed learning: it is necessary for self-assessment, eliciting and responding to feedback, reconciling feedback with one's own self-assessment, and then incorporating self and peer assessment into subsequent performance [20]. In this way, reflection extends beyond the individual and can be described as "critical reflection," defined as self-reflection that is supplemented by input from trainees (when teaching), colleagues, and theory [22].

Frameworks for Understanding the Reflection Competency

The Reflective Practitioner

Helping trainees learn from real-world settings requires a framework for choosing an effective action in complex contexts. Schon's model of the reflective practitioner defines skills to apply automatically, almost by rote, as "knowing in action." There are other skills to apply and refine while they are being put into practice ("reflection-in-action"), and yet other skills that require thought after initially experiencing it ("reflection-on-action") [20]. Further refinements of this model describe another element: anticipate and prepare

for what we are about to do ("reflection-for-action") [23].

Kolb's Cycle of Experiential Learning

Learners must develop the capacity to derive lessons from concrete clinical experiences effectively and efficiently and then apply their learning to subsequent encounters, refining their own skills in the process [17, 24].

Ahmad (he/him) is a medical student on the first day of the Neurology clerkship. On inpatient rounds, the supervisory team examines and discusses each patient very briefly; the most common diagnoses are stroke, seizure, brain tumor, and psychological factors contributing to neurologic symptoms. Seven of these patients initially presented with hemiparesis. The potential for learning from this concrete experience is immense, but Ahmad perceives this as "drinking from a fire hose." He tries to read about strokes, seizures, and brain tumors, but because of the overwhelming breadth of material available, he feels unprepared to learn efficiently in this situation. With a wellhoned and disciplined approach, he could learn how to distinguish a "basic" neurologic exam from a series of special maneuvers applied in unique contexts based on a known or suspected disease process. Well-developed critical reflection skills will enable learners to take away specific reading goals. For instance, Ahmad could spend 1 h that evening reading about the key features that differentiate among the underlying causes of hemiparesis. By actively reflecting on what he does and does not understand, he can maximize his learning from concrete experiences.

Figure 15.1 illustrates how this cycle works in clinical situations.

Fig. 15.1 Kolb's Learning Cycle adapted by Greenberg and Blatt for clinical experiences

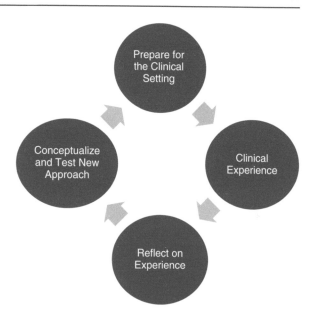

Gibbs' Reflective Cycle: Learning to "Pay Attention" to Concrete Experiences

Trainees encounter many challenging situations on clinical rotations [25–27]. They see vivid, dramatic, and shocking things that are often hard to digest emotionally.

> *I have seen entirely too many people naked. I have seen 350 pounds of flesh, dead: dried red blood streaked across nude adipose, gauze, and useless EKG paper strips. I have met someone for the second time and seen them anesthetized, splayed, and filleted across an OR table within 10 min [28].*

Paying attention during these experiences and allowing for reflective observation in the moment presents challenges and is important to learning and emotional growth. Concrete methods include promoting personal awareness, mindfulness training, and participating in Balint groups [29–31]. Gibbs' Reflective Cycle ([32]; see Fig. 15.2) provides structure and suggests a series of prompts to help facilitate trainees' reflective observation skills. If done in groups, individuals using this cycle can compare their own observation to those of peers, their teachers, or the literature [32], which promotes critical reflection skills [22].

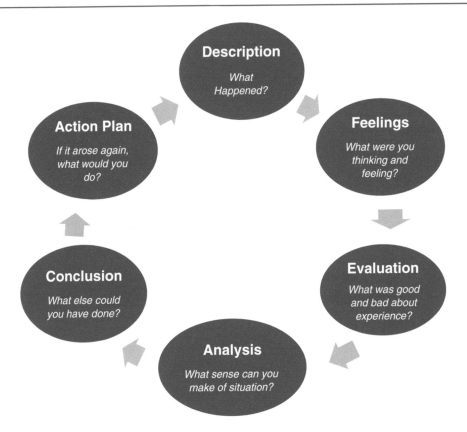

Fig. 15.2 Gibbs' Reflective Cycle provides prompts to facilitate a stepwise approach to analyzing or debriefing concrete experience. Adapted from [24]. Reproduced with permission of the author

Narrative in Clinical Education: Deepening Learning and Abstract Conceptualization

Stories have a central place in healthcare, both in hearing stories from patients and colleagues, and in telling stories [33]. The relationship between reflection and storytelling has been described in health professions literature [34–37]. Researchers have demonstrated that reflection narratives can be characterized [38] and measured [39], frameworks to analyze and give feedback on reflections can be used [40], depth of reflection can be measured, and reflective ability can improve [41]. Learners who reflect superficially encounter professionalism issues with greater frequency than those who can reflect deeply ([42]; Chap. 13).

Therefore, narratives encouraging reflection can facilitate growth in the clinician.

Additionally, utilizing illness narratives in clinical education has been proposed as a model to foster empathy, professionalism, meaning making, trust, and identification with the unfamiliar [43, 44]. Both patient and learner narratives can be part of transformative learning, helping to enhance understanding of the patient and of the provider. In this way, narrative reflection may contribute to professional identity formation (PIF) [45, 46].

Writing narratives favors depth over breadth in understanding a phenomenon [47]. Writing is a useful strategy to move from raw reflections toward formulating abstract conceptualizations needed to drive cycles of continually improving performance (Fig. 15.1). A systematic review of narrative medicine programs, involving both close reading of literature and reflective writing, showed self-reported improvement in relationship-building, empathy, perspective-taking, resilience, and burnout detection and mitigation [48]. One study demonstrated that a program where interns wrote narratives led to greater personal awareness [49]. Reading and listening to reflective writing helps prepare learners for the risk-taking and vulnerability inherent in clinical practice and promotes professional development, general well-being, and empathy [50]. This has broad applications, including promoting cultural humility and fostering professionalism and professional development [51, 52] (see Chap. 13).

There is, however, limited literature on outcomes for those who do not wish to write or are not inclined toward reflection [53]. The remainder of this chapter will focus on using narrative to enhance reflection in remediation of trainees and clinicians. Here, the goal of narrative is to serve as evidence of reflection of one's own attitudes, and to demonstrate understanding of another's perspective. It also has the potential to document improved self-awareness, performance improvement, and learning about how to think through complex clinical dilemmas.

Remediation Strategies

Let's consider several challenging cases.

- **Case 1.** *You are responsible for clinical skills remediation and meet with PM (he/him), a student who failed a clinical skills exam because he did not collect many key historical facts, did superficial physical exams, demonstrated poor clinical reasoning in his written notes, and displayed a limited number of diagnoses in his differential. PM explains that he plans a career in Emergency Medicine, and "while I know that there*

are other things that might be going on with the patient, my job is to make sure they are not going to die! Let the inpatient docs figure the rest out." His recent clinical supervisors report that he is a "nice guy," interacts well with patients, knows a lot, and is eager to be helpful, but he often "misses the boat" with patient diagnoses.

- **Case 2.** *A colleague (she/her) approaches you, a clinical rotation director, that trainee RA (he/him) has regularly interrupted her in the middle of a conversation with a patient, to disagree with what she was saying. RA explains, "the supervisor was saying something that I didn't think was accurate. We have an obligation to be honest with the patient, don't we?"*

- **Case 3.** *A peer files a professionalism complaint against SJ (she/her). In a hospital-based paired peer clinical skills exercise, SJ repeatedly interrupted her partner's conversation with the patient, asking repetitive questions. Her partner asked her to hold her questions to the end, but SJ loudly replied, "I want to make sure this isn't a heart attack," not seeming to notice the worried look on the patient's face.*

These cases illustrate, among other things, problems with premature closure (deciding too quickly on a diagnosis without considering other possibilities—see Chap. 9), professionalism, and teamwork. In each case, the learner has potential difficulty perceiving the perspectives of others and lacks awareness of their own biases or assumptions that significantly impact clinical problem solving, patient interaction, and teamwork.

How do we engage these learners in sincere and critical reflection on what happened? How do we encourage the practice of perceiving multiple perspectives simultaneously? How do we convince them to remain "open-minded," both clinically and interpersonally? I will explore how to use narrative as a practical tool to enhance reflection and learning.

Reflective Capacity and Motivation to Learn

In remediation, by definition, we are working with trainees whose initial approach has not worked. Disagreements about the presence of a learning need between the learner and others may indicate a need to develop reflective capacity. Therefore, the learner can be seen as *unconsciously incompetent*: not yet aware that they have a learning need [54].

Working with learners who need insight is challenging but critical. Theorists have proposed that transformative learning is stimulated by a "disorienting dilemma" [17, 55, 56], a situation that, upon reflection, typically guided by someone with authority, can lead to critically re-examining strongly held beliefs, ultimately leading to new insights and new ways of behaving [57]. Our job is to promote insight or point out the disorienting dilemma, while avoiding inducing shame or humiliation in the learner, which may undermine motivation to learn [58].

When we identify a learner for remediation, ideally the learner is presented with a powerful disorienting dilemma: they are off track. This facilitates the potential transformative impact of narrative reflection. Learners who previously lacked insight can be pushed to examine their own attitudes and beliefs with expert help (see Chaps. 4, 6). To deepen reflection and enhance reflective capacity, writing assignments can achieve success by encouraging perspective-taking and through narrative coherence [59].

Perspective-Taking

Clinical experts gain insight into the human condition by seeing the self in relation to others [60]. Trainees requiring remediation often have an incomplete understanding of multiple participants' viewpoints in a situation; they may think

they understand themselves, yet they are unaware of the effect that they are having on others. PM, who focused solely on "emergency" diagnoses (Case 1), risks discounting the patient's desire to know their diagnosis. It is not sufficient to explain "your chest pain does not represent a heart attack or a pulmonary embolism." RA, who interrupts a patient encounter (Case 2), may not intend to offend the supervisor, or worry the patient, but seems to be unaware of the possibility that this might occur. These trainees have a substantially different version of "what happened" (one of the first steps of the reflective cycle) and do not exert effort to see others' perspectives [60]. A writing assignment may help them accomplish this critical task but must be direct and clear. Some may perceive assignments like "write your reflections on a challenging patient" as "busy work" that forces them to be insincere (an interesting perspective in itself) [53]. With trainees who lack insight into their own learning needs, it is best to proceed in steps, guided by Gibbs' Reflective Cycle.

Seeking the Trainee's Perspective

Assigning learners to write narratives can help us understand the learner's perspective, however objectionable we might perceive their behavior to be. A first remediation assignment for PM (Case 1) is to ask him to describe his approach to a patient with chest pain in the Emergency Department, particularly the goals of care for patients who are not admitted to an inpatient unit. Sometimes simply giving a trainee time to write his actions and opinions may lead to significant insights. It also provides a baseline for the ongoing remediation work. By seeking his perspective before addressing the behavior, we also model the perspective-taking we hope to enhance.

For RA (Case 2), you might ask:

"I was curious about your interruption in the middle of the encounter. I wonder what you were hoping that would achieve."
"What effect do you think questioning antibiotic choice in front of the patient might have on the patient's willingness to take any medicines that we prescribe?"

These questions, asked with curiosity rather than judgment and followed by a pause, encourage learners themselves to pause, think about their actions, reflect on their own internal process, or speculate about intended outcomes. Their response, whether written or spoken, represents a narrative, because they are telling their story about what took place, how they reacted, and how others reacted or might react. Following this dialogue, you could assign them a written narrative to expand their reflective capacity by using Gibbs' Reflective Cycle as a guide. Clarity about the goal of the assignment is critical ("We need to deepen your perspective-taking and improve your awareness of the impact of your behavior, despite your good intentions"). It should be explicit, defined, and structured.

> **A Suggested Writing Assignment for SJ (Case 3)**
> Write a 500-word reflection on this episode. Describe what happened, and what you were thinking and feeling. Evaluate what was effective and ineffective about what happened from your perspective, that of your physical diagnosis partner, and the patient, what you make of the situation, what you might have done differently, and what you anticipate you might do differently the next time you are in a comparable situation. Email this to me by next Monday, and we will meet again Tuesday at 3.

Sharing Narratives to Reinforce and Deepen the Capacity to Learn from Reflection

There is inspiring work regularly occurring around us, and we can celebrate this by promoting positive examples of healthcare professional or trainee behavior.

In their report of professionalism narratives at Indiana University School of Medicine, Karnieli-Miller and colleagues recount narratives of both professional and unprofessional behavior written from the perspective of third-year medi-

cal students. In one example, as a patient with HIV and acute leukemia neared the end of life, multiple supervisors took extraordinary measures to ensure that the patient could be discharged from the hospital to attend her child's graduation [26]. Looking at this example, consider asking a learner, "what made it possible for this to happen?" Such a question promotes examining individual and institutional elements that support exemplary acts of professionalism and reflecting on facilitators and barriers to professional behavior for all [61].

Sharing Narratives to Address Negative Attitudes

There may be times when sharing different perspectives using published narratives might promote an alternative perspective that learners had not considered.

Consider the following situation. Supervising an inpatient team, you have had many elderly patients with delirium on your service and have noticed multiple comments made by the trainees that seem to disparage elderly patients. You could merely tell your team that you perceive these comments to be dehumanizing, or that it is unprofessional to make such comments. Alternatively, you can choose a 10-min slot during rounds to share and discuss the following poem illustrating a son's grief resulting from a mother's dementia, written by one of our students.

> **Buttered Toast**
>
> *While I tend the toaster*
> *My mother has dabbed butter*
> *On all six sides of her sourdough.*
> *I am angered by her manners.*
> *Even before her dementia, she was*
> *the immediate light to my darker passion.*
> *So I get offended at her impropriety,*
> *As if manners were a thing that mattered in my family*
> *While I really am angry at my inability*

To make her happy, to stop her from losing her
Dignity, in front of strangers on the street, to save her.
And when her brow is tense with frustration,
About food, or the plans for the rest of the day,
Or the inability to come up with any
Word at all, she really is afraid of dying
And sadly grieving the things she knew she lost though forgot the losing.
But the butter moves into the nooks,
and onto the fingers of Miss Alameda County 1960.
And her eyes widen as she says
Oh, this is so good! and I try like the butter
To melt for both of us [62].

We see that despite the losses, she still derives pleasure in eating a piece of buttered toast. This humanizes a woman whom the team may have trouble seeing as anything but a delirious and demented patient. We can see her like her son has, as a once-beautiful woman and imagine (and even inquire) about other personal and humanizing features. A brief discussion of this poem has served to create a highly memorable moment for a clinical team I have led, where they gained insight without the needing me to directly criticize their behavior.

The Perspectives of Others

Learners have high sensitivity to conflicting values in the clinical environment and exhibit distress when required to select from mutually exclusive, values-based alternatives [63]. Therefore, for Case 1, asking PM to write a series of brief essays about the same event from differing viewpoints (*How would the patient presenting to the ER with chest pain perceive your approach? How would your ER attending view this?*) may enable him to reconcile some of this distress and provide material to discuss with the

remediation coach, potentially leading to new perspectives on taking shortcuts prematurely. Subsequent assignments can include reading and writing an essay on cognitive errors in diagnosis and common cognitive biases in the Emergency Department [64] (see Chap. 9).

A Perspective-Taking Writing Prompt for SJ (Case 3)

You are seeing a patient. You feel confident that you know what is going on with the patient. As you are explaining this to your patient, a student, whom you offered to have shadow you, interrupts and contradicts what you are saying. Write a narrative detailing what you would do in this situation, what you would think and feel about the interruption, and how it might influence what the patient thought of you and what you were saying to them. Detail what you would say to the student.

An extension of this assignment might include a narrative coda: After the encounter, you look up what the student said and discover he was correct. Does this alter your thoughts and feelings about what happened? Given your thoughts about how you might act when you are interrupted, how does this situation prompt you to reconsider your actions?

Another perspective-switching approach might be to provide the learner a published narrative of a challenging situation and ask them to imagine being the faculty member asked to confer with the trainee. Stories such as William Carlos Williams' "The Use of Force" [65], in which a learner loses his composure, or a narrative in which learner takes part in a physician-assisted suicide [66], make good material for this exercise.

Collectively, these exercises allow learners to engage in critical reflection in a stepwise fashion. Initially, we ask for their version of the events and debrief this by changing the frame by asking "what if" questions. We can present them with an alternative narrative from the literature, ask them to write a narrative to illustrate another "character's" perspective, ask them to take on a faculty role through "role exchange," or share with them a series of narratives from the literature that comment on the same theme in their narrative. Saving these narratives and reviewing them in sequence provides evidence of the growing perspective-taking ability (or lack thereof).

Framing and Fostering Narrative Coherence

Language used by healthcare personnel frames the developing attitudes of our learners. In his timeless essay, "Can you teach compassion?" Lowenstein describes a common case presentation on rounds on the inpatient service. This trainee started the clinical story the way many do, using standard, impersonal language: "This is the first admission for this 35-year-old IVDA" (Intravenous Drug Abuser). On that day, Dr. Lowenstein interrupted the presenter and asked the team: "Would our thinking or care be different if you began your history by telling us that this is a 35-year-old Marine veteran who has been addicted to drugs since he served, with valor, in Vietnam?" The inpatient team was embarrassed and silent as insight grew: standard medical nomenclature can frame our thinking, and dehumanize [67].

It was the early days of the HIV epidemic. I was at the beginning of my career as a physician, and I was seeing the next in a series of HIV-infected drug-addicted patients who I was going to follow longitudinally. As I took her social history, she told me that she began drinking alcohol regularly with her parents at the age of 6. She was sexually abused by her uncle and became pregnant at the age of 14, at which time she dropped out of high school and

entered a series of increasingly challenging foster care settings. When I asked her how she had coped with all these challenges, she laughed at my "silly question" and answered: "I became a drug addict!" I was shocked at the powerful impact her laughter had on me. Because of my limited personal experience of drug use, my comparatively stable family life, and biases based on news accounts and popular press, I held beliefs that demonized drug users. In that moment, I gained insight. I was shocked out of my previously held beliefs by the fact that this woman's drug addiction made perfect sense in the context of her life.

People do things for a reason, their reasoning can be elucidated, and similar reasoning will inform subsequent actions. This concept of "narrative coherence" [68] suggests that characters act in a reliable manner; it has informed my subsequent practice, leading me to elicit information during my patient interviews to understand behavior or symptoms that at first do not make sense. This enables my therapeutic rapport building and, as a result, enhances my clinical competence.

Both these examples represent variations of PM's challenge in Case 1. The absence of a trigger to reflect leads to premature closure. While Case 1 refers to premature closure as a struggle with problem-solving or clinical reasoning, also note here a "story" or "narrative" deficit: failure to consider alternatives to reductionistic thinking.

Faculty Development

Faculty must recall the purpose of asking learners to reflect: to deepen their understanding of self and the situation and to inform subsequent action under similar circumstances. This learning experience should explicitly foster metacognitive skills essential for lifelong and self-directed learning (see Chap. 4). Therefore, design of narrative reflective assignments should be focused, structured, and clearly defined as modeled above. Additionally, faculty must create a safe learning environment, show comfort with strong emotions, and provide clear feedback and follow-up to the trainee [59, 69, 70] (see Chap. 6).

Models for evaluating written reflections provide step-by-step instructions that allow for determination of the depth of reflection and discernment between reflective writing skills and storytelling [59, 71]. The strategy should best fit the purpose of the narrative exercise. The REFLECT framework describes four hierarchical levels of reflection: (1) "habitual action," or non-reflective descriptions; (2) "thoughtful action or introspection," with more elaborate description yet limited analysis; (3) "reflection" that includes attempts to understand or analyze a situation through clear description of the conflict or challenge, or explores emotions and attempts to look for meaning; and (4) "critical reflection," which adds to simple reflection by exploring and critiquing personal assumptions and fully exploring alternate perspectives [59]. Although efforts to demonstrate psychometric reliability and validity of narrative assessments have been challenging and will require additional study, using a structured approach to defining reflective ability provides a shared language and mental model which is valuable in conducting professionalism remediation (Chaps. 13 and 14) [72–74].

While this chapter has emphasized individual reflection focused on remediation and its potential uses, additional literature suggests that narratives can be used as part of a formative evaluation system [75] or learning portfolios [76]. Additionally, qualitative reports of student narratives provide a window into broader systems that affect groups of learners beyond the individual [27]. Organizational data about how our health system is perceived undergird competencies in systems-based practice and quality improvement, both examples of processes that can trigger organizational reflection that frames health care systems as learning organizations [77, 78]. Collectively, this literature reinforces the necessity of reflection at the individual, team, and

organizational levels and highlights the need for meaningful reflection to promote learning, teamwork, and performance improvement activities, including remediation, within an organization. Clearly, reflection extends beyond the individual.

For reflection to lead to performance improvement, learners must be willing to engage deeply in thinking about situations that have gotten them into trouble. Under optimal circumstances, many clinicians and trainees can engage in this type of reflection and even enjoy writing assignments, but some do not. In fact, some are not inclined to be introspective, may resist reflection, and may refuse to write anything that reveals personal thoughts or feelings. In the end, as with all remediation activities, judgments about whether this constitutes clinical incompetence or not must be made and documented.

For faculty members interested in learning more, there are several educational strategies for developing reflection and reflective capacity [15], guided reflection, and useful faculty development resources [51]. Additional methods have been described to help clinicians enhance personal awareness through reflection [25, 29, 30, 36, 49, 79].

Conclusion

Using narrative as a form of reflection for remediation in health professions education has potentially far-reaching implications. Narratives explore the depths of an experience [40] and seek a fuller understanding of the self and of the situation, both desired outcomes of reflection [15]. Narrative is especially useful for helping to explore complex clinical situations, uncover biases and assumptions, elicit multiple perspectives, plumb the depths of our thoughts and feelings, and reinforce our choices or propose alternate actions for times when we encounter similar situations in the future. Clearer outcomes need to be delineated [41, 80, 81], but enhanced self-awareness, relationship building, empathic understanding of patients, problem solving, teamwork, and resilience/burnout mitigation are potentially demonstrable endpoints. With learners who require remediation and may not naturally be inclined toward reflection, challenging them to write clear narratives, which demonstrate the willingness to reflect, is the first step. Reflection as described in this chapter is clearly an important metacognitive skill closely related to the process of "slowing down when you have to," described in studies of expert clinicians who, when facing something unexpected or challenging consciously, switch into a more deliberate, effortful, yet mindful state that can ultimately lead to the delivery of expert, value-based, patient-centered, safe patient care [82] (see Chap. 4).

References

1. Lovecchio K, Dundes L. Premed survival: understanding the culling process in premedical undergraduate education. Acad Med. 2002;77:719–24.
2. Gunderman R, Kanter S. "How to fix the premedical curriculum" revisited. Acad Med. 2008;83:1158–61.
3. Cooke M, Irby DM, O'Brien BC. Educating physicians: a call for reform of medical school and residency, vol. 304. San Francisco: Jossey-Bass; 2010. p. 304.
4. American Medical Association Accelerating Change in Medical Education. https://www.ama-assn.org/education/accelerating-change-medical-education. Accessed 29 Dec 2022.
5. Accreditation Council for Graduate Medical Education (ACGME). ACGME 2012 Accreditation. Chicago: ACGME, 2000. https://www.acgme.org/What-We-Do/Accreditation/Milestones/Overview. Accessed 29 Dec 2022.
6. Association of American Medical Colleges. Behavioral and social science foundations for future physicians. Washington, DC: Association of American Medical Colleges; 2011. p. 45. https://www.aamc.org/download/271020/data/behavioralandsocialsciencefoundationsforfuturephysicians.pdf.
7. Braveman P, Gottlieb L. The social determinants of health: it's time to consider the causes of the causes. Public Health Rep. 2014;129 Suppl 2(Suppl 2):19–31.
8. Gonzalo JD, Dekhtyar M, Starr SR, Borkan J, Patrick B, Fancher T, Green J, Grethlein S, Lai C, Lawson L, Monrad S, O'Sullivan P, Schwartz M, Skochelak S. Health Systems Science Curricula in Undergraduate Medical Education: identifying and defining a potential curricular framework. Acad Med. 2017;92:123–31.
9. Kirch DG, Mitchell K, Ast C. The new 2015 MCAT: testing competencies. JAMA. 2013;310:2243–4.
10. Schwartzstein RM. Leveraging the medical school admissions process to foster a smart, humanistic, and diverse physician workforce. Acad Med. 2020;95:333–5.
11. Monroe A, Quinn E, Samuelson W, Dunleavy DM, Dowd KW. An overview of the medical school admission process and use of applicant data in decision making: what has changed since the 1980s? Acad Med. 2013;88:672–81.
12. Witzburg RA, Sondheimer HM. Holistic review—shaping the medical profession one applicant at a time. N Engl J Med. 2013;368(17):1565–7.
13. Grabowski CJ. Impact of holistic review on student interview pool diversity. Adv Health Sci Educ. 2018;23:487–98.
14. Conrad S, Addams A, Young G. Holistic review in medical school admissions and selection. Acad Med. 2016;91:1472–4.
15. Sandars J. The use of reflection in medical education: AMEE Guide No. 44. Med Teach. 2009;31:685–95.
16. Duffy FD, Holmboe ES. Self-assessment in lifelong learning and improving performance in practice: physician know thyself. JAMA. 2006;296:1137–9.
17. Greenberg L, Blatt B. Successfully negotiating the clerkship years of medical school: a guide for medical students, implications for residents and faculty. Acad Med. 2010;85(4):706–9.
18. Bindels E, Verberg C, Scherpbier A, Heeneman S, Lombarts K. Reflection revisited: how physicians conceptualize and experience reflection in professional practice. BMC Med Educ. 2018;18:105.
19. Miller SH. American board of medical specialties and excellence in lifelong learning: maintenance of certification. J Cont Educ Health Prof. 2005;25:151–6.
20. Schon DA. Educating the reflective practitioner: toward a new design for teaching and learning in the professions. San Francisco: Jossey-Bass; 1987. p. 355.
21. Custers EJ, Stuyt PM, De Vries Robbé PF. Clinical problem analysis (CPA): a systematic approach to teaching complex medical problem solving. Acad Med. 2000;75(3):291–7.
22. Brookfield SD. Becoming a critically reflective teacher. San Francisco: Jossey-Bass; 1995. p. 296.
23. Edwards S, Reflecting differently. New dimensions: reflection-before-action and reflection-beyond-action. Int Prac Dev J. 2017;10:58.
24. Kolb DA. Experiential learning: experience as the source of learning and development. Englewood Cliffs, NJ: Prentice-Hall; 1984. p. 256.
25. Branch WT Jr. Use of critical incident reports in medical education. A perspective. J Gen Intern Med. 2005;20:1063–7.
26. Karnieli-Miller O, Vu TR, Holtman MC, Clyman SG, Inui TS. Medical students' professionalism narratives: a window on the informal and hidden curriculum. Acad Med. 2010;85:124–33.

27. Karnieli-Miller O, Vu TR, Frankel RM, Holtman MC, Clyman SG, Hui SL, Inui TS. Which experiences in the hidden curriculum teach students about professionalism? Acad Med. 2011;86:369–77.

28. Treadway K, Chatterjee N. Into the water—the clinical clerkships. N Engl J Med. 2011;364:1190–3.

29. Novack DH, Suchman AL, Clark W, Epstein RM, Najberg E, Kaplan C. Calibrating the physician. Personal awareness and effective patient care. Working group on promoting physician personal awareness, American Academy on Physician and Patient. JAMA. 1997;278:502–9.

30. Krasner MS, Epstein RM, Beckman H, Suchman AL, Chapman B, Mooney CJ, Quill TE. Association of an educational program in mindful communication with burnout, empathy, and attitudes among primary care physicians. JAMA. 2009;302:1284–93.

31. Kjeldmand D, Holmstrom I. Balint group as a means to increase job satisfaction and prevent burnout among family practitioners. Ann Fam Med. 2008;6:138–45.

32. Gibbs G. Learning by doing: a guide to teaching and learning. London: FEU; 1988. p. 129. http://www2.glos.ac.uk/gdn/gibbs/index.htm. Accessed 25 July 2013, Created by Claire Andrew created January 2001

33. Verghese A. The physician as storyteller. Ann Intern Med. 2001;135:1012–7.

34. Charon R. Narrative and medicine. N Engl J Med. 2004;350:862–4.

35. DasGupta S, Charon R. Personal illness narratives: using reflective writing to teach empathy. Acad Med. 2004;79:351–6.

36. Hatem D, Ferrara E. Becoming a doctor: fostering humane caregivers through creative writing. Patient Educ Couns. 2001;45:13–22.

37. Epp S. The value of reflective journaling in undergraduate nursing education: a literature review. Int J Nurs Stud. 2008;45:1379–88.

38. Hanlon CD, Frosch EM, Shochet RB, Buckingham Shum SJ, Gibson A, Goldberg H. Recognizing reflection: computer-assisted analysis of first year medical students' reflective writing. Med Sci Educ. 2021;31:109–16.

39. Williams JC, Ireland T, Warman S, Cake MA, Dymock D, Fowler E, Baillie S. Instruments to measure the ability to self-reflect: a systematic review of evidence from workplace and educational settings including health care. Eur J Dent Educ. 2019;23:389–404.

40. Reiss S, Wald H, Monroe A, Borkan J. Begin the BEGAN (the Brown Educational Guide to the Analysis of Narrative)-a framework for enhancing educational impact of faculty feedback on students' reflective writing. Pat Educ Couns. 2010;80:253–9.

41. Aronson L, Niehaus B, Hill-Sakurai L, Lai C, O'Sullivan P. A comparison of two methods of teaching reflective ability in year 3 medical students. Med Educ. 2012;46:807–14.

42. Hoffman LA, Shsew RL, Vu R, Brokaw JJ, Frankel RM. Is reflective ability associated with professionalism lapses during medical school? Acad Med. 2016;91:853–7.

43. Charon R. Narrative medicine. JAMA. 2001;286:1897–902.

44. Kumagai A. A conceptual framework for the use of illness narrative in medical education. Acad Med. 2008;83:653–8.

45. Cruess RL, Cruess SR, Boudreau D, Snell L, Steinert Y. A schematic representation of the professional identity formation and socialization of medical students and residents: a guide for medical educators. Acad Med. 2015;90:718–25.

46. Hatem DS, Halpin T. Becoming doctors: examining student narratives to understand the process of professional identity formation within a learning community. J Med Educ Curric Dev. 2019;6:238212051983454.

47. Bolton G. Stories at work: reflective writing for practitioners. Lancet. 1999;354(9174):243–5.

48. Remein CD, Childs E, Pasco JC, Trinquart L, Flynn DB, Wingerter SL, Bhasin RM, Demers LB, Benjamin EJ. Content and outcomes of narrative medicine programmes: a systematic review of the literature through 2019. BMJ Open. 2020;10:e031568.

49. Levine RB, Kern DE, Wright SM. The impact of prompted narrative writing during internship on reflective practice: a qualitative study. Adv Health Sci Educ Theory Pract. 2008;13:723–33.

50. Shapiro J, Kasman D, Shafer A. Words and wards: a model of reflective writing and its uses in medical education. J Med Humanit. 2006;27:231–44.

51. Kleinman A, Benson P. Anthropology in the clinic: the problem of cultural competency and how to fix it. PLoS Med. 2006;3:e294.

52. Bolton G. Reflective practice: writing and professional development. 3rd ed. London: Sage; 2010. p. 272.

53. Campbell BH, Treat R, Johnson B, Derse AR. Creating reflective space for reflective and "unreflective" medical students: exploring seminal moments in a large group-writing session. Acad Med. 2020;95:882–7.

54. Luft J, Ingham H. The Johari window, a graphic model of interpersonal awareness. In: Proceedings of the western training laboratory in group development, Los Angeles; 1955.

55. Mezirow J. A critical theory of adult learning and education. Adult Educ Q. 1981;32:3–24.

56. Mezirow J. Transformative dimensions of adult learning. San Francisco: Jossey-Bass; 1994. p. 247.

57. Cranton P. Understanding and promoting transformative learning: a guide for educators of adults. San Francisco: Jossey-Bass; 1994. p. 252.

58. Lazare A, Levy RS. Apologizing for humiliations in medical practice. Chest. 2011;139:746–51.

59. Wald HS, Borkan JM, Taylor JS, Anthony D, Reis SP. Fostering and evaluating reflective capacity in medical education: developing the REFLECT rubric for assessing reflective writing. Acad Med. 2012;87:41–50.

60. Quirk ME. Intuition and metacognition in medical education: keys to developing expertise. New York: Springer; 2006. p. 151.

61. Inui TS, Cottingham AH, Frankel RM, Litzelman DK, Suchman AL, Williamson PR. Supporting teaching and learning of professionalism—changing the educational environment and students' navigational skills. In: Cruess RL, Cruess SR, Steinert Y, editors. Teaching medical professionalism. New York: Cambridge; 2009. p. 108–23.

62. Bonavitacola P. Buttered toast (unpublished poem). Medical Student at University of Massachusetts School of Medicine; 2013.

63. Ginsburg S, Regehr G, Lingard L. The disavowed curriculum: understanding student's reasoning in professionally challenging situations. J Gen Intern Med. 2003;18:1015–22.

64. Croskerry P. The importance of cognitive errors in diagnosis and strategies to minimize them. Acad Med. 2003;78:775–80.

65. Williams CW. The use of force. In: Williams CW, Coles R, editors. The doctor stories. New York: New Directions; 1984.

66. A piece of my mind. It's over, Debbie. JAMA. 1988;259:272.

67. Lowenstein J. Can you teach compassion? In: Coles R, Testa R, editors. A life in medicine: a literary anthology. New York: New Press; 2002.

68. Fisher WR. Narration as a human communication paradigm: the case of public moral argument. Commun Monogr. 1984;51:1–22.

69. Murdoch-Eaton D, Sandars J. Reflection: moving from mandatory ritual to meaningful professional development. J Arch Dis Child. 2014;99:279–83.

70. Aronson L. Twelve tips for teaching reflection at all levels of medical education. Med Teach. 2011;33:200–5.

71. Aronson L, Niehaus B, DeVries CD, Siegel JR, O'Sullivan PS. Do writing and storytelling skill influence assessment of reflective ability in medical students' written reflections? Acad Med. 2010;85:S29–32.

72. Learman LA, Autry AM, O'Sullivan P. Reliability and validity of reflection exercises for obstetrics and gynecology residents. Am J Obstet Gynecol. 2008;198(461):e1–8.

73. Moniz T, Arntfield S, Miller K, Lingard L, Watling C, Regehr G. Considerations in the use of reflective writing for student assessment: issues of reliability and validity. Med Educ. 2015;49:901–8.

74. Grierson L, Winemaker S, Taniguchi A, Howard M, Marshall D, Zazulak J. The reliability characteristics of the REFLECT rubric for assessing reflective capacity through expressive writing assignments: a replication study. Perspect Med Educ. 2020;9:281–5.

75. Konopasek L, Norcini J, Krupat E. Focusing on the formative: building an assessment system aimed at student growth and development. Acad Med. 2016;91:1492–7.

76. Buckley S, Coleman J, Davison I, Khan K, Zamora J, Malick S, Morley D, Pollard D, Ashcroft T, Popovic C, Sayers J. The educational effects of portfolios on undergraduate student learning: a Best Evidence Medical Education (BEME) systematic review. BEME Guide No. 11. Med Teach. 2009;4: 282–98.

77. Sim SM, Lai J, Aubrecht K, et al. CIHR health system impact fellows: reflections on "driving change" within the health system. Int J Health Policy Manag. 2019;8(6):325–8.

78. Taylor MJ, McNicholas C, Nicolay C, Darzi A, Bell D, Reed JE. Systematic review of the application of the plan-do-study-act method to improve quality in healthcare. BMJ Qual Saf. 2014;23(4):290–8.

79. Smith RC, Dwamena FC, Fortin VIAH. Teaching personal awareness. J Gen Intern Med. 2005;20: 201–7.

80. Mann K, Gordon J, MacLeod A. Reflection and reflective practice in health professions education: a systematic review. Adv Health Sci Educ Theory Pract. 2009;14(4):595–621.

81. Misra-Hebert AD, Isaacson JH, Kohn M, Hull AL, Hojat M, Papp KK, Calabrese L. Improving empathy of physicians through guided reflective writing. Int J Med Educ. 2012;3:71–7.

82. Moulton CA, Regehr G, Lingard L, Merritt C, MacRae H. Slowing down to stay out of trouble in the operating room: remaining attentive in automaticity. Acad Med. 2010;85:1571–7.

Remediation Through the Lens of Systems-Based Practice and Practice-Based Learning and Improvement

16

Kelly Williamson, Peter Moffett, and Cedric Lefebvre

Introduction

Even when learners' clinical knowledge and skills are strong, some are challenged when needing to apply this competence in the context of the healthcare system. For instance, trainees may struggle to incorporate patient safety measures into daily practice, work well within interprofessional teams, or use the electronic medical record effectively.

Systems-based practice (SBP) is broadly defined by the Accreditation Council for Graduate Medical Education (ACGME) as "an awareness of and responsiveness to the larger context and system of health care," which includes effectively calling on resources to provide optimal care [1]. Concepts such as considering costs and social determinants of health as well as working to identify and remedy quality-of-care concerns at the systems level are all a part of the domain of

K. Williamson (✉)
Department of Emergency Medicine, Northwestern University, Chicago, IL, USA
e-mail: margaret.williamson@northwestern.edu

P. Moffett
Department of Emergency Medicine, Virginia Commonwealth University, Richmond, VA, USA
e-mail: peter.moffett@vcuhealth.org

C. Lefebvre
Department of Emergency Medicine, Wake Forest University School of Medicine, Winston-Salem, NC, USA
e-mail: clefebvr@wakehealth.edu

SBP. On the other hand, the ACGME defines practice-based learning and improvement (PBLI) as "the ability to investigate and evaluate their care of patients" [1]. This includes using scientific evidence and technology to improve the care of patients as well as being self-reflective and responsive to feedback. Learners may struggle with either competency or with both as they begin to find their place in the healthcare system.

> *As an emergency department attending, you receive a report from your cardiology colleagues that a new intern, Adam (he/ him), deviated from established care algorithms for the management of patients with chest pain. Adam vociferously insisted that a patient with low-risk chest pain be admitted to the inpatient service and undergo a cardiac MRI study. Despite Adam's advocacy for admission of the patient, both requests were denied. It is unusual in your experience for an intern to behave this way. You decide to have a talk with Adam, who you know to be a very capable intern in most situations.*

As with other chapters in this section, we refer to the framework from Chap. 6 to organize the approach to learners like Adam who struggle with SBP or PBLI. While we developed this approach with emergency medicine residents, we believe it is easily generalizable to all health professions learners.

Identification

Learners needing guidance in SBP and PBLI come to the attention of faculty and program leadership in several different ways. As with Adam's example above, diagnostic or treatment plans that do not correspond to standards of care may signal a potential deficit in these competency domains. Other common examples include recurrent "near-miss" safety events, over-ordering diagnostic testing, and struggles with handoffs to colleagues. We will walk through approaches to these examples at the end of the chapter.

Clarification

In Table 16.1, we list possible explanations for Adam's perspective through the lens of SBP and PBLI deficiencies.

Upon examining Adam's file and evaluations from the other rotations, you notice a consistent theme. While Adam has always scored well on standardized tests and clerkship written exams and can answer directed medical knowledge questions, he struggles to apply this knowledge to the clinical care of his patients. Specifically, he struggles to apply clinical decision rules in real-time patient management.

In the first meeting, Adam tells you that he was trying to do the "best and safest thing for the patient" and that "this would never have happened" where he went to medical school. You make certain to hear his intentions and explore his underlying emotions.

You further learn that Adam is aware of the challenges noted on several of his evaluations. Because he had performed well in medical school clerkships, he had not anticipated any problems adjusting to residency, so he is disappointed. He is unsure how to prepare for his rotations and lacks a strategy to identify appropriate resources, such as peer-reviewed evidence-based medicine compilations and well-vetted free open-access medical education (FOAM) resources.

You let Adam know that he has an excellent fund of medical knowledge but at times struggles to translate this to the clinical care of patients. You ask Adam to describe times when he was able to successfully apply current evidence to his practice. You point out these successes as a place from which to build consistent clinical learning and adaptability approaches [2].

Table 16.1 Potential causes for challenges in SBP and PBLI

1. Lack of adaptability to new practice settings and local practice standards (SBP)
   (a) Inattentiveness to local policies and procedures. Failure to review or recall orientation documents and available resources
   (b) Lack of experience with adapting to different practice settings
2. Inflexibility in adopting new practice styles or patterns (PBLI)
   (a) Unwillingness to modify practice style
   (b) Difficulty adapting to new ways of doing things
3. Poor management of knowledge base and clinical experience (SBP and PBLI)
   (a) Failure to recognize knowledge gaps
   (b) Overconfidence in existing knowledge and/or clinical experience
   (c) Low self-confidence or embarrassment about knowledge gaps; fear of admitting/revealing inadequate knowledge or experience

Intervention

Learners like Adam clearly benefit from direct observation of both patient encounters and other aspects of workflow to provide the most appropriate feedback to support his remediation. Learners should identify areas for improvement before the direct observation and then again after the observation period. During the feedback conversations, learners should be given the opportunity to reflect upon what they did effectively, focusing first on the self-identified areas (see Chap. 6). This not only allows the educator to emphasize effective feedback but also promotes self-reflection and thereby provides tools for ongoing PBLI.

It is essential that feedback to a learner be both specific and based upon objective data. Multisource feedback is the most helpful as it may reveal different reasons as to why the learner is struggling.

Several methods can equip the learner with experiential tools during their SBP and PBLI remediation

1. **Simulation:** For learners struggling to work within an interprofessional team, a particular SBP area of focus and creation of a multidisciplinary simulation allow for direct observation and feedback [3–5].
2. **Patient encounters:** Developing a habit of obtaining patient follow-up enhances a learner's understanding of care coordination while ensuring patient safety and quality improvement. Learners should be coached to create follow-up logs and call patients after clinic visits, or discharge from the emergency department or hospital to discuss their ongoing care and review those logs with the coach [3].
3. **Departmental continuous quality improvement (QI) and other system processes:** Since almost all practices engage in formal CQI, a learner should

be encouraged to submit a case for review. Highlighting areas of improvement identified by others, and teaching the learner to identify these areas independently, can aid the learner in framing how they approach their own patient care. It may also help the learner to spend time with the department's billing and coding team. By identifying necessary components of the medical record, the exercise will help the learner frame their clinical encounters to gain this information. Finally, it may be helpful for the learner to work with a medicolegal expert to identify common pitfalls in both patient care and documentation [3].

4. **Self-assessment and reflection:** This can take several forms. As discussed with Adam, debriefing after a clinic day or emergency department shift allows the learner an opportunity for self-reflection that then gives the remediation coach an opportunity to give directed feedback. Another approach is asking the learner to write their own one-page letter of recommendation. This process engages the learner in a self-reflection process that allows them to identify perceived areas of both strengths and weaknesses. Then, the mentor can review these self-reflection exercises with the learner, give specific feedback, and help the learner deepen their capacity for self-analysis.

The competencies of SBP and PBLI encompass many domains, ranging from use of evidence-based medicine and teaching style to patient safety and quality improvement and use of technology within one's medical practice. For this reason, it is important for the learner to actively participate in creating a personal remediation plan that defines objective and achievable goals for the remediation process [6]. As with all remediation processes, program leadership (and often core faculty educator colleagues) must monitor learner progress and strict adherence to the plan.

Assessment

You continue to meet with Adam twice a month for 3 months. During this time, his evaluations begin to improve, and several faculty colleagues have noted that he is making appropriate clinical decisions in the care of his patients and applying his medical fund of knowledge well. Adam feels re-energized on his clinical rotations and continues to study to further improve his performance. In your final scheduled meeting with Adam, you highlight his achievements and recommend continued attention to this learning plan to optimize future success.

Adapting the Approach to Specific Circumstances

Learners Who Have Had Several "Near-Miss" Safety Events

Susan (she/her) is a second-year surgery resident. She is well-liked by her colleagues, and her medical knowledge is deemed to be appropriate based on her clinical performance. However, she seems to have difficulty multitasking, and several nurses have entered patient safety reports concerning "near-miss" safety events. In one instance, she ordered 100 μg of fentanyl on the wrong patient. In another instance, she ordered a medication that a patient had an allergy to. In both instances, the nursing team caught the error before it reached the patient. However, her program director is concerned about this emerging pattern.

A "near-miss" safety event is defined by the World Health Organization as "an error that has the potential to cause an adverse event (patient harm) but fails to do so because of chance or because it is intercepted" [7]. As described in our case, examples of "near-miss" safety events include an incorrect medication order that is caught by a nurse or entering an order for a diagnostic test on an incorrect patient. Involved learners may see each individual event as an isolated incident without a clear understanding of how these reflect an underlying pattern or process problem. It is imperative that the coach respectfully push through the learner's inability to recognize patterns. This is critical to ensuring patient safety and quality (SBP competency) as well as the ability to self-assess and form a learning plan (PBLI).

We recommend that, after making an effort to establish a psychologically safe relationship where difficult issues can be discussed and introducing the discussion of "near-misses," the assigned coach asks the learner to describe how the situation compares with similar cases and analyze why this safety event occurred.

Coach: *You've done this well before. Can you highlight any themes in your near-miss cases that are different than the times you've been successful?* [Clarification phase]
Learner: *No. Each of these cases is totally different. In the first case …* (goes on to detail all of the individual cases).
Coach: *I can see how they each seem unique to you. I think that sometimes it is easier for an outside observer to identify patterns.* [Intervention phase:] *I'd like you to go to two of our departmental quality meetings and help with a root cause analysis of at least two cases. Then we can meet to see what patterns you see in departmental quality cases.*

Reviewing cases from other providers helps learners appreciate that others make similar mistakes. This process also gives them a broader appreciation for common processes involved in medical errors. After reviewing several cases from others, the learner can be directed back to their cases to see if they can identify and correct similar errors in their own practice.

Learner Who Frequently Over-Orders Diagnostic Testing

John (he/him) is a first-year OB/GYN resident. His clinical preceptors have noticed that he routinely orders abdominal labs, cardiac markers, d-dimers, and chest X-rays on pregnant patients in their first and second trimesters presenting to clinic for their routine OB appointments.

Learners who struggle to apply evidence-based medicine to the clinical realm or have difficulty applying clinical decision rules to their practice may need PBLI remediation. While some learners may identify as "risk-averse," others may have difficulty synthesizing information obtained in a clinical history. It is essential to aid learners in balancing the need to provide reassurance of the absence of serious pathology with the over-ordering of tests, given its association with increased healthcare costs, the implications of false-positive testing, and false reassurance of patients [8, 9]. Understanding these as problems with SBP (economics and resource utilization, and patient safety and quality) may help coaches and learners find an effective path to remediation. While the reasons for over-ordering can be complex, the learner can be coached to curb the practice.

Coach: *I've noticed that you seem to order more tests than others at your stage. I'm curious about your reactions to my saying that.* [Clarification phase]
Learner: *I'm afraid of being sued so I need to make sure of every diagnosis before I discharge the patient.*
Coach: *It makes sense that we want to strive for certainty in our encounters.* [Intervention phase:] *I wonder if you are familiar with evidence-based decision aids and the "Choosing Wisely" campaign* [10] *that are designed to help clinicians feel more comfortable not ordering tests.*

Learner: *Yes, I know of them, but I feel like those do not always help the individual patients. They only help on a population level. I'm concerned about missing something in my patient.*
Coach: *I really appreciate your concern for your patients. We should also probably explore together the ways that over-testing can harm the individual patient. Why don't we look up the costs of some of those tests we are ordering, as well as the potential implications of false positive test results for the patients and for health care costs?*

The learner should be directed to evaluate and summarize in writing their care of a particular patient in the context of the system and reflect on how their practices can cause harm. It may also be beneficial for the resident to meet with a faculty member who is expert at applying the principles of evidence-based medicine to clinical practice. The resident may also benefit from performing follow-up logs of their patients to help the resident understand the relative trade-offs embedded in extensive workups [11].

Learner Struggles with Handoffs to Colleagues

Ben (he/him) is a third-year pediatrics resident. His chief resident approached the program director as she had received several complaints from Ben's co-residents that he was omitting pertinent details about the status of patient care, their diagnostic workups, and current medications during nightly hospital patient sign-out.

Transitions of care have been recognized as one of the most dangerous times in patient care [12] and are a major focus of patient care improvement as highlighted by the US Agency for Health Research and Quality [13]. Yet, many learners struggle with patient handoffs.

> **Coach**: *(After eliciting a few instances of faulty handoffs) Can you identify a common theme in your patient handoffs?*
> **Learner:** *I find that when I start talking about the case, I forget a lot of the important points and get lost in some of the details. I don't use any standard handoff tool because I find them challenging, it just isn't the way I think.*
> **Coach:** *That happens to all of us. [Intervention:] Let's pick a structured handoff tool and try to use it for your next few handoffs; then we will have a better sense of why using the tools is challenging for you and see if we can make adjustments to make it work.*

There are a variety of structured handoff tools available, such as Situation, Background, Assessment, Recommendation (SBAR), and the reader should consult their own hospital policy or professional society websites for suggestions specific to their area of training. There is a growing literature on training novice clinicians to perform high-quality handoffs [14]. After ensuring that the learner can utilize a structured handoff tool, they should be observed several times by faculty and other learners to ensure consistency and quality.

Conclusion

The recognition and remediation of learners struggling to achieve proficiency in the SBP and PBLI subcompetencies improves learner education and clinical care delivered to patients. Remediation itself can be a challenging process, but using a structured approach and a repertoire of strategies tailored to the individual learner's needs can lead to significant improvements in this area.

References

1. Accreditation Council for Graduate Medical Education, Common Program Requirements. https://acgme.org/What-We-Do/Accreditation/Common-Program-Requirements/. Accessed 29 Dec 2022.
2. Cooperrider DL, Whitney D. Appreciative inquiry: a positive revolution in change. San Francisco: Berrett-Koehler Publishers; 2005.
3. Williamson K, Moreira M, Quattromani E, Smith JL. Remediation strategies for systems-based practice and practice-based learning and improvement milestones. J Grad Med Educ. 2017;9:290–3.
4. Nadir N, Hart D, Cassara M, et al. Simulation-based remediation in emergency medicine residency training: a consensus study. West J Emerg Med. 2019;20:145–56.
5. Wilson S, Vorvick L. Dyspnea in a hospitalized patient: using simulation to introduce interprofessional collaborative practice concepts. MedEdPORTAL. 2016;12:10488.
6. Katz ED, Dahms R, Sadosty AT, Stahmer SA, Goyal D, CORD-EM Remediation Task Force. Guiding principles for resident remediation: recommendations of the CORD remediation task force. Acad Emerg Med. 2010;17:S95–103.
7. Larizgoitia I, Bouesseau M-C, Kelley E. WHO efforts to promote reporting of adverse events and global learning. J Public Health Res. 2013;2:e29.
8. Epner PL, Gans JE, Graber ML. When diagnostic testing leads to harm: a new outcomes-based approach for laboratory medicine. BMJ Qual Saf. 2013;22:ii6–ii10.
9. Greenberg J, Green JB. Over-testing: why more is not better. Am J Med. 2014;127:362–3.
10. https://www.choosingwisely.org. Accessed 22 Dec 2022.
11. Williamson K, Quattromani E, Aldeen A. The problem resident behavior guide. Intern Emerg Med. 2016;11:437–49.
12. https://www.acep.org/globalassets/uploads/uploaded-files/acep/membership/sections-of-membership/qips/toolbox/safer-sign-out-presentation.pdf. Accessed 29 Dec 2022.
13. https://www.ahrq.gov/topics/transitions-care.html Accessed 29 Dec 2022.
14. Gordon M, Hill E, Stojan JN, Daniel M. Educational interventions to improve handover in health care: an updated systematic review. Acad Med. 2018;93:1234–44.

Part III

Special Topics

Learning Differences and Medical Education

Antoinette Schoenthaler and Paul Yellin

"Although decisions about disabilities and accommodations must be made on a case-by-case basis, determinations ... should be underscored by some fundamental vision of what it means to be a physician ... **our real goal is to provide accommodations to otherwise qualified students so that they can become competent and socially committed clinicians**" [1].

One November, we received a call from the Associate Dean for Student Affairs, who was concerned about a first-year student, Sandy (she/her), who failed three of the first six examinations and passed the other three by uncomfortably narrow margins. Several weeks later, Sandy arrived for a consultation, wearing a white coat and appearing poised and professional. Her excellent interpersonal and verbal skills were evident. She said, "Listen, nothing personal, but I must tell you that I was mortified when Dr. Ovid suggested that I call your office. I mean, to think that I could have a learning disability ... I put off coming. I was pretty sure that I was going to pass the next test. Wrong again. Here I am."

Sandy attended public schools and excelled, always participating in the "Gifted and Talented Program" and qualifying for the magnet high school with participation in a special "gateway to medicine program." As a competitive athlete and high school valedictorian, she was accepted to a highly regarded college and continued to excel. Looking back, Sandy noted, "I never had any difficulties. Through high school, I did my work, but I never really had to study very much. I could just pay

A. Schoenthaler
Department of Population Health, New York University Grossman School of Medicine, New York, NY, USA

Department of Medicine, New York University Grossman School of Medicine, New York, NY, USA
e-mail: Antoinette.Schoenthaler@nyulangone.org

P. Yellin (✉)
Department of Pediatrics, New York University Grossman School of Medicine, New York, NY, USA

Yellin Center for Mind, Brain, and Education, New York, NY, USA
e-mail: pyellin@yellincenter.com

attention and remember. Just to be safe, I would read over my notes before tests. Even when I didn't remember something on the test, I could almost always figure it out." College was not much different. Asked about reading, Sandy acknowledged rarely reading for pleasure and avoiding college courses with extensive reading lists, saying, "I wouldn't say it's a problem, but I've never considered myself the fastest reader."

Since starting medical school, though, everything has been a struggle. There is "so much information and barely enough time to get through it all. I wake up at least an hour before class in the morning to study, go to class, study as soon as I get home, break for dinner, and then study until I pretty much pass out." When asked to describe her approach to work, Sandy goes to class and writes down everything possible but often finds that on rereading notes at the end of the day, it is like encountering the information for the first time. Each evening, Sandy rewatches the video-recorded lectures, stopping frequently to annotate. As tests approach, Sandy rewrites all the notes and then rereads them several times.

Sandy acknowledged being perplexed and frustrated. She was studying at least as hard as her classmates, and yet her efforts were not reflected in her performance. Sandy's eyes started to well up, saying, "Maybe I just don't belong in medical school."

Introduction

Have you met this student? Sandy's test scores are discordant with her apparent intellectual capacity and level of effort. With this presentation, there is a high index of suspicion for an underlying learning problem. Still, it is premature to reach any conclusions; all that we know is this student's overall problem, some elements of the history, and informal observations. We might describe the situation as "poor academic performance in a previously successful first-year medical student" with an extensive differential diagnosis. Presuming that we have ruled out significant medical, emotional, systemic, and other concerns and convinced ourselves that the difficulty is specific to learning and academic performance, we need a process for clearly delineating the problem and making a diagnosis. Is this a true "learning disability" or a milder "learning difference"? Is this something that will respond to a conservative approach (i.e., refining study strategies), or will it require a more aggressive one (i.e., accommodations, interventions, and treatment)?

Our goals in this chapter are to:

- Provide a conceptual framework to understand and describe learning variations in health professions trainees
- Describe an approach to academic difficulties
- Share helpful diagnostic tools and processes
- Share specific strategies, approaches, interventions, and accommodations to support learners with learning difficulties.

Our Experience

Since 2003, we have provided consultations and comprehensive evaluations to medical students referred due to concerns about academic performance. Typically, referrals were made only after students had experienced repeated failure or poor performance on National Board of Medical Examiners Shelf Examinations, despite having received some remediation and/or counseling. We describe the common patterns in the learning profiles of the referred students below.

Key Findings from the Analysis of Case Reports and Student Interviews

- The overwhelming majority of students did not report significant academic challenges prior to entering medical school. Most indicated that they had excelled academically without a methodical approach to their studies.
- Overall, the students did not fit a model typical of a student with a learning disability. Most commonly, they gave a history of minor challenges in reading speed, attention, and organization.
- Medical school presented an unprecedented educational stressor. Students found that they needed to devote increasing amounts of time to prepare for standardized multiple-choice exams, struggling with the volume of information, attention control, and their ability to distinguish important from unimportant information.
- Relying almost entirely on their exceptionally strong memories, they did not have a systematic approach to organizing and retrieving information and therefore, despite a great fund of knowledge, performed poorly on exams.
- Students were exhausted, devoting more time to their studies and sacrificing social interaction, sleep, and general health maintenance. Many of these students also reported suffering from mental health problems.

Learning Disabilities vs. Learning Differences

Historically, learning disabilities have been defined as discrepancies between cognitive potential and academic performance. However, this approach assumed that cognitive potential was fixed and measurable, and that academic failure reflected some deficiency on the part of the learner. As neuroscientists increasingly elucidate the cognitive underpinnings of learning processes, a different picture has emerged: there is a wider range of normal developmental variation and greater potential and longer window for neuroplasticity than was previously recognized. Also, minor dysfunctions or relative weaknesses in specific functions are highly prevalent. Based on this emerging understanding, educators can create learning environments that enable more students to succeed. Learning disabilities, then, represent extreme positions along a continuum [2–7].

We use two different perspectives to approach learners who struggle. First, it is important to determine whether the challenges are severe enough to meet the formal definition of a learning disability, where reasonable accommodations are legally required. We call this "looking through an LD lens."

The second perspective is more consistent with our clinical training and the emerging neuroscience. Here, the learner's academic difficulty is considered as a "chief complaint" with a corresponding differential diagnosis; we must help the learner understand why they are having trouble and what they can do to overcome their difficulties. We usually can elucidate these challenges within the context of a profile of strengths and challenges, which becomes the basis for a comprehensive learning plan that will prepare them to become successful, lifelong learners [3, 8, 9]. We call this "looking through a mind, brain, and education lens."

Looking Through an LD Lens

While consensus about definition and diagnostic criteria is elusive, learning disabilities are generally considered as a group of disorders, likely of neurologic origin, characterized by difficulties in acquiring and applying listening, reading, speaking, writing, reasoning, or math skills in the face of normal hearing, vision, intelligence, and conventional instruction. Typically, learning disabilities (Table 17.1) are diagnosed when otherwise able students exhibit disproportionate difficulty in acquiring specific academic skills [4, 5, 10].

Table 17.1 Examples of common diagnoses

There is no universally accepted taxonomy to describe learning disorders. Most learning disorders are categorized based on the academic skill that is problematic. As such, these "diagnoses" frequently resemble chief complaints rather than discrete disorders. The following list includes common diagnoses associated with significant learning challenges:

- Reading disorder (dyslexia)
- Mathematics disorder (dyscalculia)
- Disorder of written expression (dysgraphia)
- Language disorders (receptive and/or expressive)
- Attention deficit/hyperactivity disorder
- Executive function deficit
- Autism spectrum disorder/nonverbal learning disorder (see Chap. 12)

Pursuing a formal diagnosis of a learning disability can provide legal protections and access to accommodations. The label may validate life-long struggles previously dismissed or viewed harshly. In contrast, without perspective on their implications, a new diagnosis of a learning disability can be a very bitter pill to swallow for learners. A learner who identifies themselves as academically successful may find that having a "disability" can be devastating, undermining self-esteem and generating self-doubt and shame. Therefore, those making the diagnosis must be extremely sensitive to these concerns [8, 9] and must contextualize learners' challenges as discrete elements within a broader profile of strengths and challenges, coupled with specific, credible, and feasible strategies to address these challenges. Emphasizing that the "disability" refers to a discrete area of dysfunction (e.g., slow reading) can reassure the learner that it need not impact their ultimate career trajectory.

Hopefully, the learner can emerge from the diagnostic process understanding that this information can help them significantly. One student stated, *"No medical student wants to hear that they have a learning disability. Now, if I knew that the goal was to understand how I learn and identify more effective approaches, I would have come running."*

The Americans with Disabilities Act (ADA) and the Health Professions

Health professions trainees, employees, schools, and hospitals in the USA are all covered by the Americans with Disabilities Act (ADA) [11], most recently amended in 2009 to expand and extend the scope of its coverage and to further its purpose of eliminating discrimination against individuals with disabilities.

> The ADA defines disability as "(a) a physical or mental impairment that substantially limits one or more major life activities of such individual; (b) a record of such an impairment; or (c) being regarded as having such an impairment" [11].

The specific "major life activities" covered by the ADA include basic tasks relevant to health professions education and practice, such as learning, reading, concentrating, thinking, and communicating, as well as such physical tasks as seeing, hearing, standing, and lifting. Furthermore, the statute, only part of which is included here, was not intended to be exhaustive; the meanings of "disability" and "substantially limits" are to be considered broadly. Furthermore, when conditions that are episodic or in remission become active, they become disabilities.

The ADA also specifically notes that the "determination of whether an impairment substantially limits a major life activity shall be made without regard to the ameliorative effects of mitigating measures," which include nearly every conceivable accommodation, behavioral modification, and assistive technology except for eyeglasses [12, 13].

Once past the broad definitions of "disability," we next must examine the obligation of institutions and their employees to accommodate individuals with disabilities. The accommodation process starts with disclosure by the disabled individual of their disability and requirement for accommodation. The institution does not bear responsibility to determine, for example, which of its learners has ADHD or a reading disorder. Further, the institution can require documentation of such disability from a duly qualified professional. The documentation should indicate areas where the individual will require accommodation and the kinds of remedial measures that may help the disabled individual to perform the expected activities. The nature of the disability need not, and usually should not, be disclosed to each supervisor; they simply need to know that the individual will be entitled to receive, for example, extended time on examinations or will have the right to use certain assistive technology while making rounds.

The ADA is clear that a trainee must otherwise meet standards for admission or training; the right to be free from discrimination due to disability is not a free pass for an unqualified individual to gain admission to a program. A "'qualified individual' means an individual who, with or without reasonable accommodation, can perform the essential functions of the … position that such individual holds or desires … Due consideration shall be given to the employer's [or school's] judgment as to what functions of a job are essential, and if [there is] a written description before … interviewing applicants … this description shall be considered evidence of the essential functions of the [position]" [14]. A student whose grades do not meet the general standards for admission to a school need not be admitted, even if impacted by a disability. Nor is it necessary to promote or retain those who are unable to manage the demands required of all learners, if they have been given appropriate accommodations to address their disclosed disabilities.

Appropriate accommodations will differ for each individual. The institution need not implement any accommodation that will cause "undue hardship," defined as an action that causes significant difficulty or expense. So, although modified schedules and job restructuring are all examples included in the statute of potential accommodations, if reducing hours will impact the coverage of a clinical service, it would be considered an undue hardship and will not be required. Still, many accommodations can assist an individual without impacting the nature of their academic or clinical education, including use of handheld reading pens (text-to-speech translators for dyslexia and other reading disorders) and smartpens, which record lectures or rounds and link it to notes in a notebook. Textbooks now have multiple formats, and tablet computers and smartphones can access video demonstrations or active calendars for those with executive function challenges.

Regarding testing: many trainees with reading or attention challenges may simply require additional time or a quiet testing location (or both). Some individuals require more extensive testing support. For example, legal precedent shows that for a learner with both a visual impairment and a learning disability, an institution is required to provide accommodations to "best ensure" that the exam measures not their disabilities but their knowledge of professional responsibility [15–20].

Looking Through a Mind, Brain, and Education Lens

Researchers in the cognitive neurosciences are increasingly elucidating the structural and functional correlates of the components of academic performance and learning. For example, more is known of pathways and processes associated with the acquisition of numeracy and the mechanisms that enable humans to integrate several parts of our primate brains to construct reading pathways [21–25]. What we describe as distinct skills (e.g., reading and math) are made up of multiple components or sub-skills, commonly requiring neurons to acquire functions other than those presumably driven by evolutionary forces. Learning a skill involves developing multiple such sub-skills and then linking them to coordinate their functions. All told, human cognition appears to encompass a complex mosaic of strengths and vulnerabilities that vary greatly between individuals, like fingerprints. However, unlike our fingerprints, our cognitive or neurodevelopmental profiles can change over time [21–28].

The field of mind, brain, and education provides a mechanism for applying this emerging knowledge to educational practice and policy. For example, understanding that reading requires the acquisition of several discrete sub-skills, we now know that "dyslexia" has multiple possible causes. Therefore, not every child with dyslexia responds to the same reading program [10, 27]. Educators can identify specific areas for improvement in individual students and customize interventions accordingly [27, 28]. Because of the wide range of normal variation in developing these sub-skills among "typical learners," an approach called Universal Design for Learning has emerged, acknowledging and addressing this learning diversity by providing multiple means of representation, expression, and engagement [6, 29].

To optimize learning environments, traditional labels (e.g., "gifted," "learning disabled") and standard psychoeducational and neuropsychological assessments (see Table 17.1) will be replaced by an approach that identifies an individual's neurocognitive profile and tailors instruction to maximize expertise development in clearly articulated outcome areas. This shift has already gained traction in general educational domains [6]. While health professions education has developed significant innovations in theory-driven curriculum innovations (e.g., problem-based learning, competency-based assessment), development of individualized learning processes and standardized learning outcomes, necessary for optimal results, has lagged [30]. This is a wide open field of collaborative research agendas for neuroscientists, clinicians, and educators [21, 31–34].

It is beyond the scope of this chapter to describe and explore the relative merits of the numerous taxonomies that have been developed to describe learning variations. Rather, we will describe our approach, based on the conceptual framework and clinical model developed at the All Kinds of Minds Institute, a nonprofit institute affiliated with the University of North Carolina

Table 17.2 Neurodevelopmental constructs and definitions

Attention	Maintaining mental energy for learning and work, absorbing and filtering incoming information, and overseeing the quality of academic output and behavior
Higher order cognition (complex thinking)	Comprehending concepts, generating original ideas, and using logical approaches to address complex problems
Language	Understanding incoming oral and written information and communicating ideas orally and in writing
Memory	Briefly recording new information, mentally juggling information while using it to complete a task , and storing and then recalling information at a later time
Neuromotor functions (controlling movement)	Using large muscles in a coordinated manner, controlling finger and hand movements, and coordinating muscles needed for handwriting
Social cognition (making and keeping friends)	Knowing what to talk about, when, with, whom, and for how long; working and playing with others in a cooperative manner; and nurturing positive relationships with influential people
Spatial ordering (visual thinking)	Understanding information that is presented visually, generating products that are visual, and organizing materials and spaces
Temporal sequential ordering (keeping track of time/ order)	Understanding the order of steps, events or other sequences; generating products arranged in a meaningful order; and organizing time and schedules

School of Medicine [7, 24]. The model facilitates diagnostic specificity by first "task analyzing" each element of academic or clinical performance and then linking them to a series of eight neurodevelopmental functions or constructs. Table 17.2 includes a broad overview of these eight constructs to provide perspective.

In our work with medical students, we have focused on the following six factors:

1. Attention [35, 36]
2. Language [10, 27, 37, 38]
3. Memory [21, 39–45]

4. Temporal-sequential ordering [46–48]
5. Spatial ordering [25, 49, 50]
6. Higher order cognition [51–53]

We can then target our neuropsychological testing and clinical assessment to examine those cognitive functions most relevant to the task at hand.

Reframing Struggles

We last left Sandy on the verge of tears, wondering, "Maybe I don't belong in medical school." She wondered if the results would get back to the medical school, which then might move to dismiss her. I (PY) reminded her that federal law protects personal health information and provides general standards regarding confidentiality. I reassured Sandy that any information that comes out of the assessment will belong to her. In fact, even if the medical school bore the cost for the assessment, nothing could be shared without her consent.

Before beginning an assessment, to mitigate negative impacts on learners' self-perception of being academically "gifted," I typically will say something like, *"You don't know me and have no reason to trust me, but in my extensive experience, the issue of whether or not you belong in medical school is not even on the table."* I explain that learning is more complex and that our learning processes are more dynamic than once believed.

I have been told of a tennis player at the top of his profession despite having a relatively weak backhand. His success is based on his capacity to compensate using self-awareness of his strengths and vulnerabilities to his strategic advantage. He could excel through the early parts of his career without awareness that his backhand was a liability; only when moving to the highest levels of competition will this heightened self-knowledge provide a competitive edge. Similarly, many medical students can succeed through earlier schooling based on their strengths and sheer force of will, without the need for explicit strategies. However, when medical school places unique demands on their cognitive abilities, like the tennis player, they can succeed, but only if they evolve their strategies based on understanding their specific strengths and challenges [54].

When we share a visual representation of the Neurodevelopmental Framework for Learning (NDFL) and reassure Sandy that our goal is to work with her to discover how she learns best, she smiles and is eager to move forward.

Sandy's Assessment

We began our assessment with a structured interview probing her perception of her neurodevelopmental abilities. We discovered that when she studied, she had trouble discerning the most important information; to remember things, she reviewed them many times. In class, she had less difficulty recalling facts, but when taking a test, it took her much longer to remember those same things. She could not identify strategies to facilitate remembering what she was learning. When studying, she made detailed diagrams, added notes, and then repeatedly reviewed the diagrams and notes.

Three assessment instruments yielded important information. The Wide Range Assessment of Memory and Learning includes a Story Memory subtest where she summarized two narrative passages immediately after hearing them. After a delay, she retold the stories before answering multiple-choice questions about specific details in the passages. We then asked Sandy whether she did anything to help remember the stories as she was listening. She described focusing on individual details that she thought important (e.g., character names, important numbers, other facts) and then attempted to reconstruct a narrative around them. She took advantage of her superb reasoning and logical think-

ing capacity to recall the critical elements of the narrative. However, her summaries omitted important details. She answered multiple-choice questions more successfully, suggesting that she had stored more information than she had been able to access.

On the Rey-Osterrieth Complex Figure Test and Recognition Trial, Sandy first copied a complex figure that consisted of a large rectangle with various subdivisions, internal details, and shapes on the external surface. Rather than first copying the rectangle, subdividing it, and then placing the various components within this larger structure, she drew four separate rectangles adjacent to each other and then added details line-by-line and chunk-by-chunk. While her initial copy was accurate, when she attempted to draw the figure from memory, after a brief delay, she sighed. She again approached the task in a piecemeal fashion, struggling to recall many of the details and where to place them. When asked to draw the figure after a longer delay, she recalled even fewer details. However, on the recognition trial, in which she was asked to scan an array of 24 geometric shapes (12 of which had been included in the original figure and 12 looked like they might have been but were not) and circle the 12 that had been part of the original figure, she correctly identified 22 of the 24 figures. Once again, she demonstrated that she had stored much more information than she had been able to access or organize.

Providing further insight, the Reading Comprehension subtest of the Scholastic Abilities Test for Adults (SATA) is a challenging reading assessment commensurate with the high level of complexity and density typical of medical text. Sandy was correct on most of her responses but completed only one-half of the items in the standard allotted time, placing her reading comprehension at the 50th percentile for her age. With 50% increased time, her performance reached the 95th percentile, which was more consistent with her otherwise superior verbal skills. In direct observation and interview, we learned that she had to reread each passage more than once and then still had to look back to find the answers to many of the questions. She also found herself agonizing over each question, able to eliminate all but two choices and then finding herself going back and forth between the last two choices.

Synthesis

Sandy's challenges were primarily limited to two aspects of attention, common sources of difficulties for medical students: saliency determination and processing depth. She also had a limited repertoire of strategies for encoding information in her long-term memory (i.e., creating stable, accessible representations of information and processes). We could now provide her with strategies that would fit her learning profile better than the approaches she had been using.

Saliency Determination and Processing Depth

Saliency determination refers to the ability to distinguish between important and less relevant information. Students rely on saliency determination to prioritize when studying and to avoid becoming overwhelmed by the sheer volume of information. Saliency determination is also important for managing multiple-choice questions (i.e., comparing the relative merits of each choice) and for organization (i.e., discarding unnecessary materials to avoid becoming bogged down in clutter). Health professions students with weak saliency determination, like Sandy, often find examinations particularly difficult because clinical vignettes include extraneous details, and differences between the best response and the next-best choice are often subtle.

Processing depth refers to the intensity with which we attend to specific details. As with a camera's telephoto lens, we can process information deeply and focus intently on specific details to imprint them for optimal understanding and memory. We can also process information more superficially, as with a wide-angle lens, to appreciate the bigger picture and overarching themes. Saliency determination plays a critical role in regulating processing depth, enabling us to identify the main idea (i.e., overarching themes, the big picture), the most relevant details, and the linkages among all these elements (i.e., part-to-whole processing). We are continuously adjusting our processing depth so that we can see how all the elements relate to each other. Sandy struggled with this process of moving between detail (processing deeply) and big picture (processing superficially). She missed important details in her readings, required repetition to fully process what she read or heard, or made minor errors on her examinations.

At times, Sandy glossed over details and did not notice important pieces of information, misread questions, or made minor errors in her responses (processing depth). When Sandy did attend to details, she tended to process them individually, without fully appreciating how they related to each other or to the big picture. This tendency is called "bottom-up" processing.

Memory Strategies and Bottom-Up Processing

Over the course of our assessment, Sandy approached memory tasks without first developing an effective strategy. Her bottom-up approach made studying challenging for her. Without a stable infrastructure for linking stored information, Sandy had difficulty retrieving what she stored when taking examinations or presenting in class or on rounds, particularly in high-stakes settings where she felt anxious. Mentally organizing details and linking them to each other and to the bigger picture before encoding the information would help her feel less overwhelmed and process details more deeply, specifically, accurately, and efficiently.

Encoding details individually is like storing individual pieces of information on a computer's hard drive without organizing or cataloging them. The most effective way to ensure that information is available when needed is to organize it or transform it into larger meaningful "chunks" of information, in "schemas" or "scripts" (see Chap. 9).

Reading and Word Retrieval

Though we have now identified several areas for Sandy's performance challenges, it is important to consider further possible contributors. Reading is an academic skill that consists of numerous sub-skills, including processing visual information on the page, recognizing letters, recalling the sounds associated with each letter and letter combination, mentally holding and blending those sounds in the correct order, efficiently accessing the corresponding word, appreciating the word's meaning in the specific context, and so on. Each of these sub-skills is associated with specific parts of the NDFL.

When Sandy read aloud, her cadence was not smooth but included pauses, false starts, and occasional repetitions. In interviewing her, she shared that words frequently are "on the tip of her tongue," but she cannot recall them. We administered a standardized rapid object naming task; she scored at the 12th percentile. We also probed other elements of her reading processes to satisfy ourselves that her other sub-skills were intact.

Given Sandy's performance at the 50th percentile on reading comprehension, it seems logical that she should be granted extended time for testing, to best ensure that examinations measure her knowledge and abilities rather than her disabilities.

The Assessment Process

Anyone experiencing significant academic difficulties will need to undergo a formal assessment. We will describe the assessment process and some of the common terms.

Psychoeducational Testing

The most administered core assessment is called "psychoeducational testing" and typically includes cognitive and academic testing. The cognitive battery most used in adults is the Wechsler Adult Intelligence Scale-Fourth Edition (WAIS-IV). Other cognitive batteries include the Woodcock-Johnson IV Tests of Cognitive Abilities (WJ-IV Cognitive) and the Stanford-Binet Intelligence Scales-Fifth Edition (SB-5). The most common academic assessment batteries include the Woodcock-Johnson IV Tests of Achievement (WJ-IV Achievement), Wechsler Individual Achievement Test-Fourth Edition (WIAT-4), and the SATA, mentioned above. We also have used the Nelson-Denny Reading Test (NDRT) because it includes a

series of paragraphs, followed by multiple-choice questions that one can administer under standard time constraints as well as with extended time. Therefore, the NDRT can document the need for extended testing time. However, we prefer the Reading Comprehension subtest of the SATA because it includes more questions (60 vs. 38), and the passages tend to be more challenging. We believe that those factors make it more sensitive to subtle reading challenges in adult learners.

Neuropsychological Testing

The next level of assessment is commonly known as neuropsychological testing. Not a specific battery of tests, it includes a broad array of instruments that enable assessment of different cognitive functions, such as language, memory, temporal-sequential ordering, spatial ordering, and higher order cognition. While some clinicians continue to administer multiple, full neuropsychological batteries, we prefer to select specific subtests, as we would select specific blood tests or imaging studies, as we work our way through our "differential diagnosis." In addition to the instruments mentioned above, we typically include portions of the following batteries and questionnaires in our assessments:

- Comprehensive Test of Nonverbal Intelligence—Second Edition
- Delis-Kaplan Executive Function System
- Kaufman Brief Intelligence Tests—Second Edition
- Behavior Rating Inventory for Executive Function-Adult Version (BRIEF-A)
- Adult ADHD Self-Report Scale

However, we often learn as much from informal or structured qualitative observations and interactions as we do from the "results" of the standardized testing. The assessor must have a deep understanding of the NDFL in the context of medical learning and neuropsychological testing. They must link the various components of medical education and individual assessment tasks with the relevant neurodevelopmental constructs. Therefore, even clinicians with significant prior experience in neuropsychological testing typically require several months to master our approach. The assessment also moves beyond problematic functions to provide a complete picture of the student's profile of strengths and challenges as they relate to academic performance, clinical practice, and other relevant functions.

Sharing the Assessment with the Learner

Once elucidated, the profile serves as the anchor for a series of actions that we have found critical to helping students overcome their difficulties: "demystification," sharing a learning plan, and implementing accommodations.

Demystification

In our clinical practice, we refer to the feedback session following assessment as "demystification." Here, we present each element of an individual's learning profile, first their strengths and then their challenges. Each element is contextualized, in terms of the assessment findings supporting our conclusions and within their daily experience. We hope to build metacognition, self-awareness and insight into their own learning processes (see Chap. 4). This process is critical for learners who struggle, particularly those who have never experienced significant academic difficulties in the past.

Here, we typically revisit our tennis player analogy and remind the student that even world-class athletes have stronger aspects of their game than others, and we all have imperfect brains. Most people do not know their specific profile of strengths and challenges. Students who understand their learning profile are in a much better position to choose strategies that fit their kind of mind.

Starting the discussion on the trainee's inevitably highly developed cognitive abilities helps reassure them that previous successes were not illusory and that their intellectual resources are

sufficient for success. Next, identifying a small number of challenges within this larger context of numerous strengths helps them understand that their problems are also real but not insurmountable. This feedback session should occur as soon as possible, optimally on the day of the assessment [1, 3, 8, 9].

Sandy was heartened to hear of the magnitude and number of strengths that she exhibited across many areas, including her higher thinking skills, both receptive and expressive language, memory (short-term, long-term, and active working memory), her ability to process both sequential and spatial information, her interpersonal skills, and her capacity for working for long periods of time (mental work stamina). Her challenges were limited to word retrieval, saliency determination, and processing depth. She also appreciated that her specific attention challenges contributed to her bottom-up processing. These relatively minor challenges were exacerbated by her limited repertoire of strategies for learning, test preparation, and test taking.

Once we shared our findings with Sandy, she realized that her weak word retrieval was also causing problems on inpatient rounds. With a rich vocabulary and extensive fund of knowledge, she was able to express herself most of the time. However, she realized that when she experienced a supervisor as intimidating, she found it difficult to find words quickly enough to respond to questions even though she almost always knew the answers (which is true for many even without specific word retrieval challenges). Once Sandy spoke to her supervisor about her difficulty, he started giving Sandy a moment to organize her thoughts, allowing her to feel less anxious and more articulate when he did ask questions [55, 56].

Learning Plan

After elucidating a student's learning profile, we compose a learning plan, selecting strategies based on a student's profile. Particularly critical is the early implementation of strategies that leverage strengths or external resources to work around an area of weakness. For example, enabling slow readers access to audiobooks or other text-to-speech resources will predictably have an immediate impact on the efficiency and effectiveness of their study sessions.

It is beyond the scope of this chapter to provide an exhaustive overview of the constantly changing landscape of strategies and resources to support clinical learning. In addition, just as we would never write a prescription before making a diagnosis, we are reluctant to make specific recommendations without first elucidating that trainee's profile of strengths and challenges. Nonetheless, there are some resources that are compatible with a wide range of learning profiles. We find ourselves including many of these in our learning plans.

- **The landscape of websites, apps, and other digital tools to support medical learning is continuously changing.** The goal of each is to help learners create stable and readily accessible mental representations of the many concepts, details, and processes they need to learn. We recommend familiarizing themselves with a few and then focusing on the one or two that they find helpful. We list examples below that students have shared with us. (We have no financial interest in any of these resources.)
    - Sites like Picmonic (https://www. picmonic.com/) and Sketchy Medical (https://sketchy.com/) provide highly engaging visual representations of a variety of topics.
    - The Clinical Odyssey website includes exercises that allow students to test their diagnostic ability using simulated clinical cases. For exam-
    ple, Prognosis: Your Diagnosis (clinicalodyssey.com/title/ prognosis-your-diagnosis) includes clinical cases with short, but in-depth analyses of the diagnostic process, as well as a discussion on the specific condition.
    - Resources like Amboss (https:// www.amboss.com/us) and USMLE-Rx (https://www.usmle-rx. com/) provide practice questions linked to different learning tools.
    - Clinical Odyssey (www.prognosisapp.com) allows students to test their diagnostic ability using simulated clinical cases. Each case has a short but in-depth analysis of the diagnostic process, as well as a discussion on the specific condition.
    - Firecracker (https://firecracker.lww. com/) provides customized flash cards and other tools to support clinical learning and test preparation.
- **Many students benefit greatly from learning and utilizing "front-loading" strategies.**
  Front-loading is the process of preparing oneself before engaging in reading or attending a lecture by doing such things as scanning the material for main ideas, salient details, themes, structure, and tone; researching unknown vocabulary; accessing or building background knowledge connected to the topic at hand; and creating or locating related visuals. If available, we encourage students to scan through slides, notes, or other background materials prior to attending lectures. Many of the resources listed above can be used for front-loading as well as for review and test preparation.
- **Many students believe that they need to "study" before taking practice tests.**

However, there is strong evidence that answering questions and taking practice tests, also called retrieval rehearsal, may be more effective than traditional studying strategies [41–44], (Chap. 7).

- **Students whose minds wander or find that they have trouble listening and taking notes** at the same time may want to consider resources like Livescribe or Notability. These tools allow the student to record and digitize entire lectures, so they can be organized.
- **Time management is a significant challenge for many medical students.** Many find the Pomodoro technique in conjunction with the Eisenhower method helpful for organizing time and tasks. The Pomodoro timer is free and available for both iOS and Android devices. It enables users to set a timer for 25 min during which they are prompted to focus on one specific task before taking a short break. The Eisenhower task management method works through apps such as My Effectiveness (Android) or Focus Matrix (iOS) and helps the user categorize tasks as Important/Not Important and Urgent/Not Urgent. In addition to helping students structure their time and avoid distractions, the combination of these apps can help students learn how long tasks typically take them, allowing them to plan more effectively in the future. For more information about the Pomodoro technique, it may be helpful to watch a video at cirillocompany.de/pages/pomodoro-technique.
- **Students who find that they lose large amounts of time on social media or surfing the internet may benefit from tools that help them monitor and manage their digital activity.** RescueTime (https://www.rescuetime.com/) tracks website use and allows users to view how much time they spend on certain websites and can block certain websites for specific increments of time.

Implementing Accommodations

Beyond the legal obligation to provide accommodations for those with diagnosed disabilities, institutions may decide to go further. For example, within the context of the population at large, a reading fluency at the 30th percentile would be considered normal. However, it may not be sufficient for getting through all clinical vignettes and questions on shelf examinations. Therefore, we believe that it would be reasonable to offer extended time for students who might not meet strict criteria for the diagnosis of a disability. Sandy received extended time for medical school examinations, and we encouraged her to apply for accommodations for the USMLE.

Additional Barriers

Attention Deficit Disorder (ADD) and Executive Function Disorder (EFD)

Health professions schools place enormous stress on student's attention and organizational skills. Therefore, some students previously diagnosed with ADHD and/or EFD and having succeeded may experience exacerbation of their challenges during their transition to professional school. In addition, some students are not diagnosed with ADHD and/or EFD until after matriculation [55].

ADHD and EFD may be the primary cause(s) of a student's academic difficulties, or they may be present with other learning problems. Therefore, ADHD and EFD must be part of the differential diagnosis for any student who presents with academic difficulty. Conversely, when students are found to meet diagnostic criteria for either ADHD or EFD, there should be a high index of suspicion for comorbid learning problems [56].

Anxiety and Depression

Nearly half of the students referred to us for academic struggles also presented with varying degrees of anxiety and depression. It is difficult to learn when anxious or depressed. Conversely, students may experience anxiety or depression in response to their academic struggles. Often, they are intimately intertwined and must both be addressed. We believe that it is critical to maintain communication and collaboration between our team and other colleagues caring for our patients. Mental health providers can play a critical role in helping students develop a healthy perspective in understanding their strengths and challenges. In addition, mental health providers frequently tell us that the insights they derived from reading our reports were helpful in their work with our mutual patients.

Faculty and Learner Attitudes and Frustration

Traditional psychoeducational assessments can be expensive and not sufficiently sensitive or specific to identify the most common dysfunctions that undermine performance. Effective interventions are not always readily available and can become quite expensive. Who funds the assessment and remediation is highly variable across schools. However, beyond these real logistical and financial obstacles, the attitudes of faculty, administrators, other students, and students who struggle themselves create the most significant barriers to the effective management of academic difficulties. Recent developments in the mind, brain, and education world rarely find their way into the journals commonly read by health professions faculty. Therefore, many are unaware of the wide range of normal variation in learning processes, the high prevalence of minor dysfunctions even among high performers, the extent and duration of neuroplasticity over the course of adulthood, and the increasing availability of accessible instructional materials. Some may still believe that learning differences and disabilities are synonymous with intellectual disabilities and therefore

are inconsistent with safe clinical practice. Some continue to see learning challenges as "problems of motivation."

We have also encountered faculty members and students who "intellectually" understand the various bases of learning variations but continue to believe that providing support or accommodations affords an unfair advantage to students with disabilities or enables otherwise unfit physicians to practice medicine. This is emphatically untrue. When applied appropriately, academic support and accommodations level the playing field by removing arbitrary barriers that might prevent otherwise qualified students from accessing the curriculum and acquiring and demonstrating requisite knowledge and skill. At a minimum, faculty members have both a legal and moral obligation to provide reasonable accommodations to medical students with diagnosed learning disabilities. Effective teaching also requires faculty members to understand the high prevalence of low-intensity learning variations that prevent many students from fully accessing the curriculum and participating in assessments that provide an accurate measure of their knowledge and skills. With this understanding, they can embed more inclusive educational strategies in their instruction (e.g., allowing students to access videos, PowerPoint slides, and practice questions in advance of their lectures), ensure that students have reasonable opportunities to demonstrate their knowledge and skills, and help them choose among the increasing number of resources available to support medical learning.

Conclusion

We have provided a conceptual framework and vocabulary for understanding and describing the wide range of normal variations in cognitive abilities in all students. We have listed the important parameters that describe when learning variations become "disabilities" within the context of the Americans with Disabilities Act (ADA) and the legal obligations when working with students with diagnosed disabilities. We have also provided potential ways of appreciating each student's unique profile of strengths and challenges and integrating that understanding into approaches to education and assessment. Finally, for those working more actively with struggling students, either in the diagnostic process or in providing ongoing support, we have provided practical advice to add effectiveness in this work.

References

1. Hafferty FW, Gibson GG. Learning disabilities and the meaning of medical education. Acad Med. 2001;76:1027–31.
2. Butterworth B, Kovas Y. Understanding neurocognitive developmental disorders can improve education for all. Science. 2013;340(6130):300–5. https://doi.org/10.1126/science.1231022.
3. Dweck CS. Mindset: the new psychology of success. New York: Random House; 2006. 276 p.
4. Francis DJ, Fletcher JM, Stuebing KK, Lyon GR, Shaywitz BA, Shaywitz SE. Psychometric approaches to the identification of LD: IQ and achievement scores are not sufficient. J Learn Disabil. 2005;38(2):98–108. PubMed PMID: 15813593.
5. Kavale KA, Forness SR. What definitions of learning disability say and don't say: a critical analysis. J Learn Disabil. 2000;33(3):239–56. https://doi.org/10.1177/002221940003300303.
6. Rose DH, Meyer A, Strangman N, Rappolt G. Teaching every student in the digital age: universal design for learning. Alexandria: Association for Supervision and Curriculum Design (ASCD); 2002. 216 p.
7. Levine MD. Developmental variation and learning disorders. 2nd ed. Cambridge: Educators Publishing Service; 2001. 671 p.
8. Griffin E, Pollack D. Student experiences of neurodiversity in higher education: insights from the BRAINHE project. Dyslexia. 2009;15(1):23–41. https://doi.org/10.1002/dys.383.
9. Hall CW, Webster RE. Metacognitive and affective factors of college students with and without learning disabilities. J Postsecond Educ. 2008;21(1):32–41.
10. Aaron PG, Joshi RM, Gooden R, Bentum KE. Diagnosis and treatment of reading disabilities based on the component model of reading: an alternative to the discrepancy model of LD. J Learn Dis. 2008;41:67–84. https://doi.org/10.1177/0022219407310838.
11. Americans with Disabilities Act (ADA) of 1990, 42 U.S.C. Annotated, Sect. 12101 et seq.
12. 154 Cong Rec. S.8840-01 (daily ed. Sep 16, 2008) (Statement of Managers-S 3460).
13. Americans with Disabilities Act (ADA) of 1990, 42 U.S.C. Annotated, Sect. 12102.
14. Americans with Disabilities Act (ADA) of 1990, 42 U.S.C Annotated, Sect. 12111(8).
15. 28 Code of Federal Regulations Section 36.309.
16. Bagenstos SR. Technical standards and lawsuits involving accommodations for health professions students. AMA J Ethics. 2016;18:1010–6.
17. Bernstein S, Atkinson AR, Martimianakis MA. Diagnosing the learner in difficulty. Pediatrics. 2013;132:210–2.
18. Francis L, Silvers A. Perspectives on the meaning of "disability". AMA J Ethics. 2016;18:1025–33.
19. Meeks LM, Jain NR, Moreland C, Taylor N, Brookman JC, Fitzsimons M. Realizing a diverse and inclusive workforce: equal access for residents with disabilities. J Grad Med Educ. 2019;11:498–503.
20. Romberg F, Shaywitz BA, Shaywitz SE. How should medical schools respond to students with dyslexia? AMA J Ethics. 2016;18:975–85.
21. Ansari D, De Smedt B, Grabner RH. Neuroeducation—a critical overview of an emerging field. Neuroethics. 2012;5:105–17. https://doi.org/10.1007/s12152-011-9119-3.
22. Dehaene S. Reading in the brain. New York: Penguin Group; 2009. 388 p.
23. Dehaene S, Pegado F, Braga LW, Ventura P, Nunes Filho G, Jobert A, Dehaene-Lambertz G, Kolinsky R, Morais J, Cohen L. How learning to read changes the cortical networks for vision and language. Science. 2010;330(6009):1359–64. https://doi.org/10.1126/science.1194140.
24. Amalric M, Dehaene S. A distinct cortical network for mathematical knowledge in the human brain. Neuroimage. 2019;189:19–31.

25. Matejko A, Ansari A. Shared neural circuits for visuo-spatial working memory and arithmetic in children and adults. J Cogn Neurosci. 2021;33:1003–19.

26. Kirchoff BA, Buckner RL. Functional-anatomic correlates of individual differences in memory. Neuron. 2006;51(2):263–74. PubMed PMID: 16846860.

27. Heim S, Tschierse J, Amunts K, Wilms M, Vossel S, Willmes K, Grabowska A, Huber W. Cognitive subtypes of dyslexia. Acta Neurobiol Exp. 2008;68(1):73–82.

28. Shaywitz BA, Shaywitz SE, Blachman BA, Pugh KR, Fulbright RK, Skudlarski P, Mencl WE, Constable RT, Holahan JM, Marchione KE, Fletcher JM, Lyon GR, Gore JC. Development of left occipitotemporal systems for skilled reading in children after a phonologically-based intervention. Biol Psychiatry. 2004;55(9):926–33. PubMed PMID: 15110736.

29. Rose DH, Dalton B. Learning to read in the digital age. Mind Brain Educ. 2009;3(2):74–83. https://doi.org/10.1111/j.1751-228X.2009.01057.x.

30. Cooke M, Irby DM, O'Brien BC. Educating physicians: a call for reform of medical school and residency. Hoboken: Wiley; 2010. 323 p.

31. Fischer KW. Mind, brain and education: building a scientific groundwork for learning and teaching. Mind Brain Educ. 2009;3(1):3–16. https://doi.org/10.1111/j.1751-228x.2008.01048.x.

32. Fischer KW, Daniel DB. Need for infrastructure to connect research with practice in education. Mind Brain Educ. 2009;3(1):1–2. https://doi.org/10.1111/j.1751-228X.2008.01054.x.

33. Fischer KW, Goswami U, Geake J, Task Force on the Future of Educational Neuroscience. The future of educational neuroscience. Mind Brain Educ. 2010;4:68–80.

34. Ronstadt K, Yellin PB. Linking MBE to clinical practice: a proposal for transdisciplinary collaboration. Mind Brain Educ. 2010;4(3):95–101.

35. Fan J, McCandliss BD, Sommer T, Raz A, Posner MI. Testing the efficiency and independence of attentional networks. J Cogn Neurosic. 2002;14(3):340–7. PubMed PMID: 11970796.

36. Waszak F, Li SC, Hommel B. The development of attentional networks: cross-sectional findings from a life span sample. Dev Psychol. 2010;46(2):337–49. https://doi.org/10.1037/a0018541.

37. Immordino-Yang MH. The stories of Nico and Brooke revisited: toward a cross-disciplinary dialogue about teaching and learning. Mind Brain Educ. 2008;2(2):49–51.

38. MacWhinney B, Snow C. The child language data exchange system: an update. J Child Lang. 1990;17(2):457–72. PubMed PMID: 2380278.

39. Ackerman PL, Beier ME, Boyle MO. Working memory and intelligence: the same or different? Psychol Bull. 2005;131(1):30–60.

40. Legge ELG, Madan CR, Ng ET, Caplan JB. Building a memory palace in minutes: equivalent memory performance using virtual versus conventional environments with the method of loci. Acta Psychol. 2012;141:380–90.

41. Butler AC. Repeated testing produces superior transfer of learning relative to repeated studying. J Exp Psychol Learn Mem Cogn. 2010;36(5):1118–33. https://doi.org/10.1037/a0019902.

42. Deng F, Gluckstein JA, Larsen DP. Student-directed retrieval practice is a predictor of medical licensing examination performance. Perspect Med Educ. 2015;4:308–13.

43. Karpicke JD, Bauernschmidt A. Spaced retrieval: absolute spacing enhancing learning regardless of relative spacing. J Exp Psychol Learn Mem Cogn. 2011;37:1250–7.

44. Ecker UK, Lewandowsky S, Oberauer K, Chee AE. The components of working memory updating: an experimental decomposition and individual differences. J Exp Psychol Learn Mem Cogn. 2010;36(1):170–89. https://doi.org/10.1037/a0017891.

45. Regeher G, Norman GR. Issues in cognitive psychology: implications for professional education. Acad Med. 1996;71(9):988–1001. PubMed PMID: 9125988.

46. Creel SC, Dahan D. The effect of temporal structure of spoken words on paired-associate learning. J Exp Psychol Learn Mem Cogn. 2010;36(1):110–22. https://doi.org/10.1037/a0017527.

47. Dominey PF. A shared system for learning serial and temporal structure of sensori-motor sequences? Evidence from simulation and human experiments. Cogn Brain Res. 1998;6(3):163–72. https://doi.org/10.1016/j.bbr.2011.03.031.

48. Planton S, Dehaene S. Cerebral representation of sequence patterns across multiple presentation formats. Cortex. 2021;145:13–36.

49. Schneps MH, Rose LT, Fischer KW. Visual learning and the brain: implications for dyslexia. Mind Brain Educ. 2007;1(3):128–39.

50. Stull AT, Hegarty M, Mayer RE. Getting a handle on learning anatomy with interactive three-dimensional graphics. J Educ Psychol. 2009;101:803–16.

51. Cole MW, Yarkoni T, Anticevic A, Braver T. Global connectivity of prefrontal cortex predicts cognitive control and intelligence. J Neurosci. 2012;32(26):8988–99. https://doi.org/10.1523/JNEUROSCI.0536-12.2012.

52. Stein Z, Dawson T, Fischer KW. Chapter 10. Redesigning testing: operationalizing the new science of learning. In: Khine MS, Saleh IM, editors. New science of learning-cognition, computers, and collaboration in education. New York: Springer; 2010.

53. West DC, Pomeroy JF, Park JK, Gerstenberger EA, Sandoval J. Critical thinking in graduate medical education: a role for concept mapping assessment? JAMA. 2000;284(9):1105–10. PubMed PMID: 10974689.

54. Sack W, Gale J, Gulati S, Gunther M, Nesheim R, Stoddard F, St. John R. Requesting accommodation for a disability: a telephone survey of American medical schools. J Postsecond Educ Disabil. 2008;20(2):93–9.

55. Liston C, McEwen BS, Casey BJ. Psychosocial stress reversibly disrupts prefrontal processing and attention control. Proc Natl Acad Sci U S A. 2009;106(3):912–7. https://doi.org/10.1073/pnas.0807041106.

56. Brown TE, Reichel PC, Quinlan DM. Executive function impairments in high IQ adults with ADHD. J Atten Disord. 2009;13(2):161–7. https://doi.org/10.1177/1087054708326113.

Trainee Well-Being and Remediation

18

Kendra Moore, Sarah Williams, and Larissa Thomas

Introduction

Caring for patients is a meaningful and rewarding vocation. It is a tremendous privilege to accept patients' secrets, decode their symptoms, heal their ailments, and empower them to change their lives for the better. Yet our professions have also grown more stressful, with increasing productivity expectations, higher documentation and bureaucratic burdens, sicker patients, and rapidly expanding medical knowledge and technology.

Unsurprisingly, then, healthcare professionals are suffering from significant work-related distress [1–3]. Burnout is extremely common: 44% of practicing US physicians reporting at least one symptom of burnout [3], with indications that trainees experience similar or even higher rates of distress [1]. Asking our learners directly about how they are doing, normalizing the distress and stress that accompany training, and listening closely will often reveal well-being challenges.

In this chapter, we will discuss stress and distress in health professions trainees and review common "presentations" of well-being issues. We will then review some of the evidence-based interventions that have been shown to reduce burnout and promote well-being and share our approach to improving well-being for distressed, poorly functioning, or troubled learners. Admittedly, the literature cited in this chapter is physician and United States-centric, as most of the research in this area has focused on American physicians, residents, and medical students. However, we believe that the general principles apply broadly to healthcare trainees. We also recognize that well-being is deeply tied to cultural context, and we look forward to learning more about the well-being of trainees throughout the world.

K. Moore (✉) · L. Thomas
Department of Medicine, University of California, San Francisco, CA, USA
e-mail: kendra.moore@ucsf.edu; larissa.thomas@ucsf.edu

S. Williams
Department of Psychiatry, New York University Grossman School of Medicine, New York, NY, USA

> **Case 1**
>
> *Toward the end of Jim's (he/him/his) intern year, his residency adviser, Marjorie (she/her/hers), asked him to come in for a meeting. She asked him how he was doing with the pressures of intern year and listened to him tell her how tired and discouraged he was. Jim had started residency optimistic and excited but felt more powerless and fatigued the longer the year stretched on. He felt that teams of doctors were torturing patients in the hospital, without attention being paid to quality of life or futility of care. He had worked with so many patients where he felt as if nothing he could do or say would make any impact on their health, because they were experiencing homelessness, repeated trauma, or substance use disorders.*

Influences on Trainee Well-Being

We list three important influences on healthcare professional distress below.

Practical and Emotional Challenges of Early Clinical Experience: As they are beginning to deal with all the daily stresses of being a healthcare worker, trainees encounter, for the first time, many of the most emotionally challenging experiences of healthcare practice, such as witnessing suffering, physical and mental trauma, and challenging ethical dilemmas. Often, trainees face these experiences alone, with few opportunities to share their experiences and emotions in an environment that generally discourages vulnerability.

Personal and Professional Development: Younger trainees also face the central developmental tasks of early adulthood: forming personal and professional identity (see Chap. 13), building healthy relationships, and finding meaning and engagement. Some may also undergo ongoing neurological development, for example, in executive functioning (see Chap. 11). These factors, combined with a lack of control over their daily lives and insufficient time to engage in self-care, can eat away at emotional reserve [4].

Social Determinants of Health: Many trainees, and indeed practicing healthcare professionals, are troubled and frustrated by working in a system where the broad range of caring and sophisticated techniques seem useless in the face of societal problems such as homelessness, discrimination, substance use disorders, lack of access to education and healthcare, and all the other negative social determinants of health.

Presentations of Distress

Pressures on clinicians and trainees can manifest in several ways, ranging from a low-grade, vague unhappiness to clinical psychological problems and competency issues. Such troubles may appear differently in different people: one trainee experiencing burnout may become socially withdrawn, another may become disorganized and inefficient, still another may begin acting disruptively. It is therefore important to identify when something is wrong and how problematic and urgent it is.

> **Box 18.1: Defining Terms**
>
> **Stress**: the body's reaction to a change that requires a physical, mental, or emotional adjustment or response. It is an adaptive response, which may not be experienced as abnormal or upsetting.
>
> **Distress**: a negative stress response that results from being overwhelmed by demands, losses, or perceived threats that generates physical and psychological maladaptation [6].
>
> **Burnout**: a psychological syndrome (not a psychiatric diagnosis) characterized by depersonalization (feelings of cynicism or detachment from one's work), emotional exhaustion, and a diminished sense of personal accomplishment in a professional setting. Engagement, the opposite state, is characterized by energy, involvement, and a feeling of self-efficacy in the workplace.

Driver Dimensions

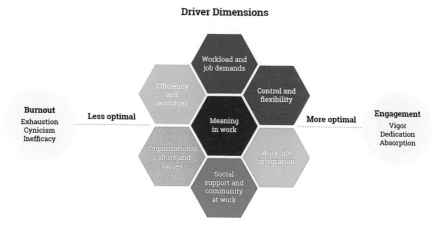

Fig. 18.1 Drivers of burnout. It is important to note that the drivers of burnout are complex and largely out of control of the trainee or health professional; they include individual, team, organizational, and cultural/societal factors, represented in this schema [8]

While *stress* is a normal, and in many cases necessary, growth-promoting aspect of medical training and practice, *distress* is an unhappy, dysfunctional condition that can have a wide variety of physical, psychological, and behavioral consequences, as described below. These consequences do not remain at the individual level: they can translate into significant problems for patients, colleagues, and healthcare systems [5].

Burnout

When Jim spoke about his feelings of powerlessness and fatigue, Marjorie remembered the same feelings during her intern year. In fact, she remembered some of those feelings from her last time on service. She normalized Jim's feelings and shared his despair over the magnitude of factors that affect patients' health that doctors cannot control.

After discussing his feelings, she told him that she was concerned about tasks dropping off his list and his cynical comments on rounds. She wondered if he was experiencing burnout. Jim teared up as he acknowledged that he felt as though he did not have any more to give.

Burnout is a manifestation of the enduring cumulative workplace stressors present in healthcare practice over time and consists of three major components [7]. In addition to its deleterious effects on dedicated clinicians, burnout may associate with, or lead to, other forms of distress, such as depression, suicidality, or alcohol and substance use. Drivers of burnout are delineated in Fig. 18.1.

Burnout and depression can look similar; however, depression usually manifests in all areas of life (see below), whereas burnout is generally confined to reactions, feelings, and behaviors around work, though overlaps occur. Overall, burnout is best conceived as a response to the cumulative effect of workplace factors on the individual, rather than symptoms caused by a psychiatric condition or personal weakness.

Compassion Fatigue

As a result of repeated exposure to traumatized patients, trainees may experience *compassion fatigue*, a state of physical and mental exhaustion caused by a depleted ability to cope with one's everyday environment [9]. Those suffering from compassion fatigue often feel that they have nothing left to give, resulting in existential pain and questioning of their identity and purpose [10].

Work-Life Tension

Excessive workload, limited control over sched-ules and workflows, limited financial resources, and tension between work responsibilities and per-sonal lives can lead to significant stress for train-ees. Personality traits common in healthcare (e.g., perfectionism) can contribute to these challenges.

Presentations Related to Background and Identity

Trainees come to the health professions from all sorts of backgrounds, which may inform their experience of healthcare training and practice. We list some well-being challenges related to trainee identity.

Imposter Syndrome

"Imposter syndrome" is characterized by chronic feelings of self-doubt and fear of being discovered as a fraud. Between 25 and 50% of medical students experience imposter syndrome, with women being twice as likely to face these feelings [11]. Trainees are particularly vulnerable to imposter syndrome at times of transition and uncertainty [12].

Stereotype Threat

Trainees who identify as being part of a social group or background that has been subject to negative stereotypes may feel that they must work harder and perform better to disconfirm those stereotypes. This "stereotype threat" causes stress and anxiety that can impede performance [13]. Individual discussion of performance issues must be undertaken with care so as not to rein-force these fears (see Chap. 3).

Perfectionism

Healthcare professions often attract perfection-ists. Perfectionism can drive distress, particu-larly when coupled with low self-compassion [14, 15]. Perfectionists fear that they are never good enough, a misconception supported by an aggressively achievement-oriented healthcare culture.

Presentations Related to Mental Health

Depression and Suicide

Depression is more common, and suicide is 2–4 times more common, in physicians than in the general population [16]. Up to 30% of residents experience depression [17].

Alcohol and Substance Use

Up to one in five American physicians abuse alcohol [18]. Other healthcare professionals are also at increased use of substance misuse, with 30% of dentists reporting high-risk alcohol use in the past month and 13% of pharmacists reporting the use of non-prescribed controlled substances in the past year [19].

Other Psychiatric Concerns

The years of health professions training coincide with the age of onset of several serious mental illnesses, which can be exacerbated by the stresses of training and practice. These include unipolar depression and bipolar disorder, anxiety disorders, eating disorders, attention deficit dis-order, schizophrenia and other psychotic disor-ders, and obsessive-compulsive disorder. In addition, we suspect that subclinical post-traumatic stress disorder is more common among health professionals and trainees than generally recognized. Unless they compromise patient care, most psychiatric illnesses, if properly treated and monitored, do not preclude complet-ing training and achieving competence. In deal-ing with psychiatric illness (as with any other illness), it is very important to distinguish between "illness" and "impairment" and to care-fully assess "fitness for duty" (see Chaps. 20, 26, 29) in addition to simply considering their diag-noses [20, 21].

Approach to Trainee Well-Being

Becoming a healthcare professional is a demand-ing and profound developmental process, which involves acquiring vast knowledge and skill, developing professional responsibility, making difficult decisions, witnessing suffering, and even holding others' lives in one's hands. As teachers and mentors, our job is to educate and support trainees in their efforts to move through this process in a healthy and successful way.

Since the last edition of this book, the literature around interventions that may reduce burnout and promote well-being has exploded. Several different models of drivers of well-being and the interventions that facilitate it have been developed (Table 18.1); this is not an exhaustive review but a collection of some examples with citations for further reading.

Two important revelations have emerged from this body of research. First, well-being is a shared responsibility between individuals and the systems in which they work, requiring systemic change in addition to support and education for individuals [24]. However, mandatory, individually focused interventions for self-care are less likely to make a significant impact [25]. The most effective well-being programs offer a range of resources that trainees can choose from to best meet their needs (Table 18.2).

Based on these frameworks, we detail our five-pronged comprehensive approach to promoting well-being in medical training (summarized in Box 18.2). This conceptual and practical approach encompasses efforts that can be made today, as well as broader, ongoing efforts toward

Table 18.1 Frameworks for conceptualizing physician well-being

Framework	Description
Shanafelt-Noseworthy Model [8]	Workplace driver dimensions of burnout
National Academy of Medicine Model [22]	Detailed conceptual framework for drivers of well-being
Stanford University WellMD Professional Fulfillment Model [23]	Conceptual model for domains of comprehensive well-being
Charter on Physician Well-Being [24]	Framework for ideal future state

Table 18.2 Examples of well-being issues and linkage to interventions

Domain of well-being [23]	Driver of engagement [8]	Manifestation of well-being issue (Lack of driver can lead to …)	Example intervention by domain of well-being	
			System level	Individual level
Culture of well-being	Organizational culture and values	Burnout	Established health system boundaries for expectations of after-hours work	Role modeling of self-care by educational leaders
	Social support and community at work	Imposter syndrome	Institutional peer support programs	Processing groups that normalize experiences and struggles of training
	Work-life integration	Work-life tension	Paid parental leave	Contingency plans for personal crises
	Control and flexibility	Burnout	Programs with built-in redundancy to allow for flexible time off policies for trainees	Ability to trade schedules for important personal events
Efficiency of practice	Workload and job demands	Perfectionism	Highly functioning interprofessional teams with clear responsibilities	Open communication between trainees and supervisors about demands
	Efficiency and resources	Compassion fatigue	Investment in technological solutions to efficiency challenges (e.g., laptops for rounds)	Individualized mentorship on managing work-related demands
Personal resilience	Meaning in work	Compassion fatigue	Schwartz Center Rounds for interprofessional teams to reflect on meaningful experiences [26]	Mindfulness courses, Balint groups

individual/group wellness and culture/systems change. Please note that interventions occur in at least one of the three categories, following the Stanford Model of Professional Fulfillment [23]: culture of well-being, efficiency of practice, and personal resilience.

> **Box 18.2: Five-Pronged Approach to Promoting Well-Being in Health Professions Trainees**
>
> - **Advocate:** Advocate for legislation and organizational policies that enhance physician well-being
> - **Prevent:** Create supportive, health-promoting programmatic structures (schedules, coverage arrangements, and social interactions) and challenge institutional cultural and personal attitudes that impede well-being.
> - **Teach:** Offer trainees skill-building curricula and ongoing processing opportunities
> - **Monitor:** Establish open, supportive relationships with trainees and be available, be observant, and reach out; consider well-being issues when problems with competency are identified
> - **Act:** Practice humble inquiry when issues are identified, support trainees to connect with appropriate treatment, reflect and make programmatic changes based on feedback

Advocate

As teachers, mentors, and supervisors, we must advocate for legislation and organizational changes (several of which we describe in the next sections), that will enhance our trainees' well-being and engagement. Problems are perceived as less overwhelming when we have some con-

trol or agency over our circumstances. In addition, we must also support and protect our learners when they advocate for themselves in schools and residencies, or around broader healthcare issues.

Prevent

Rather than waiting to "remediate" burned-out trainees, we strongly believe that both prevention of distress and burnout and promotion of engagement and flourishing should be our goals. Prevention includes both changes to our clinical culture and systems and preventive health measures for individuals and groups.

Create a Culture of Well-Being

While changing culture can be a difficult endeavor, teachers and educational leaders have the opportunity to influence culture within their programs and at the health system and societal levels [27]. The first and most essential goal is to establish trainee well-being as a core priority of training programs, departments, and healthcare organizations. We should establish wellness champions, who, along with students and residents, can be included in all decisions and planning that affect their well-being.

Build a supportive learning climate: A positive learning climate has a significant impact on trainees' work-related well-being [28]. It should normalize emotion and anticipate the emotional challenges that arise when learning to be (and ultimately practicing as) a healthcare professional [21]. Role modeling by educational leaders reinforces this culture; in particular, showing vulnerability around sharing challenges or past mistakes can be extremely impactful. A supportive learning climate also requires integration of curricula designed to raise awareness of well-being issues and promote recognition of those in crisis by their peers [29]. When in the hands of individual teachers, setting a positive learning climate is also a critical facet of the third prong of our approach, i.e., teach (see below).

Preserve control and flexibility: The lack of control and flexibility around work lives is one of the biggest causes of distress and poor satisfaction for trainees as well as practicing physicians. Program structures that preserve as much control and flexibility as possible for trainees result in successful and satisfied trainees [30]. We highly recommend allowing trainees to make day-off requests, trade schedules, and attend to personal obligations during work hours.

Develop crisis plans: Because of the nature of both our work in healthcare and our lives as human beings, crises will arise. Some crises will be personal, affecting an individual trainee (e.g., the death of a loved one, personal illness). Others will be institution- or society-level events (death of a colleague, natural disasters, social unrest, the COVID-19 pandemic) that deeply and broadly affect the well-being of trainees, as well as patient care needs and arrangements. As educators, we should expect that both personal and societal crises will happen and plan for them. For individual crises, programs should have a protocol that includes information on practical concerns and accessing resources, as well as a coverage system allowing trainees to take time off as needed. For institutional or societal crises, programs should prepare for rapid deployment of support and resources to trainees, focused on providing for basic needs, such as food, lodging, safety, and support [31].

Address financial needs of students and residents: Many medical students and residents have limited socioeconomic resources. They may need help accessing funding such as loans or grants, help with financial management, and opportunities to earn extra income through training-relevant work.

Promote Efficiency of Practice

Despite two decades of efforts to rehabilitate work hours for trainees, health professions training maintains an exhausting schedule. Reducing absolute hours alone is not enough due to work compression (expecting trainees to complete the same amount of work in less time while maintaining expectations to meaningfully connect with patients). Programs must attend to working conditions and the tension between service and education [32]. Practical approaches include reducing time spent on noneducational, non-patient care activities; use of scribes and administrative coordinators/assistants; and offering flex time and job sharing [33]. Efforts can include leveraging technological solutions that streamline care (e.g., messaging and sign-out tools) and coaching trainees on using them.

Encourage Enhanced Personal Resilience

Mind-body techniques can confer physical and psychological benefits.

- Breathing techniques are particularly helpful as they can be easily and unobtrusively used in challenging situations. These, in concert with other training such as guided imagery, progressive relaxation, and autogenic training, improve distress tolerance [34].
- Mindfulness and mindfulness meditation affect major elements of burnout (depersonalization and emotional exhaustion) in trainees, although mandatory mindfulness programs may not be effective [22, 35]. Mindfulness-based cognitive therapy may also prove to be helpful in trainees; studies suggest that it reduces suicide and hospitalizations in veterans with PTSD and recurrent depression [36].
- Yoga has been shown in numerous studies to promote physical health; promote recovery from and treatment of addiction; reduce stress, anxiety, depression, and chronic pain; improve

sleep patterns; and enhance overall well-being and quality of life [37].

Cognitive-behavioral therapy (CBT) has been shown to reduce suicidal ideation and anxiety in trainees and can be effective using Web-based strategies [38, 39]. CBT helps participants recognize and change fixed, dysfunctional thoughts and reactions and have a healthier perspective on difficult situations [40].

Opportunities for *group processing* should be regularly scheduled, ideally with a trusted facilitator, since it is not always possible to address difficult events right when they happen. These meetings work best with naturally occurring groups (e.g., students at the same training level; trainees working together in the ICU). Such groups can allow and encourage self-exploration and awareness, to validate experiences, to support and feel support, and to enhance empathy and understanding toward others. There are a variety of group formats that are useful in the setting of health professions training and practice, including open-ended groups [41], Balint groups [42], narrative medicine groups (see Chap. 15), and Schwartz Rounds [26].

Teach

Appropriate teaching and training are essential to promote and maintain well-being and excellence in our trainees. In addition to its intrinsic value, quality education helps trainees learn the knowledge, understanding, and skills necessary to prepare them for the stresses and challenges that lie ahead. Increasingly refined educational approaches, including hands-on, participatory, and collaborative learning, give teachers the opportunity to work with and observe trainees in their "natural habitat," to identify signs of distress or impaired functioning.

Though seemingly distant from explicit teaching about wellness, addressing specific topics can provide trainees with important knowledge, understanding, and skills to navigate common challenges of training and practice. These topics include understanding our own feelings, reactions, and behaviors (see group processing section above); communicating effectively, especially in tough situations; coping with disturbing events, including disability, suffering, and death; addressing difficult clinical, moral, and ethical quandaries; and medical errors and bad outcomes.

Education for Well-Being

The Accreditation Council for Graduate Medical Education (ACGME) now requires that residency programs provide educational content related to well-being [43]. An increasing number of health professions schools are also incorporating this training.

Clinicians who have deliberate self-care strategies are less likely to experience burnout. Those who focus on the meaning in their work, foster positive emotions, attempt to integrate work with their personal lives, and tend to their physical health have higher quality of life [44]. Lowering barriers and creating protected time to pursue these and other strategies (such as exercise, engaging in hobbies or avocations, and spiritual and religious practices) will set them up for satisfaction and success in their careers.

Monitor

Despite the help of preventive interventions and education, trainees will continue to experience distress and functional deficits. Therefore, we must remain alert to how our learners are doing, identify problems early, and intervene as soon as problems occur. There are several evidence-based approaches to monitoring; we encourage braiding techniques together to support learners with different personalities and coping styles.

Educators recognize that "on-the-ground" observation and intervention can be a valuable approach to identifying trainees in distress.

Regularly checking in with learners in various educational venues conveys care about how they are doing and coping and acknowledges that emotionally difficult situations arise every day in clinical practice. Check-ins also acknowledge that clinical practice is rife with difficult situations and that maintaining well-being is critical. Preexisting processing groups (see above) can provide regular opportunities for these check-ins, which may also take place in passing.

Some programs have found success with coaching/advising programs in which trainees can feel comfortable discussing tough issues openly, either with near-peer leaders or trained faculty who provide longitudinal coaching [45, 46]. Creating protected time to visit a therapist may reduce stigma and encourage participation in needed mental healthcare [47].

Most trainees are well versed in the "hidden curriculum" of medical training and may be reluctant to acknowledge problems or perceived weakness. Supervisors and respected clinician-teachers need to model honest, but boundaried, discussions of the issues (perhaps including their own) and make it routine to check in with all trainees. While some will have little trouble letting you know how they are, others will be more guarded and will require a more indirect approach.

To identify trainees who are not reaching out for help, some programs use regular online well-being screening. One commonly used tool is the Well-Being Index (WBI) (https://www.mededwebs.com/well-being-index), validated in various professions and stages of training [48]. Other options for screening include the Maslach Burnout Inventory (the most commonly used instrument in research studies), the Copenhagen Burnout Inventory, and the Stanford Professional Fulfillment Index.

Act and Intervene

Marjorie told Jim that she had some ideas about things they could do to help him get through the rest of the year, but she wanted his perspective and ideas. He told her that he just wanted time to sleep. Marjorie arranged for Jim to have a couple of days of coverage so that he could take some space to breathe. She offered him an appointment with the Faculty and Staff Assistance Program during that time, and he accepted.

Once a problem is identified, sit down with the trainee and address the situation by listening, normalizing reactions and emotions, and, potentially, troubleshooting. Consider their emotional and functional state, and pitch your questions and conversation appropriately. As health professionals, we may wish to step in immediately to "fix" things; however, it is most beneficial to begin the intervention process with sincere curiosity, an open mind, and authentic, nonjudgmental inquiry. As we seek to understand, we can build a trusting, collaborative relationship before rushing in with advice and solutions. When counseling learners who are struggling, we find it helpful to acknowledge the extent to which well-being is impacted by factors outside of the learners' control. Further counseling or interventions may include those shown in Table 18.3 and Fig. 18.2.

Table 18.3 Escalating interventions

- Explore problems and provide counseling
- Refer for peer support
- Refer for therapy
- Plan with dean of students, residency directors, and department chairs to create program modifications
- On-site physician/student wellness programs.
- Statewide (medical society) physician health committee
- Regulatory bodies, such as the Office of Professional Medical Conduct

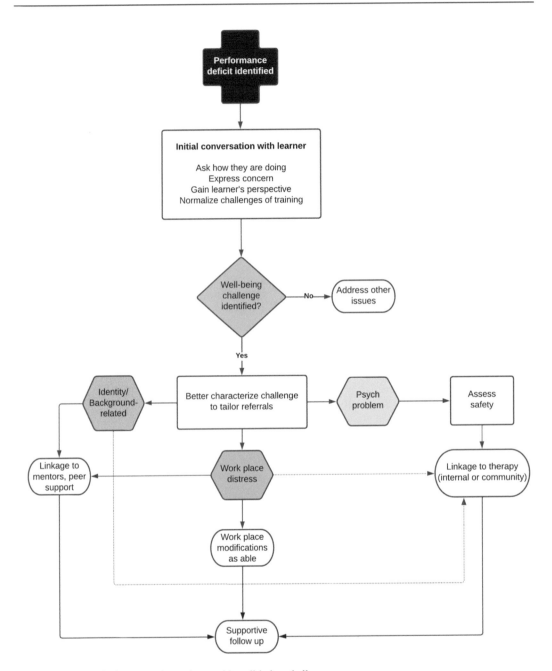

Fig. 18.2 Schematic for supporting trainees with well-being challenges

Consider referring the trainee to your health system's peer support program. When clinicians are in distress, they may prefer to speak with a peer who understands what they are going through [49]. Referral to mentors for support can also be helpful, particularly when trainees are struggling with identity-related well-being issues. Regularly scheduled groups, mentioned above, are also excellent options for ongoing support.

If you are able, and the trainee feels that it would be helpful, explore the possibility of time off or modifications to the trainee's schedule. Given the stress of healthcare profession training, an extra day or two off can sometimes provide the space needed to process emotions or understand distress. Space may need to be made for attention to these issues on an ongoing basis. When considering options, the trainee's supervisor (dean of students, program director, etc.) should be involved. To preserve trust, always inform the trainee prior to divulging information to their supervisor, and remember that, in this context, you are serving as the trainee's educator, not their treating clinician.

At any point, if it sounds like the trainee would benefit from dedicated time with a professional to process emotions and/or build skills, consider connecting them with psychotherapy. Most institutions now have a counseling program dedicated to faculty and staff: an easy place to start.

The immediate space helped Jim take a little time to process and connect with support. After 3 days, he felt well enough to go back to work. His burnout was not "cured," but he had had time to think about his own self-care plan. Over time, he was able to integrate psychotherapy, more time with friends outside of medicine, exercise, and mindfulness into his routine. At the beginning of his second year, he realized that he no longer felt dread on waking on a work day morning.

Impaired and Disruptive Trainees

Mark (he/him), a well-regarded junior faculty hospitalist, was found to be misusing alcohol: he often showed up on the hospital wards with alcohol on his breath, slurred speech, and being unable to clearly articulate his thoughts. The day after this problem was identified, he was evaluated by the hospital's medical staff committee, and the decision was made to refer him for alcohol abuse treatment. Mark walked out of the meeting to find the chief of his department with a limousine waiting to take Mark to a

"professionals-only" alcohol treatment center some distance away.

When he returned, sober and well-functioning, arrangements were made with the State Committee on Physician Health for 3 months of monitoring and supervision; after this time, he was able to continue his work without monitoring and without further incident.

In rare cases, concerns for impairment in clinical practice arise. According to the Joint Commission, the healthcare system's accreditation organization (https://www.jointcommission.org), clinicians with significant concerns about impairment, or dangerous disruption, may be required to be evaluated (and hopefully helped), by a series of boards and committees, each with somewhat different goals and practices. These bodies include the following:

- The healthcare system's clinical staff committee: designed to gather and evaluate the information on the clinician and decide if further evaluation or remediation is needed. These clinical staff committees are separate from any disciplinary proceedings.
- State Committees on Physician Health (CPH): A step-up in power from hospital committees, but still oriented toward helping healthcare professionals with their problems, working with the professional's program to make remediation plans, and getting the provider back to work, often with temporary supervision and monitoring. Referrals to CPH can be made anonymously.

The above programs are designed to help, support, and remediate. They are places where trainees and clinicians can discuss their problems with a knowledgeable, empathic professional and get help in a safe and confidential environment. In most cases, trainees can complete their training program after engaging in this remediation process. Dismissal is only considered after extensive efforts to support return to training and practice have been exhausted.

- State Offices of Professional Misconduct (OPMC): These are powerful boards whose stated mission is to protect the profession and the public from providers who are significantly impaired or engaging in serious misconduct. Their processes can seem harsh, including publishing alleged misconduct online, or even taking away licenses. Generally, significant efforts have been made by programs and institutions to address the problem before an individual clinician's case is raised to an OPMC.

Many trainees have concerns that seeking mental health treatment will have negative effects on future licensure and career opportunities. In states where questions on licensure applications ask about the history of diagnosis or treatment of mental illness (rather than asking only about current *impairment*), clinicians are more likely to be reluctant to seek care for a mental health condition [50]. The Federation of State Medical Boards has recently affirmed that application questions should focus on current issues and impairments [51]. Although not all states have yet changed their applications, these new policies represent progress in destigmatizing help-seeking for mental illness.

Conclusion

> **Case 1, Epilogue**
> *A few months later, Jim reached out to Marjorie to ask about becoming a peer supporter for the residency program. He knew so many people who were burned out, and he wanted to help.*

We strive to train clinicians who are whole and can prioritize their own and each other's well-being as well as that of their patients. We must teach them to take satisfaction in a job well done, a patient well cared for, a staff member supported, or teamwork accomplished; to be proud

of their achievements, humble in the face of all the things we do not know and cannot fix, resilient enough to roll with the punches when they come, and to know when to stand up and fight for what they need. We have a long way to go, as a healthcare community and as a society, to address the well-being of healthcare professionals. We hope that the approaches laid out in this chapter will help us do so.

References

1. Dyrbye LN, West CP, Satele D, et al. Burnout among U.S. medical students, residents, and early career physicians relative to the general U.S. population. Acad Med. 2014;89(3):443–51. https://doi.org/10.1097/ACM.0000000000000134.
2. Shanafelt TD, Boone S, Tan L, et al. Burnout and satisfaction with work-life balance among US physicians relative to the general US population. Arch Intern Med. 2012;172(18):1377. https://doi.org/10.1001/archinternmed.2012.3199.
3. Shanafelt TD, West CP, Sinsky C, et al. Changes in burnout and satisfaction with work-life integration in physicians and the general US working population between 2011 and 2017. Mayo Clin Proc. 2019;94(9):1681–94.
4. Moore KA, O'Brien BC, Thomas LR. "I wish they had asked": a qualitative study of emotional distress and peer support during internship. J Gen Intern Med. 2020;35:3443–8.
5. West CP, Dyrbye LN, Shanafelt TD. Physician burnout: contributors, consequences and solutions. J Intern Med. 2018;283:516–29.
6. American Psychological Association Dictionary. https://dictionary.apa.org/distress. Accessed 3 Jan 2022.
7. Zalaquett CP, Wood RJ. Evaluating stress: a book of resources. Lanham: Scarecrow Press; 1997.
8. Shanafelt TD, Noseworthy JH. Executive leadership and physician well-being: nine organizational strategies to promote engagement and reduce burnout. Mayo Clin Proc. 2017;92(1):129–46. https://doi.org/10.1016/j.mayocp.2016.10.004.
9. Cocker F, Joss N. Compassion fatigue among healthcare, emergency and community service workers: a systematic review. Int J Environ Res Public Health. 2016;13(6):1–18.
10. Pfifferling J-H, Gilley K. Overcoming compassion fatigue. Fam Pract Manag. 2000;7(4):39.
11. Villwock JA, Sobin LB, Koester LA, Harris TM. Impostor syndrome and burnout among American medical students: a pilot study. Int J Med Educ. 2016;7:364–9. https://doi.org/10.5116/ijme.5801.eac4.

12. Ladonna KA, Ginsburg S, Watling C. "Rising to the level of your incompetence": what physicians' self-assessment of their performance reveals about the imposter syndrome in medicine. Acad Med. 2018;93:763–8. https://doi.org/10.1097/ACM.0000000000002046.

13. Spencer SJ, Logel C, Davies PG. Stereotype threat. Annu Rev Psychol. 2016;67:415–37. https://doi.org/10.1146/annurev-psych-073115-103235.

14. Flett GL, Hewitt PL. Perfectionism and maladjustment: an overview of theoretical, definitional, and treatment issues. In: Perfectionism: theory, research, and treatment. American Psychological Association; 2004. p. 5–31. https://doi.org/10.1037/10458-001.

15. James K, Verplanken B, Rimes KA. Self-criticism as a mediator in the relationship between unhealthy perfectionism and distress. Pers Individ Dif. 2015;79:123–8. https://doi.org/10.1016/j.paid.2015.01.030.

16. Center C, Davis M, Detre T, et al. Confronting depression and suicide in physicians: a consensus statement. JAMA. 2003;289:3161–6.

17. Mata DA, Ramos MA, Bansal N, et al. Prevalence of depression and depressive symptoms among resident physicians a systematic review and meta-analysis. JAMA. 2015;314(22):2373–83. https://doi.org/10.1001/jama.2015.15845.

18. Oreskovich MR, Shanafelt T, Dyrbye LN, et al. The prevalence of substance use disorders in American physicians. Am J Addict. 2015;24(1):30–8. https://doi.org/10.1111/ajad.12173.

19. Kenna GA, Wood MD. Prevalence of substance use by pharmacists and other health professionals. J Am Pharm Assoc. 2004;44(6):684–93. https://doi.org/10.1331/1544345042467281.

20. Miller L. Doctors, their mental health and capacity for work. Occup Med (Lond). 2009;59(1):53–5. https://doi.org/10.1093/occmed/kqn111.

21. Anfang SA, Faulkner LR, Fromson JA, Gendel MH. The American Psychiatric Association's resource document on guidelines for psychiatric fitness-for-duty evaluations of physicians. J Am Acad Psychiatry Law. 2005;33(1):85–8.

22. Brigham T, Barden C, Legreid Dopp A, et al. A journey to construct an all-encompassing conceptual model of factors affecting clinician well-being and resilience. NAM Perspect. 2018;8(1) https://doi.org/10.31478/201801b.

23. Bohman B, Dyrbye L, Sinsky CA, et al. Physician well-being: the reciprocity of practice efficiency, culture of wellness, and personal resilience. New Engl J Med Catal. 2017;April:1–17. https://catalyst.nejm.org/doi/full/10.1056/CAT.17.0429. Accessed 25 Jan 2021.

24. Thomas LR, Ripp JA, West CP. Charter on physician well-being. JAMA. 2018;319(15):1541. https://doi.org/10.1001/jama.2018.1331.

25. Dyrbye LN, Shanafelt TD, Werner L, Sood A, Satele D, Wolanskyj AP. The impact of a required longitudinal stress management and resilience training course for first-year medical students. J Gen Intern Med. 2017;32(12):1309–14. https://doi.org/10.1007/s11606-017-4171-2.

26. Taylor C, Xyrichis A, Leamy MC, Reynolds E, Maben J. Can Schwartz Center Rounds support healthcare staff with emotional challenges at work, and how do they compare with other interventions aimed at providing similar support? A systematic review and scoping reviews. BMJ Open. 2018;8(10):e024254. https://doi.org/10.1136/bmjopen-2018-024254.

27. Sinsky CA, Biddison LD, Mallick A, et al. Organizational evidence-based and promising practices for improving clinician well-being. NAM Perspect. Published online November 2, 2020. https://doi.org/10.31478/202011a.

28. Lases LSS, Arah OA, Busch ORC, Heineman MJ, Lombarts KMJMH. Learning climate positively influences residents' work-related well-being. Adv Health Sci Educ Theory Pract. 2019;24(2):317–30. https://doi.org/10.1007/s10459-018-9868-4.

29. Zabar S, Hanley K, Horlick M, et al. "I cannot take this any more!": preparing interns to identify and help a struggling colleague. J Gen Intern Med. 2019;34(5):773–7. https://doi.org/10.1007/s11606-019-04886-y.

30. Linzer M. Working conditions in primary care: physician reactions and care quality. Ann Intern Med. 2009;151(1):28. https://doi.org/10.7326/0003-4819-151-1-200907070-00006.

31. Shanafelt T, Ripp J, Trockel M. Understanding and addressing sources of anxiety among health care professionals during the COVID-19 pandemic. JAMA J Am Med Assoc. 2020;323(21):2133–4. https://doi.org/10.1001/jama.2020.5893.

32. Ludmerer KM. Resident burnout: working hours or working conditions? J Grad Med Educ. 2009;1(2):169–71. https://doi.org/10.4300/jgme-d-09-00077.1.

33. Weinstein L, Wolfe HM. The downward spiral of physician satisfaction: an attempt to avert a crisis within the medical profession. Obstet Gynecol. 2007;109(5):1181–3. https://doi.org/10.1097/01.AOG.0000260390.52029.f4.

34. Kraemer KM, Luberto CM, O'Bryan EM, Mysinger E, Cotton S. Mind-body skills training to improve distress tolerance in medical students: a pilot study. Teach Learn Med. 2016;28:219–28.

35. Lebares CC, Coaston TN, Delucchi KL, et al. Enhanced stress resilience training in surgeons. Ann Surg. 2021;273(3):424–32. https://doi.org/10.1097/sla.0000000000004145.

36. Interian A, Chesin MS, Stanley B, Latorre M, et al. Mindfulness-based cognitive therapy for preventing suicide in military veterans: a randomized clinical trial. J Clin Psychiatry. 2021;82:20m13791.

37. Cocchiara RA, Peruzzo M, Mannocci A, Ottolenghi L, et al. The use of yoga to manage stress and burnout in healthcare workers: a systematic review. J Clin Med. 2019;26:284.

38. Guille C, Zhao Z, Krystal J, Nichols B, Brady K, Sen S. Web-based cognitive behavioral ther-

apy intervention for the prevention of suicidal ideation in medical interns. JAMA Psychiatry. 2015;72(12):1192. https://doi.org/10.1001/jamapsychiatry.2015.1880.

39. Howell AN, Rheingold AA, Uhde TW, Guille C. Web-based CBT for the prevention of anxiety symptoms among medical and health science graduate students. Cogn Behav Ther. 2019;48(5):385–405. https://doi.org/10.1080/16506073.2018.1533575.

40. Greenberger D, Padesky CA. Mind over mood: change how you feel by changing the way you think. 2nd ed. New York: The Guilford Press; 2016.

41. Chou CL, Johnston CB, Singh B, Garber JD, Kaplan E, Lee K, Teherani A. A "safe space" for learning and reflection: one school's design for continuity with a peer group across clinical clerkships. Acad Med. 2011;86:1560–5.

42. Yazdankhahfard M, Haghani F, Omid A. The Balint group and its application in medical education: a systematic review. J Educ Health Promot. 2019;8(1):124. https://doi.org/10.4103/jehp.jehp_423_18.

43. Accreditation Council for Graduate Medical Education. Common program requirements, Section VI, with background and intent. 2017;9(6):1–19. https://www.acgme.org/Portals/0/PFAssets/ProgramRequirements/CPRs_SectionVI_with-Background-and-Intent_2017-01.pdf. Accessed 19 Dec 2022.

44. Shanafelt TD, Oreskovich MR, Dyrbye LN, et al. Avoiding burnout: the personal health habits and wellness practices of US surgeons. Ann Surg. 2012;255(4):625–33. https://doi.org/10.1097/SLA.0b013e31824b2fa0.

45. Fischer J, Alpert A, Rao P. Promoting intern resilience: individual chief wellness check-ins. MedEdPORTAL. 2019;15(15):10848. https://doi.org/10.15766/mep_2374-8265.10848.

46. Palamara K, Kauffman C, Chang Y, et al. Professional development coaching for residents: results of a 3-year positive psychology coaching intervention. J Gen Intern Med. 2018;33(11):1842–4. https://doi.org/10.1007/s11606-018-4589-1.

47. Sofka S, Grey C, Lerfald N, Davisson L, Howsare J. Implementing a universal well-being assessment to mitigate barriers to resident utilization of mental health resources. J Grad Med Educ. 2018;10(1):63–6. https://doi.org/10.4300/JGME-D-17-00405.1.

48. Skrupky LP, West CP, Shanafelt T, Satele DV, Dyrbye LN. Ability of the well-being index to identify pharmacists in distress. J Am Pharm Assoc. 2020;60(6):906–914.e2. https://doi.org/10.1016/j.japh.2020.06.015.

49. Hu Y-Y, Fix ML, Hevelone ND, et al. Physicians' needs in coping with emotional stressors. Arch Surg. 2012;147(3):212. https://doi.org/10.1001/archsurg.2011.312.

50. Dyrbye LN, West CP, Sinsky CA, Goeders LE, Satele DV, Shanafelt TD. Medical licensure questions and physician reluctance to seek care for mental health conditions. Mayo Clin Proc. 2017;92(10):1486–93. https://doi.org/10.1016/j.mayocp.2017.06.020.

51. Workgroup on Physician Wellness and Burnout. Physician wellness and burnout. Fed State Med Boards. 2018;(April):1–22. https://www.fsmb.org/siteassets/advocacy/policies/policy-on-wellness-and-burnout.pdf. Accessed 19 Dec 2022.

Faculty Development: Preparing to Conduct Remediation

Adina Kalet and Sondra Zabar

Introduction

Ideally, every health professions educator's job description would include conducting remediation. After all, we rely almost entirely on the judgment and skills of frontline educators to identify and remediate our trainees. Usually, though, only a few individuals take up this challenge with the enthusiasm, knowledge, skills, and compassion required to be effective. Moreover, institutions provide highly variable support and at times may hinder remediation by casting it as fundamentally regulatory and punitive rather than educational.

Health professions educators are unique among other faculty members in higher education in that we routinely "live" with the learners we supervise. We engage in patient care with trainees at our sides. As trainees gain our trust, we gradually allow them more independent practice until they can conduct patient assessments and make high-stakes decisions. Therefore, we are exceptionally motivated to ensure that our trainees are trustworthy. We are also uniquely qualified to conduct remediation because the clinical reasoning model (see Chap. 9) corresponds to clinical skill remediation practices: both use evidence to determine diagnosis and prognosis, implement therapies, and monitor outcomes. Additionally, clinicians manage complex high-stakes problems, combine rigorous critical thinking with skillful communication, and inhabit a culture of maintaining confidentiality and working within a clear code of ethics. Possibly, the most important reason healthcare professionals should vigorously take on the responsibility of conducting remediation is that in doing so, we fulfill our professional obligations to society. However, given the intellectual and emotional challenges of working with learners who struggle, many prefer to avoid confrontation or identify and empathize with the trainee and therefore "cut them some slack." Some faculty blame the trainee or the system for allowing this problem to go unaddressed. Others remain dubious that effective, practical remediation strategies exist. For these reasons and more, we frequently abdicate our responsibility and do not identify learners who struggle early enough to intervene effectively.

In contrast, many institutions have a few dedicated educators who have developed the needed expertise and deeply enjoy the work of remediation. Increasingly, institutions are moving from *ad hoc* remediation interventions—rooting out

A. Kalet
Kern Institute for the Transformation of Medical Education, Medical College of Wisconsin, Milwaukee, WI, USA
e-mail: akalet@mcw.edu

S. Zabar (✉)
Department of Medicine, New York University Grossman School of Medicine, New York, NY, USA
e-mail: sondra.zabar@nyulangone.org

"bad apples"—toward systematic programmatic approaches, which at their best are continuous quality improvement efforts that sustainably engage all learners and teachers (see Chap. 2). Most trainees, whether identified as struggling or not, deeply appreciate the opportunity to address a vexing weakness in a supportive and confidential manner. Even when the outcome is not ideal for the learner, the remediation process can clarify and satisfy, and long-term outcomes are likely to be optimistic. But without faculty development in this domain, our institutions will lack adequate capacity to address the need to get learners back "on course" when required.

In this chapter, we assert that effective faculty development for remediation is an organizational capacity-building process that requires both individually and institutionally focused approaches. We propose a set of specific competence areas for individual faculty development and briefly discuss attributes of teachers, theories of learning, and teaching strategies that affect the ability to remediate effectively. We discuss the importance and specifics of developing judgment, facilitation skills, emotional intelligence, courage, and attitudes consistent with effective remediation work. Finally, we propose the need to organize these activities with the intention of creating a community of practice in remediation, integrated with other important communities of practice (e.g., education and workplace), to ensure healthcare systems that are optimally "competent" and continuously learning.

Who Should Conduct Remediation?

As discussed above, the most effective facilitators of clinical competence remediation are likely to be educators deputized by educational pro-gram leaders who are responsible for making promotion, graduation, and dismissal decisions. We feel strongly that educators should be in charge during two critical stages of remediation: initial identification and summative assessment (see Chap. 6). Once specific issues are identified, a variety of specialists can add value. These experts most often include communication coaches, experienced standardized patient trainers (who often have additional training, for example, in feedback or drama therapy), learning specialists, study skills and executive function coaches, mental health professionals (such as psychiatrists and psychologists), and respected faculty members who function as professionalism role models and/or clinical skill coaches.

Faculty Development for Remediation

Specific Competencies for Faculty

The institutional capacity to remediate struggling trainees is dependent on the number, commitment, and expertise of available faculty members. While not every member of the teaching faculty must lead remediation efforts, the more competence there is in the faculty as a whole, the better the community can manage struggling learners. Faculty members who have a talent for working with trainees one-on-one and commit to developing learners' clinical competence are ideally suited for this work (see Chaps. 4 and 6). Table 19.1 lists learning objectives for faculty development in clinical skill remediation. Appropriately, many of these attributes align closely with those identified for effective clinician-educators [1].

Table 19.1 Specific competencies and objectives and suggested reading in this book

Clinical educators conducting remediation should be able to ...

1. Explore personal perspectives, attitudes, and beliefs that inhibit identification of learners who struggle (see Chaps. 2 and 6)
2. Articulate how current learning theories apply to routine medical teaching and assessment practice as well as remediation (see Chaps. 2, 4, and 19 below)
3. List common and uncommon areas of difficulty for trainees who struggle (see Chaps. 7–18)
4. Discuss the role of adaptive learning in assessing clinical competence (see Chap. 4)
5. Collaborate with learners on useful individualized remediation plans with proper accountability, based on critical review of objective and subjective assessment data for an individual learner (Chaps. 4, 6–17)
6. Discuss the underlying assumptions of various assessment strategies and common misunderstandings (e.g., including psychometric and sociopsychological frameworks, the evidence for reliability and validity of assessment measures, the impact of context on performance) (see Chap. 19 below)
7. Participate enthusiastically in setting standards for trainees and other performance assessment experiences including Performance Dimension, Frame of Reference, and Behavioral Observation training in order to improve skills and understand relevant aspects of "rater cognition" (see Chap. 19 below)
8. Define clinical competence in a behaviorally specific and measurable manner (Chaps. 7–16)
9. Identify and design authentic complex tasks in which trainees can demonstrate competence (Chaps. 7–17)
10. Articulate expectations for professional behavior, appropriate attitudes, needed attributes, and character traits of excellent physicians (Chaps. 13 and 14)
11. Recognize, describe, categorize, and address common lapses in professionalism (Chap. 14)
12. Discuss the impact of bias and prejudice on achievement (see Chaps. 2 and 3)
13. Demonstrate taking an educational history from a trainee, including addressing clues suggesting the presence of a Verbal or NonVerbal Learning Disability or Attention Deficit Disorder (see Chap. 17)
14. Demonstrate the ability to screen for common psychiatric issues that may manifest as or coexist with clinical incompetence (see Chaps. 7 and 18)
15. Demonstrate exceptional metacognitive awareness (see Chap. 4)
16. Give effective reinforcing feedback as well as direct and difficult-to-receive constructive feedback (see Chap. 6)
17. Demonstrate the courage, intellectual rigor, and compassion to make defensible judgments of clinical competence in borderline cases (see Chap. 19 below)
18. Document a concise, useful remediation process that addresses legal and regulatory requirements (see Chaps. 20, 26, 29)

What Is Learning? Theories 101

Learning Theory
A well-substantiated, research-based, coherent group of tested general propositions commonly regarded as correct, defining, and explaining learning, which serve as a framework to guide educational practice and explain and predict outcomes.

Learning is a fundamental aspect of human life. Anyone who has lived with an infant can attest to the unstoppable human drive to explore, discover, and master their world. However, this drive toward competence can also be dangerous unless we have guidance in learning and protection from doing harm. While a working knowledge of learning theory is foundational for trained general educators, most health professions educators do not formally prepare for their teaching role and therefore cannot connect what they do with learning theory. Yet, we each have our own theory of learning or beliefs about what it means to teach [2] (see http://teachingperspectives.com/drupal/ to take the Teaching Perspectives Inventory). These beliefs, combined with the desired outcomes for learning, available resources, and practical conditions of learning (e.g., bedside rounds, morning report), guide how we organize or structure learning experiences (e.g., by discipline, organ system, problem, team, or case) and the tactics we use to facilitate learning (e.g., observation, guided problem-solving, lectures, seminars).

Health professions educators must examine and critique our own beliefs about learning and teaching, since we often base these beliefs on our own unique experiences in formal and informal learning settings and only sometimes compare these with well-substantiated theories. Therefore, health professions education is often disorganized, confusing, unacceptably idiosyncratic, and inconsistently effective in leading to learning. What follows is a brief and selective discussion of the intertwining, coevolving threads of learning theory that currently have significant influence on health professions education: behaviorism, cognitivism, and constructivism. Extensive appraisals of this subject are available elsewhere [3–7].

Behaviorism. Classical *behaviorism*, the predominant learning theory in the late nineteenth century, held that all learning could be described as a response to a stimulus. In the first decades of the twentieth century, with the advent of experimental psychology, *Gestalt theory* proposed that learning occurs as a "flash of insight" produced by experiencing something unfamiliar and actively analyzing the new experience in the context of the learner's prior knowledge until the underlying patterns and generalizable principles become apparent. The teacher supports this active process of discovery, a radical departure from the then-prevailing view that learning was passive and received from teachers.

Neo-behaviorists working in the 1920s saw learning as an operant conditioning of observable behaviors, proposing that reinforcement by reward or punishment was the most important factor in learning. Probably, the most iconic example of this *"programmed learning"* technique in medical education is the best-selling book *Rapid Interpretation of EKG's* [8], continuously published since 1972 and well known to healthcare professionals as a very effective introduction to EKG reading. The behaviorist view is also apparent in much of the work to define competence and learning objectives as observable behaviors in the second half of the twentieth century [9].

Cognitivism. In the 1930s, Jean Piaget studied child development and suggested that the most important factor influencing learning is the individual's stage of cognitive development. This *stage theory* had far-reaching impact on education in general. It also stimulated similar work in adults, which influenced higher and professional education. For example, Kohlberg [10] proposed a staged theory of moral development in adults, which provides a backbone for our modern understanding of moral reasoning, ethical decision-making, and professional identity formation (see Chap. 13).

From the 1950s through the mid-1970s, following breakthroughs in the neurosciences, the information processing capacities of the human mind began to be described in terms such as encoding, storing, retrieving, and transferring. Deep learning, which can be retrieved and applied as needed to solve novel problems, requires active information processing. The rich and dynamic field of cognitive psychology, which has dominated learning science since then, provides innumerable relevant insights and tools. Among the most important for health sciences education and practice has been the idea that learning consists of building symbolic cognitive representations in what are called scripts or schemas. Therefore, most adult learning is seen as the process of adding new information to existing networks. Experts have rich schemas arranged in semantic networks, which include many variations built through experience. In this paradigm, the most important factor influencing learning is what someone already knows. This *cognitivist theory* greatly influences the work done to understand how novices learn clinical reasoning (by constructing and improving on illness scripts) and how to best measure it [11–13]. This paradigm also provides a rich foundation for the decision sciences and further refines our understanding of clinical reasoning, impact on patient outcomes and safety [14], and technology-based systems of learning. It also provides a framework for learning or experience curves, which illustrate how deliberate practice produces and sustains expertise [15].

Constructivism. In *social constructivism*, a current dominant learning theory, meaningful learning is actively constructed by an individual or a group of individuals through social interaction. A social construct is a concept or practice that is created by a particular group. For example, competency frameworks define individual competence because we say they do, not because there is an inherent truth about professional competence. In fact, sociological (as contrasted with psychological) theories tend to situate the focus of learning in a social interpersonal environment (e.g., team, unit, department, institution, profession) rather than as a capacity of a single individual. Theorists challenge us to consider collective competence as highly contextualized or situated within a network of complex interactions among clinicians, the patient and family members, and the organizational setting rather than in any one of those individuals [16]. The impact of this view on education practice is reflected in the emerging focus in health sciences education on quality and safety, workplace learning, learning communities, and interprofessional education.

Through the lens of *social cultural theory* which underlies problem-based learning and other activity-based instructional models, learning occurs when a learner internalizes their interaction with others. Teachers construct learning experiences partially by identifying and manipulating the "zone of proximal development" [17]—the knowledge and skills that learners cannot yet understand or perform on their own but are capable of learning with guidance from teachers or with peers.

Many other important learning, psychological, and sociological theories are relevant to remediation in medical education. For instance, theories that help us understand motivation to learn, such as self-determination and self-efficacy theory, apply to remediation work [18]. Emerging complex conceptual models integrate theories from multiple disciplines and perspectives to provide frameworks for learning in rapidly changing environments, such as the Master Adaptive Learner model proposed by Cutrer and colleagues [19] (see Chap. 4) or competency-based education which redefines and provides guidance for structuring curriculum and assessment (see Chap. 2).

Faculty Skills for Remediation Work

The Teacher as Facilitator of Learning

Facilitation of learning is a simple idea: in "learner-centered learning," the teacher sincerely and fundamentally values that individual students focus on their own learning rather than on the teacher's teaching. This approach is often especially challenging in the context of remediation, where trainees have underperformed or behaved badly. Both learner and teacher must embrace a growth mindset, believing that learning occurs through persistent, effortful pursuit of competence rather than being committed to notions of fixed characteristics such as inherent talent [20]. Importantly, learner-centered learning should not be confused with teacher passivity or indulgence of the learner. An effective facilitator can be fierce, active, and demanding. A facilitative teacher tends to have an exceptional ability to ask frank questions and actively listen to the answers. This type of teacher tends to be highly emotionally intelligent and has the capacity to actively maintain what the humanist psychologist Carl Rogers termed *unconditional positive regard* for learners [21]: regardless of what learners say or do, or how well or poorly they perform, they deserve basic acceptance and support as individual people. Rogers believed that unconditional positive regard is essential to healthy psychological development and to individuals accepting and taking responsibility for themselves.

For remediation to be effective and meaningful, there must be trust in the relationship between teacher and learner. This trust is dynamic and is threatened whenever someone "makes trouble" (e.g., a teacher unleashes criticism, or a learner refuses to engage in remediation). Repair of trust occurs when it becomes clear that the trouble does not destroy the positive regard: the relationship is maintained through interacting "nonjudgmentally" and expressing fundamental respect for and acceptance of the learner even when needing to confront and correct performance [22] (see Chap. 6). These skills of facilitation can be learned and refined; one of the longest running and most successful approaches to professional development in this domain is the Faculty Training Program of the Academy of Communication in Healthcare [23] (https://achonline.org/Programs/Faculty-in-Training-Program).

Coaching

In an article in the New Yorker magazine, surgeon Atul Gawande related his experience of having a very senior surgeon observe him in the operating room and provide highly specific feedback on his technical performance [24]. This article is often cited as having brought the term "coaching" into the discourse of health professions education. The rise of "coach" as a distinct role of educators parallels the rise of competency-based and time-variable structures within health professions programs and has been included in many of the recent "future of medicine" conversations [25].

Frameworks for the role of the coach in learning medicine, derived from the extensive literature in sports, music, and business, have been proposed and studied [26]. Proponents of the coaching model emphasize its collaborative nature, focusing on learner goal-setting, developing solutions, goal attainment, and development of self-directed learning. Coaching differs from traditional teaching, role-modeling, and mentoring in being more explicitly structured, learner-centered, and data-driven. Coaches also do not provide advice or focus on providing general psychosocial support ("therapy"). Coaching models that incorporate both transactional (external motivators such as rules, standards for performance data) and transformational (intrinsic motivators such as career aspirations) approaches appear to be most effective. Several faculty development programs both train health professions educators as coaches and use a coaching framework to conduct faculty development.

Cognitive Apprenticeship

Apprenticeship is an ancient and well-worn instructional method, still highly valued in health professions education, in which novices learn by doing real-world work alongside experts. The critique of this model in practice has been that the master teacher often fails to share all the tacit processes involved in carrying out complex skills, making what they do seem mysterious or magical to novice learners. *Cognitive apprenticeship* is an instructional model that explicitly and deliberately brings tacit processes into the open, where learners can observe, enact, and practice them with help from the teacher, thereby acquiring expertise [27]. This framework for instruction is based on several learning theories, including situated learning, in which the context of the learning is inextricable from the learning (e.g., people who cannot do simple arithmetic on a math quiz may still have skills to make change expertly in the supermarket). Below is a sample of specific teaching strategies suggested by this framework that are especially useful in remediation work.

Cognitive Apprenticeship: Teaching Strategies

Modeling: Demonstrate the task so that learners can build their own internalized schema or script. Narrate the underlying thinking and decision-making behind key steps in the task.

Coaching (see prior section): Observe the learner's performance and offer feedback along the way to guide the development of the learner's ability. Adjust the task so that it is just beyond the learner's current abilities.

Scaffolding: Support learning by analyzing the learner's current ability and providing just enough support to allow the learner to practice the task. Initially, this may include doing part of the process. Scaffolding should fade away as learner expertise grows.

Articulation: Ask questions that enable the learner to state what they know, think, or can do already. Then follow this by asking the student to "think aloud" or narrate the process. Guide learners in groups to help each other articulate the underlying factual knowledge and concepts needed to conduct the skill.

Reflection: Have the learner analyze their performances to develop awareness of the similarities and differences between their own thought processes and that of an expert. The goal is to have the student develop an internalized model of expertise. Ask students to list "take-home points" verbally or in writing.

Exploration: Create opportunities for students to define an interesting problem within the domain for themselves and take the initiative to solve these problems.

Judgment

In health professions education, it is not acceptable to promote someone just because they do not fail a knowledge exam or upset someone enough to instigate a complaint. When working with a struggling trainee, one must take responsibility to make difficult affirmative judgments about competence and promotion.

Judgment: the ability to make considered decisions or come to sensible conclusions.

Within a psychometric framework, faculty competence judgments are rarely of high quality because of inconsistency and unreliability, due to halo effects, leniency in grading, and range restriction [28]. Achieving an acceptable level of reliability when using faculty as raters, if possible at all, requires significant investment of resources, and such efforts are frequently frustrating and unsuccessful. Often, we unfairly blame faculty for this inconsistency.

The Best Use of Faculty Raters: In-Training Assessment

Real-life performance assessment is less about measurement and more about reasoning, problem-solving, and decision-making in a dynamic environment, akin to clinical reasoning and decision-making in medical practice.—Norman [29]

While standardized assessments of aspects of clinical competence (e.g., knowledge, procedures, basic communication) provide valuable feedback to trainees, educators understand that the performance that matters most cannot be defined independently of a real clinical context. For this reason, we recommend emphasis on in-training (or workplace-based) assessment (ITA), defined as multiple observations and assessment of performance in the setting of day-to-day practice using direct observation and simplified tools [30]. ITA has become an invaluable tool in comprehensive and valid assessment of clinical competence because it approximates measuring the most relevant clinical performance when training healthcare professionals. Although this approach also suffers from considerable limitations in accuracy and reliability, it has the distinct advantage of explicitly valuing the expert judgment of faculty raters, who actively process information in a complex environment and can continuously assess a trainee's performance for different contexts (i.e., performance rating, formative feedback).

At its best, ITA is an active give-and-take between trainee and assessor. In this relational context, goals and performance criteria are negotiated and responsive to the particulars of the situation. Therefore, in clinical settings, assessment is embedded in the larger context of teaching, shaped by the demands of patient care and often with the direct involvement of the patient. In contrast to standardized assessments, in which inconsistent ratings between teachers can become problematic, disagreements between trainee and assessor may be the most valuable aspects of ITAs [31]. The experience, expertise, unique opinions, biases, and idiosyncrasies of the teacher provide rich and relevant information about performance, especially when compared with those of other individual teachers. For example, a clinical preceptor with extensive expertise in working with "somatizing" patients (those who experience psychological stress as physical distress) might be uniquely and consistently harsh in his or her assessment of learners who do not show interest in such patients. Understanding this context provides program directors with important discriminating data about these learners.

Measurement vs. Judgment

Faculty involved in assessment of competence and remediation must understand the underlying assumptions of various assessment approaches (e.g., psychometric, objective, constructivist). It is also important to distinguish between a measurement (an objective and incontrovertible rating) and a judgment, a more flexible decision-making process in which the faculty rater considers the individuals involved and the social context in which assessment occurs. Emerging research in "rater cognition" has identified that experts form instantaneous impressions of a trainee's performance and categorize the trainee, often in very idiosyncratic ways [32]. Using a constructivist framework, a member of the faculty may appropriately assess the same trainee performance differently based on the purpose of that judgment. In our assessment and remediation practice, we have stopped using faculty raters when highly consistent measurements are needed (e.g., assessment of foundational physical exam skill in OSCEs) but save these valuable teachers to make judgments where needed (e.g., assessment of decision-making when simultaneously managing multiple acute medical issues in an understaffed clinical setting).

Understanding how an expert faculty member judges the competence of a trainee helps deepen our capacity to make considered decisions and draw sensible conclusions. However, no matter how sophisticated or high-quality we make assessments and the judgments based on them, it will always require courage and conviction to act definitively once a trainee or colleague is judged to be incompetent (see Chap. 29).

Effective Models of Faculty Development for Remediation

There have been calls for a unified set of expectations and effective faculty development approaches [33]. As practiced, the term "faculty development" applies to a broad range of activities that institutions use to assist faculty members in their multiple roles and includes a variety of structures (e.g., single session, episodic, longitudinal, train-the-trainer, fellowships). Although evaluation methodology is flawed, faculty development activities generally are satisfying to participants; have positive impact on attitudes, knowledge, and teaching behaviors as reported by learners; and lead to the establishment of networks among colleagues. Features of effective faculty development include the use of experiential learning, provision of feedback, effective peer and colleague relationships, well-designed interventions following principles of teaching and learning, and use of a diversity of educational methods within single interventions [34]. Yet, other evidence suggests that faculty are almost always reluctant to change educational practice. What is clear from the literature is that while faculty development programs have focused on providing participants with strategies, approaches, and best teaching practices, they have succeeded less well at supporting participants in implementing these practices in their institutional contexts.

Current faculty development tends to compartmentalize (e.g., a lecture or workshop on remediating professionalism), de-emphasizing critical relationships among objectives essential to mastering complex skills (e.g., remediating lapses in professionalism). Consequently, participants have difficulty transferring their learning to new complicated situations. This "transfer problem" is of great interest to education researchers and practitioners and has emerged at the forefront as medical education embraces simulation centers [35]. As a result, health professions education is moving toward holistic models of curriculum and instructional design, intended to support complex learning and avoid fragmentation of learning [36]. Rather than breaking down learning tasks into knowledge, skills, and attitudes [37], these models depend more on performing tasks as meaningful wholes (e.g., conduct an effective, data-driven professionalism remediation process with residents) and introducing variation that challenges learners to compare different "presentations," building richer and more accurate schemas in the process [38]. These approaches emphasize coherence, relationships, and coordination of learning in authentic real-life tasks. In this model, a coach defines and prioritizes the tasks in all its meaningful variations, developing supportive and just-in-time material and judging competence. The process of this training parallels the recommended process of remediation with learners. Research has shown that this approach to curriculum design, while potentially slowing short-term learning, produces better retrieval and transfer (Chaps. 6 and 7).

Case Example of a Holistic Faculty Development Curriculum

A surgeon, Susan (she/her), must address the consistently unprofessional behavior of one of her residents, Tim (he/him). Susan has never performed this task. She requests that you coach her to effectively address Tim's unprofessional behavior and to learn the needed knowledge and skills to be competent at professionalism remediation in the future.

Step One. *Susan negotiates a simple individualized learning contract with you: breaking down this complex task into a series of steps, committing to practicing each step, and discussing her progress with you. She lists the following activities:*

A. *Writing a concise summary of Tim's unprofessional behavior, labeling behaviors using the 4 I model (Chap. 14), and analyzing the seriousness of the situation from the perspective of key stakeholders*

B. *Seeking demonstrations of experts addressing learners like Tim, e.g., a Web-based module or book chapter, reviewing the important steps of remediation coaching (Chaps. 4, 6, and 14)*

C. *Creating just-in-time information to assist her learning, e.g., a pocket card listing key elements of the program's expectations for professionalism [39] and an example remediation plan*

D. *Practicing subsets of the skills with an expert, e.g., interpreting and discussing a series of Defining Issues Test (DIT-2) results and Professional Identity Essays reflecting typical and atypical variation in these measures (see Chap. 13)*

E. *Supervising Susan's real-time remediation coaching with Tim*

Step Two. *Susan would then demonstrate increasing competence by performing the whole complex task repeatedly, applying the task to different situations (e.g., an Ob-Gyn resident who walked out of a difficult delivery, a hematology fellow who falsified research results), until she demonstrates the ability to assess and address unprofessional behavior at a consistently competent level as judged by both her coach and herself.*

A Proposal to Support Effective Faculty Development for Remediation in "Communities of Practice"

O'Sullivan and Irby critique the current state of faculty development in medical education and propose that we move toward considering it as a

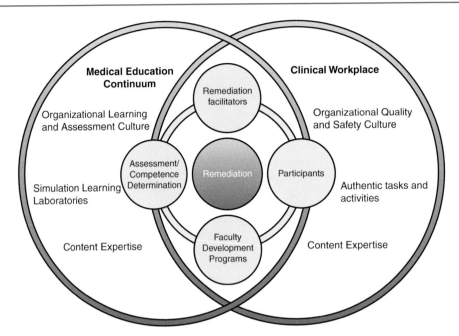

Fig. 19.1 This model for faculty development to support remediation suggests that remediation practice is embedded within two communities of practice: the clinical workplace and the educational space. The work of remediation requires interaction among facilitators, faculty development programs, assessment programs, and participants in remediation. The critical aspects of these communities of practice include organizational culture, availability of practice opportunities, and content expertise. Strong relationships and alignments among these elements are needed to support effective remediation to maximize healthcare and educational outcomes. (Adapted from [40])

"social enterprise" embedded in and tightly linked to the larger educational and clinical environments—rather than emphasizing individual events which take participants out of their daily experience. They argue that using more complex frameworks and moving away from episodic models of workshops and events, which tend to attract those least likely to benefit, will more likely lead to better patient outcomes [40].

A "community of practice" (CoP) is a group of people deeply engaged in a joint enterprise to develop a shared social structure, common values, and shared resources and emerges from constructivist theory [41]. As proposed by O'Sullivan and Irby, effective faculty development ideally is embedded in other important CoPs. We agree with this embedded strategy. Incorporating the views of Holmboe et al., who call for developing a team of faculty development experts to raise the bar on faculty training in assessment [42], we propose further that remediation practice should situate across two highly linked CoPs (Fig. 19.1).

First, it overlaps the "education space," including leadership and administrative structures for educational programs across the continuum of medical training communities (undergraduate, graduate, and continuing education). Second, it overlaps the clinical workplace where training occurs. Remediation faculty development programs are situated in both communities and highly linked with the organizational cultures, available content expertise, and learning resources. Leadership of and relationships around this shared CoP must be strong to ensure that the work is effective.

In conclusion, to expand our profession's capacity to engage in effective remediation in clinical skills and professionalism, we propose the following:

1. Programs create multidisciplinary, interprofessional teams of remediation experts through longitudinal fellowship or train-the-trainer and "just-in-time" models. Members

of this team will coach others in their remediation work and lead remediation and faculty development efforts.

2. Institutions continue to conduct episodic small and large group events in the relevant communities of practice sparingly to define domains of remediation practice, and identify medical educators with a special interest in these domains (grand rounds, brief workshops).

3. Leaders garner institutional support for remediation including championing efforts and financial resources (see Chap. 2).

4. Workplace learning strategies infuse remediation practice competence into authentic work environments

5. Ongoing study of these efforts informs policy and best practices and make faculty development relevant, efficient, and effective.

Conclusion

Faculty development programs are outward signs of the inner faith that institutions have in their workforce.—Bligh [43]

In a perfect learning environment, remediation activities might rarely be needed. The environment would be organized to support high-quality, excellent healthcare practice, centered on the needs of patients and communities served. Individual practitioners would be highly valued and held to clearly articulated high standards, agreed upon by all members of the community of practice. We would all be expected to engage in continual and effortful expertise development (Chap. 4). Each of us would occasionally be required to make a "course correction" and would do so without shame and with the support of members of the relevant communities of practice.

Until then, we must ensure that committed team members identify and work effectively with those of us who do not meet professional standards. We must also develop the capacity in the systems of education and clinical practice to support remediation efforts. Faculty development programs would interact in overlapping communities of practice to ensure awareness of learning and assessment theories, develop skills to work effectively with colleagues and trainees who are struggling, and support courageous acts of judgment that ensure the excellence and safety of the healthcare enterprise.

References

1. Hatem CJ, Searle NS, Gunderman R, Krane NK, Perkowski L, Schutze GE, Steinert Y. The educational attributes and responsibilities of effective medical educators. Acad Med. 2011;86:474–80. https://doi.org/10.1097/ACM.0b013e31820cb28a.

2. Pratt DD, Arseneau R, Collins JB. Reconsidering "good teaching" across the continuum of medical education. J Contin Educ Heal Prof. 2001;21:70–81. PubMed PMID: 11420868.

3. Kaufman D. Applying educational theory in practice. BMJ. 2003;326:213–6. PubMed PMID: 12543841.

4. Kaufman D, Mann K. Chapter 2: Teaching and learning in medical education: how theory can inform practice. In: Swanwick T, ed. Understanding medical education: evidence, theory and practice. 1st ed. Hoboken: Wiley; c2010. 446 p.

5. Taylor DC, Hamdy H. Adult learning theories: implications for learning and teaching in medical education: AMEE guide no. 83. Med Teach. 2013;35:e1561–72.

6. ten Cate O, Snell L, Mann K, Vermunt J. Orienting teaching toward the learning process. Acad Med. 2004;79(3):219–28. PubMed PMID: 14985194.

7. Baker LR, Phelan S, Woods NN, Boyd VA, Rowland P, Ng SL. Re-envisioning paradigms of education: towards awareness, alignment, and pluralism. Adv Health Sci Educ Theory Pract. 2021;26:1045–58.

8. Dubin D. Rapid interpretation of EKG's: an interactive course, 6th ed. Tampa: Cover Publishing Company; c2000. 368 p.

9. Mager R. Preparing instructional objectives. 3rd ed. Atlanta: CEP Press; c1997. 197 p.

10. Kohlberg L, Levine C, Hewer A. Moral stages: a current formulation and a response to critics. Basel: Karger; 1983. isbn:978-3-8055-3716-2.

11. Charlin B, Tardif J, Boshuizen HP. Scripts and medical diagnostic knowledge: theory and applications for clinical reasoning instruction and research. Acad Med. 2000;75:182–90. PubMed PMID: 10693854.

12. Eva KW. What every teacher needs to know about clinical reasoning. Med Educ. 2005;39:98–106. PubMed PMID: 15612906.

13. Bordage G. Elaborated knowledge: a key to successful diagnostic thinking. Acad Med. 1994;69:883–5. PubMed PMID: 7945684.

14. Croskerry P. A universal model of diagnostic reasoning. Acad Med. 2009;84:1022–8. https://doi.org/10.1097/ACM.0b013e3181ace703.

15. Pusic MV, Kessler D, Szyld D, Kalet A, Pecaric M, Boutis K. Experience curves as an organizing framework for deliberate practice in emergency medicine learning. Acad Emerg Med. 2012;2012(19):1476–80.

16. Lingard L. Paradoxical truths and persistent myths: reframing the team competence conversation. J Cont Educ Health Prof. 2016;2016(36):S19–21.

17. Vygotsky LS. Mind and society: the development of higher psychological processes. Cambridge: Harvard University Press; 1978. c1980.159 p.

18. Bandura A. Social cognitive theory. In: Van Lange PAM, Kruglanski AW, Higgins ET, editors. Handbook of theories of social psychology, vol. 1. 1st ed. Thousand Oaks: SAGE Publications; c2012. 556 p.

19. Cutrer WB, Miller B, Pusic MV, Mejicano G, Mangrulkar RS, Gruppen LD, et al. Fostering the development of master adaptive learners: a conceptual model to guide skill acquisition in medical education. Acad Med. 2017;2017(92):70–5.

20. Yeager DS, Dweck CS. Mindsets that promote resilience: when students believe that personal characteristics can be developed. Educ Psychol. 2012;47(4):302–14.

21. Rogers C. On becoming a person: a therapist's view of psychotherapy. 3rd ed. New York: Houghton Mifflin Harcourt; c1989. 420p.

22. Rogers C, Freiberg HJ. Freedom to learn. 3rd ed. Pearson; c1994. 352p.

23. Chou CL, Hirschmann K, Fortin AH 6th, Lichstein PR. The impact of a faculty learning community on professional and personal development: the facilitator training program of the American Academy on Communication in Healthcare. Acad Med. 2014;89:1051–1056.

24. https://www.newyorker.com/magazine/2011/10/03/personal-best.

25. Simpson D, Marcdante K, Souza KH, Anderson A, Holmboe E. Job roles of the 2025 medical educator. J Grad Med Educ. 2018;10:243–6.

26. Orr CJ, Sonnadara RR. Coaching by design: exploring a new approach to faculty development in a competency-based medical education curriculum. Adv Med Educ Pract. 2019;10:229–44.

27. Lyons K, McLaughlin JE, Khanova J, Roth MT. Cognitive apprenticeship in health sciences education: a qualitative review. Adv Health Sci Educ Theory Pract. 2017;22:723–39.

28. Kalet A, Earp J, Kowlowitz V. How well do faculty evaluate the interviewing skills of medical students? J Gen Intern Med. 1992;7:499–505. PubMed PMID: 1403205.

29. Norman G. Research in clinical reasoning: past history and current trends. Med Educ. 2005;39:418–27. PubMed PMID: 15813765.

30. Norcini JJ, Blank LL, Duffy FD, Fortna GS. The mini-CEX: a method for assessing clinical skills. Ann Intern Med. 2003;138:476–81. PubMed PMID: 12639081.

31. Govaerts MJ, van der Vleuten CP, Schuwirth LW, Muijtjens AM. Broadening perspectives on clinical performance assessment: rethinking the nature of in-training assessment. Adv Health Sci Educ Theory Pract. 2007;12(2):239–60.

32. Gingerich A, Regehr G, Eva KW. Rater-based assessments as social judgments: rethinking the etiology of rater errors. Acad Med. 2011;86:S1–7. https://doi.org/10.1097/ACM.0b013e31822a6cf8.

33. Searle NS, Thibault GE, Greenberg SB. Faculty development for medical educators: current barriers and future directions. Acad Med. 2011;86:405–6. https://doi.org/10.1097/ACM.0b013e31820dc1b3.

34. Steinert Y, Mann K, Anderson B, Barnett BM, Centeno A, Naismith L, Prideaux D, Spencer J, Tullo E, Viggiano T, Ward H, Dolmans D. A systematic review of faculty development initiatives designed to enhance teaching effectiveness: a 10-year update: BEME Guide No. 40. Med Teach. 2016;38:769–86.

35. Norman G, Dore K, Grierson L. The minimal relationship between simulation fidelity and transfer of learning. Med Educ. 2012;46:636–47.

36. Vandewaetere M, Manhaeve D, Aertgeerts B, Clarebout G, Van Merriënboer JJ, Roex A. 4C/ID in medical education: how to design an educational program based on whole-task learning: AMEE guide no. 93. Med Teach. 2015;37:4–20.

37. van Merriënboer JJG, Kirschner P. Ten steps to complex learning: a systematic approach to four-component instructional design. 2nd ed. London: Lawrence Erlbaum Associates, c2013. 306p.

38. Bowen JL. Educational strategies to promote clinical diagnostic reasoning. N Engl J Med. 2006;355:2217–25.

39. Blank L, Kimball H, McDonald W, Merino J, ABIM Foundation; ACP Foundation; European Federation of Internal Medicine. Medical professionalism in the new millennium: a physician charter 15 months later. Ann Intern Med. 2003;138:839–41.

40. O'Sullivan PS, Irby DM. Reframing research on faculty development. Acad Med. 2011;86:421–8. https://doi.org/10.1097/ACM.0b013e31820dc058.

41. Wenger E. Communities of practice: learning, meaning, and identity. Cambridge: Cambridge University Press; 1998, c1998. 336p.

42. Holmboe ES, Ward DS, Reznick RK, Katsufrakis PJ, Leslie KM, Patel VL, Ray DD, Nelson EA. Faculty development in assessment: the missing link in competency-based medical education. Acad Med. 2011;86:460–7.

43. Bligh J. Faculty development. Med Educ. 2005;39:120–1. PubMed PMID: 15679676.

Part IV

Systems, Legal, and Ethical Considerations: Undergraduate Medical Education and Interprofessional Schools

The View from the Medical School Dean's Office

20

Lynn Buckvar-Keltz, Allison Ludwig, and H. Carrie Chen

Remediation Concerns During a Day in the Dean's Office

8:30 am: Review of data on students to be discussed at the preclinical board meeting tomorrow reveals that one of the students who failed an exam last week is already currently repeating the first academic year. This will automatically trigger a discussion regarding dismissal. A meeting will be required with the student to assess his recent difficulties and prepare him for potential consequences.

10:00 am: Phone call from a clerkship director concerned that BD (they/them) is "odd" and does not relate well to patients, nurses, or the clinical team. Their peers seem to lose patience with them quickly, and the residents report that BD has not integrated into the clinical team after 3 weeks on the rotation. The director observed BD interview a patient and found them to have difficulty with developing rapport and eliciting the narrative thread of the patient's history. The director does report that BD seems to be working hard and "has a good heart." Nobody has given this feedback to BD verbally or in writing. When it is suggested that BD's performance may be in the failing range, the director immediately states, "Oh, I don't want to fail them. I just want the Dean's Office to be aware so you can do something for BD." The director then asks, "Has BD had problems like this in other clerkships?"

11:15 am: A student pops in, presumably to say hello, and then becomes tearful. She expresses worry that she will fail another exam and that she does not belong in medical school. Upon questioning, she reveals that she is isolated, does not feel connected to her classmates, has difficulty sleeping, and feels exhausted all the time.

12:00 pm: Meeting with a third-year student who just failed his second NBME shelf exam during his core clinical clerkships.

L. Buckvar-Keltz
Department of Medicine, New York University Grossman School of Medicine, New York, NY, USA
e-mail: Lynn.Buckvar-Keltz@nyulangone.org

A. Ludwig
Department of Medicine, Albert Einstein College of Medicine, Bronx, NY, USA
e-mail: allison.ludwig@einsteinmed.edu

H. C. Chen (✉)
Department of Pediatrics, Georgetown University School of Medicine, Washington, DC, USA
e-mail: carrie.chen@georgetown.edu

1:30 pm: Review the neuropsychological report of a second-year student sent by the consultant learning specialist (with the student's permission) that includes a new diagnosis of ADHD and recommendation for test accommodations.

3:30 pm: Email from first-year course director concerned that MR has been late to small group several times, did incomplete jobs on two assignments, and now has a second unexcused absence from lab today. The director, who has tried speaking to the student multiple times, believes that MR may be struggling because of pressure from home and some ambivalence about being in medical school.

5:30 pm: Chair of the professionalism disciplinary committee comes by to personally update the dean's office on the results of the afternoon's committee meeting. Based on the evidence provided, the committee has determined that NH did deliberately alter the results on an assessment in an attempt to boost his grade. He has been suspended, and the "suspension due to a professionalism violation" will be included on his transcript and on his Medical School Performance Evaluation (MSPE, also known as the "Dean's Letter"), a required part of residency program applications.

Introduction

It is the role of a medical school dean's office to balance the dual responsibilities of advocating for students and upholding the integrity of the curricular program. This work is especially challenging when working with students who struggle and require remediation. Given the diverse portfolio of responsibilities in the medical school dean's office, which include overseeing the academic progress of students, disciplinary processes, mentoring and advising, student health and wellness programs, student experience, extracurricular activities, and admissions, deans are often the first to identify and intervene with students who struggle. In addition to working with students and faculty to identify the underlying causes of a student's challenges, the dean's office needs to be concerned about resource availability for and the cost of remediation, legal and privacy issues, and final competency decisions. In this chapter, we will discuss the issue of medical student remediation from pre-admission until graduation through the lens of the school's interests and obligations to students, faculty, and society.

Before embarking on the challenges of remediation as medical school deans, it is important to note that the responsibilities of the dean's office listed above may be housed within one position/person or shared among multiple people. Traditionally, and in many institutions, all or most of the responsibilities above fall under the purview of a student affairs dean. More recently, there has been some recommendations to separate the oversight of academic progress and therefore student remediation from that of other student support functions (e.g., advising, student well-being) to prevent potential conflicts of interest. Some institutions have created a competency or assessment arm of the dean's office to oversee academic progress and remediation, while others have housed these functions under curricular affairs. Regardless of the approach to delegating responsibilities within an institution, there are key issues and challenges to address regarding student remediation. We will first delineate common underlying causes of student difficulty and then discuss potential resources as well as contextual and other important considerations.

Common Causes of Student Difficulties

By definition, a student who struggles does not meet the expectations of medical school because of at least one of many underlying reasons having to do with knowledge, skills, or attitudes [1]. The more common causes as viewed from the dean's office are discussed below.

Academic Issues

Academic Concerns Arising in the Pre-clerkship Curriculum

Deficits in foundational knowledge are usually identified via poor performance on knowledge examinations and small group discussions and come to attention within the first few months of school. Some students may be less academically prepared in general (see Chap. 7). There are also students who have difficulty acclimating to the type of studying and testing common in medical school, for example, if students have taken time away or are accustomed to more conceptual testing from prior studies in fields such as engineering. Finally, some students will benefit from neuropsychological evaluation by a learning specialist to assess for an underlying undiagnosed learning disability (see Chap. 17).

At times, substandard performance in foundational knowledge may merely be a symptom of a problem with motivation. Some students may not have been prepared to sit through or be able to see the relevance of the pre-clerkship curriculum to their goal of providing excellent patient care. Other students have difficulty articulating their reasons for wanting to become a physician and sometimes voice the pressure put upon them by external expectations, such as from parents and other family members. It is important to identify an unmotivated student, as the usual remediation approaches will not help them. These students may appear to be sabotaging their own success and require culturally sensitive coaching that leads to insight and help with practical career planning. Serious reflection on the part of the student is necessary (see Chap. 15). For students who are motivated for clinical but not classroom education, arranging for clinical shadowing can remind them why they chose medical school. For students who express ambivalence about becoming a physician, a leave of absence to pursue other interests can be helpful. Some of these students will choose a different career path with better personal fit, which should be viewed as a successful outcome for the student.

Academic Concerns Arising in the Clinical Curriculum

The transition from pre-clerkship to clerkship curriculum is often the time that difficulties with interpersonal skills and professional behavior are noted and begin to have a greater impact on academic performance. The clinical setting requires students to rapidly gain and apply a new set of skills. Workplace-based learning has been described as "learning as participation" [2]. Students who have difficulty participating and engaging in teams and with others in the clinical workplace experience negative impacts on their knowledge and clinical skill development. These difficulties may be due to shyness and not knowing how to engage proactively or to a range of deficits in interpersonal or professionalism skills. Some of these students may be identified in the pre-clerkship curriculum because of early clinical exercises in which interpersonal, communication, and professionalism skills are practiced and/or assessed. The more significant behavioral challenges are addressed next.

Professionalism Issues

What most often keeps deans up at night are students' high-profile unprofessional acts. Though most students behave professionally all the time, unsavory behavior by a student is long remembered by faculty and classmates. Unfortunately, deans can recount stories of egregious behavior: student arrests for breaking the law, collusions between students to cheat or lie about absences from didactic sessions, etc. Naturally, there are often several different issues that may intercalate to produce those behaviors, including many of the forces listed above and below. Academic dishonesty, patient privacy violations, and failure to meet academic responsibilities in a timely manner are the more common instances of unprofessional behavior.

Schools vary in their policies regarding the reporting, investigation, and remediation versus dismissal for unprofessional behavior. Several schools utilize honor codes, which have been shown to lower the rates of academic integrity violations. Honor codes often delineate expectations, provide examples of violations, and detail judiciary procedures including reporting, proceedings, penalties, and/or appeals. In many cases, the judiciary body includes student members, so that peers are engaged determining whether a violation has occurred, the severity of the violation, and the appropriate penalty [3].

More frequently, unprofessional behavior may be minor and investigated and remediated without the formal activation of a disciplinary committee. However, this can become problematic if a pattern of relatively "low-level" inappropriate behaviors develops. Systems should be in place to identify these patterns, provide early intervention, and appropriately escalate to a disciplinary committee when necessary [4, 5]. This may occur at the level of the student affairs dean and/or course/clerkship director committees where records are kept of minor issues. Regardless of the system used, it should be transparent to students that a pattern of behavior will trigger an official complaint to the disciplinary committee (see Chap. 14).

Psychological Distress and Mental Health Issues

Some students become anxious regarding their academic performance in medical school, hindering their success. Because medical students are academically gifted and have typically been at the top of their classes throughout their education, adjustment to being "average" in medical school is a challenge for some. Many of these students become disappointed and question their abilities. Impostor syndrome and stereotype threat run rampant throughout medicine [6] (see Chaps. 3, 18). Support and encouragement can be very helpful in this circumstance. Simply pointing out the obvious fact that 90% of medical students cannot be in the top 10% of their medical school class often helps students adjust expectations. A pass/fail curriculum may lower the anxiety level for students and importantly may particularly help underrepresented

minority students in the clerkships, where implicit bias among supervising staff in a subjectively graded milieu further reinforces anxiety [Chap. 3; 7].

Most medical schools preemptively encourage students to attend to stress management and their wellness, providing support through formal and informal programming. Student health psychiatrists have extensive experience with medical students and can be helpful with specific issues such as "test anxiety" (see Chap. 7). Learning specialists can speak to students about neurocognitive profiles and study strategies (see Chap. 17). Many schools have embraced a range of formal or informal sessions and tools that address healthy eating, mindfulness meditation and stress management, yoga and other exercise, sleep, acupuncture and other complementary and alternative health strategies, and other activities that reinforce resilience. Attendance at voluntary events can increase if, rather than focusing on "self-help," they emphasize how activities may help their peers or future patients (see also Chap. 18).

Mental Health Disorders

Anxiety, Mood, and Thought Disorders

Academic stress can trigger an episode of an underlying mental health disorder or uncover significant previously undiagnosed illness, such as depression, bipolar disorder, anxiety, and thought disorders. Thought disorders also show an increased prevalence in people in their 20s, exactly when most are in medical school. Faculty and deans must be vigilant in identifying medical students at risk for developing mental health issues and have mechanisms for intervention in place. Mental health professionals at student health services represent an important adjunct. These resources must be confidential and accessible outside the medical student workday. In addition, schools need the ability to regularly refer students to outside mental health professionals for ongoing treatment.

When mental illness is diagnosed for the first time in medical school, students exhibit a range of insight into their illness and willingness to undergo treatment. Extra difficulty may present when there are coexisting substance use disorders (see Substance Use below). Recent data on suicides in medical students and residents heighten the importance of detection and treatment [8, 9]. Balancing the student's personal safety and ability to get through their clerkships with the safety of the patients they care for remains one of the dean's office's greatest challenges.

Personality Disorders

In general, the persistence of personality traits or disorders and their relative lack of responsiveness to treatment make working with students who exhibit these traits challenging. Careful monitoring and follow-up throughout medical school are important. We describe three personality types that present particular difficulty: antisocial, borderline, and schizotypal.

Students with antisocial personality traits demonstrate socially irresponsible and exploitative behaviors, disregard for school policies and professionalism expectations, lack of remorse, and inability to learn from the consequences of their actions. These students need clear expectations outlined for them. A national criminal background check for applicants at the time of their acceptance to medical school, currently used by most schools, may help reduce the number of medical students with antisocial personality disorder in the future.

Students with borderline personality traits are emotionally labile, have unstable relationships with others, are impulsive, and often have coexisting mood, anxiety, and substance use and eating disorders. Support teams working with these students should be aware of the student's common tendency to "split" the team members into extreme groups of "good" and "bad" and pit them against each other, which makes remediation very challenging.

Students with schizotypal personality traits are often described as "odd" or "eccentric" and have difficulty interacting with their clinical teams and with patients. It can be challenging to ascertain whether a thought disorder is present.

For such students, it is essential to have access to formal psychiatric evaluation.

Autism Spectrum Conditions

Students with previously identified or suspected autism spectrum disorders (ASDs), including those identified as having what has been referred to as high-functioning Asperger's syndrome (ASD without language or intellectual deficits), are often viewed as competent but quirky in the classroom setting. Their inaccuracy in reading social and emotional cues of others can lead to challenges in interacting in clinical teams and with patients. While these students commonly engender significant sympathy from classmates and faculty because of their good intentions and earnestness, their communication behaviors can alienate patients or clinical supervisors. Ideally, many would arrive at medical school already with the diagnosis and clear action plans. For those who do not, clinical exposures in the pre-clerkship years can identify students and allow early social skill training. Intensive coaching and role-play practice focused on clinical interviewing can help students gain and demonstrate the ability to function as effectively as their more "neurotypical" medical student peers (see also Chap. 12). The best predictor of success in these cases is the student's level of motivation and awareness of their own challenges.

Substance Use

Students may be impaired due to use of legal or illegal substances. Peers are usually the most knowledgeable about a classmate's substance use and may come forward to a faculty member or the dean's office to share this information. Care should be taken to be supportive of classmates' concerns and privacy while also obtaining accurate, reliable, and complete information. The school should confront the impaired student with information (test scores, evaluative comments, informal comments) that supports the conclusion that the student is unfit in their role as a medical student. The school may require an individual student undergo random blood and urine testing. Students found to be impaired are required to undergo treatment and monitoring. In New York State, medical students can be enrolled in the Committee on Physician Health (CPH) for ongoing monitoring and treatment. Students should be required to allow communication between CPH or similar monitoring/treatment programs and the medical school for the duration of their time as a student. CPH requires continued random drug testing and therapy as conditions of their program and reports periodically to the medical school regarding ongoing compliance with their requirements.

> The mission of the New York State Medical Society's Committee for Physician Health is to promote quality medical care by offering "non-disciplinary confidential assistance to physicians, residents, medical students, and physician assistants experiencing problems from stress and difficult adjustment, emotional, substance abuse, and other psychiatric disorders, including psychiatric problems that may arise as a result of medical illness. We recommend evaluation, treatment, and/or other assistance to our participants and monitor for progress in recovery from illness. In this way, we can also provide strong advocacy on behalf of the participant to continue their practice as a physician or physician-in-training" [10].

Fitness for Duty Evaluation

Occasionally, a student's psychiatric illness or suspicion of impairment will call into question their fitness to continue as a medical student. While fitness for duty issues may be more common at the GME level and in clinical practice, where physician impairment must be reported to the state medical boards, the same concerns for patient safety also apply to students on clinical rotations. Some schools may have an administra-

tive psychiatrist who conducts fitness evaluations using primary and sometimes ancillary data to make a determination. Other schools may need to rely on determinations made by the psychiatrist to whom the student has been referred or who is treating the student. Schools should place students found to be "unfit" on a leave of absence and require students to address their issue before being considered for return to the school. Students on leave who request a return should be evaluated for fitness to return by either the school's administrative psychiatrist or the student's treating psychiatrist. Where available, students should be strongly encouraged to participate in monitoring and support programs such as the New York State CPH.

Dean's Office Resources for Remediation

Schools develop their own resources to remediate students and vary widely on what is available and on who pays for the remediation. Philosophically, schools need to determine whether their supports (i.e., offering and paying for remediation) are helpful to the student or enabling a lack of responsibility and ownership on the student's part. Table 20.1 lists resources that schools may commonly make available for remediation, a list of "Dream Resources" (those that would be of great help but unavailable to most schools), and an estimate of the cost of remediation per student at this point in time.

An example of student use of resources follows, using New York University (NYU) as a case study. At NYU, unlimited peer tutoring is offered to all students who request it. Peer tutors are selected based on faculty nomination, undergo training as coaches of medical knowledge learning and assessment, and are required to develop goal-directed learning plans with the students they work with and submit progress reports regularly. Out of about 730 students enrolled, approximately 100 students will use tutoring services in an academic year. Students do not need to fail an exam or have "marginal" exam performance to obtain peer tutoring. Approximately 10–15 students undergo a

Table 20.1 Remediation resources

Resources commonly available for remediation:
1. Learning specialist (expenses related to neuropsychiatric testing and diagnosis may or may not be covered; expenses related to treatment typically not covered)
2. Academic tutoring
3. Student mental health services with staff psychiatrists and/or psychologists (the insurance accepted, and number of visits covered varies)
4. Course faculty
5. Faculty with expertise in remediation
6. Simulation experiences with expert faculty
7. Resident/Physician support programs open to medical students offered by the affiliated hospital/healthcare system, state medical society, etc.

"Dream resources" that are not typically available:
1. Targeted remediation programs, including simulation, developed and delivered by expert faculty
2. Administrative psychiatrist
3. Comprehensive mental health services with expanded coverage (e.g., unlimited number of visits, support for intensive psychotherapy)
4. Professionalism coaches and assessment tools to remediate and reassess students who have failed due to professionalism concerns
5. Social skills coach/therapist to work one-on-one with students who struggle with interpersonal and communication skills (e.g., students with autism spectrum conditions) to observe behaviors in clinical settings, develop intervention plans, and remediate the students

Examples of the costs associated with remediation per student (as of December 2022):
1. Complete learning specialist evaluation: ~$5000/student
2. Peer tutoring: $26/h
3. Private tutoring: $150 and up/h
4. Student health psychiatrist: typically included in student health service budget
5. Administrative psychiatrist: $20,000/year and an additional $2000/student evaluation
6. Course faculty: no additional cost
7. Faculty with expertise in remediation: no additional cost
8. Comprehensive clinical skills exam (CCSE) remediation: ~$400/student excluding faculty time
9. Outside professionalism programs: $2500–$7500

detailed learning evaluation each year. Approximately 20 students undergo remediation for skills exams each year, which includes students remediating within preclinical modules (such as after failing an Objective Structured Clinical Examination, or OSCE) or failure in a comprehen-sive clinical skills exam, which is an eight-station, high-stakes, end-of-clerkship-year OSCE.

Each school has its own method of remedia-tion of medical students. While the remediation often occurs within a course or clerkship struc-ture, it can be helpful to also have faculty with expertise in remediation of clinical skills and pro-fessionalism lapses. For some schools, there may be resources available within their affiliated health systems/hospitals such as communication training programs for residents and physicians willing to accept medical students. Finally, there are also available outside resources for remedia-tion of professionalism issues such as the Vanderbilt Comprehensive Assessment Program for Professionals at Vanderbilt University Medical Center and Acumen Assessments in Kansas.

Considerations for Admissions

Academic and Nonacademic Attributes

The policy for medical school admissions is the most important factor determining who becomes a physician. In the United States, the competition for a spot in medical school is daunting: in 2020, the AAMC reported that there were 50,030 applicants, 22,239 of whom matriculated to US medical schools. This is a 44% acceptance rate for students having undergone grueling premedical coursework and the MCAT, both of which cull out lower performing students. The good news for these matriculants to US medical schools is that they will most likely graduate with a degree to practice medicine. For 20 years, starting with the 1997–1998 school year, an average of 3.2% of students left medical school for any reason; from 2007–2008 to 2017–2018, approximately 1.2% of all medical students left for academic reasons [11]. Thus, admissions committees and officers are more influential in determining who becomes a physician than others in the dean's office. Given this, the question is whether we are giving our admissions committees/officers the tools to make the most informed decisions.

The first time a student's ability to succeed in medical school may be questioned is during review of his or her application to medical school. Academic concerns arise when students have grade point averages and MCAT scores significantly below the school's mean for accepted students. Studies suggest that these academic indicators correlate, but without statistical significance, with learning foundational medical knowledge and USMLE scores [see Chap. 2; 12].

Much attention is paid to an uneven academic record or fluctuating grades, as this may be a sign of lack of motivation, lack of interest, or emotional difficulties. Withdrawals from coursework, especially repeatedly, raise concerns. Additionally, the record is scanned for certain patterns. Has the student been fully engaged in the extracurricular life at their undergraduate school? If not, why not? Is all their nonclass time already devoted to studying, suggesting that the student may not have "additional reserve" to handle medical school? A leave of absence may be another sign of some underlying difficulty. Indication of disciplinary action is a concern. Supporting materials such as a Dean's Letter (supplied by some undergraduate schools), the student's personal statement, or letters of recommendation may help explain any unevenness in performance without raising red flags. Unfortunately, the value of these specific application-based variables as predictors of success in medical school has not been well studied. However, studies have shown that unprofessional behavior of practicing physicians reported to state boards is correlated with a history of certain unprofessional behavior in medical school [13].

While academic attainment is a predictor of early performance in medical school, it becomes a less important predictor as students advance into clinical training and practice [14]. In order to assess nonacademic qualities of applicants such as ethical judgment, communication skills, and problem-solving capabilities, some US schools have adopted McMaster University's model of multiple mini-interviews (MMIs) with standard scenarios to be discussed by the applicant. Others have added situational judgement tests (SJTs), which have been used in the United Kingdom for selection in graduate medical education and other health professions. In SJTs, written or video-based scenarios are followed by a list of response options that can be administered online to generate a score or used as part of an MMI. Both MMIs and SJTs have been shown to be valid and reliable methods for assessing nonacademic qualities, and more effective as selection tools than traditional interviews and personal statements [15]. The data thus far also show that the MMI predicts success on national licensing examinations in Canada [16]. Some of this approach may depend on one's philosophical stance regarding whether certain characteristics are static and should be selected for or against, whether the same or other characteristics are dynamic and responsive to coaching, and the availability of a school's resources to devote to coaching.

Since the last edition of this book, many medical school admissions offices have adopted at least some elements of "holistic admission": de-emphasizing traditional markers of achievement (e.g., school grades and standardized testing performance) in favor of a broader definition of achievement: distance traveled, underrepresentation, etc. This shift has importantly amplified attention to how graduating medical students may develop to meet the evolving needs of the population as a whole. This broader definition of "achievement" brings a greater range in student academic backgrounds as well as differences in student preparation for the academic rigor of medical school, adding some uncertainty to determining admissions decisions. This new approach raises many questions. Are a history and conviction that the candidate will make a wonderful physician for interpersonal reasons enough to overcome the possibility that the demands of medical school may overwhelm a student who is incompletely prepared? How might schools meet promising students where they are and better support their learning?

Schools can provide support prior to, at, and/or after matriculation. Georgetown University offers a postbaccalaureate program specifically designed to equip underrepresented and disadvantaged students for future success in medical school. The program exposes students to a rigorous curriculum comparable to the experience of first-year medical students and adds customized advising and a parallel curriculum focused on the development of academic skills ("learning how to learn"). Many schools offer programs prematriculation or immediately at matriculation for students who have a gap between college and medical school and/or did not have an undergraduate major in science. With the increased use of online platforms for delivering this content, these programs can be offered to all students. Additional methods of supporting students both before and after matriculation must consider the common experiences of impostor syndrome, stereotype threat, bias, and microaggressions that disproportionately affect underrepresented minority students (see Chap. 3). Schools should attend to student stories of their experience and, particularly if they have dedicated deans of diversity, work closely with them to develop support programs.

Technical Standards in Admissions

Schools are expected to assess applicants based on their ability to complete the educational program. Occasionally, an applicant will apply to medical school but may not possess the functional ability to perform as a medical student. The Americans with Disabilities Act (ADA) protects citizens with disabilities from discrimination. The purpose of the ADA is to provide opportunities for persons with disabilities to compete with other applicants based on their ability. The ADA requires medical schools to provide accommodations to disabled persons to enable them to access the benefits, services, and opportunities available to the nondisabled (see Chap. 17). This means that suitable applicants must be able to perform the "essential functions" and meet the "essential eligibility requirements" of the program once provided with the appropriate accommodation. Each school is free to determine the "essential functions" or "essential eligibility requirements" of its own educational program. While schools cannot inquire about a disability prior to admission, they can seek information to ensure that an applicant can perform these essential functions [17]. In recent years, many schools have developed *technical standards* to clarify and communicate those essential functions and eligibility requirements.

We share a sample set of technical standards from Georgetown University in Table 20.2 [18]. The technical standards at each school will vary

Table 20.2 Sample technical standards [18]

Guided by the Jesuit tradition of *cura personalis*, care of the whole person, Georgetown University School of Medicine will educate a diverse student body, in an integrated way, to become knowledgeable, ethical, skillful, and compassionate physicians and biomedical scientists who are dedicated to the care of others and health needs of our society. An applicant for the M.D. degree, and an enrolled student seeking the M.D. degree, must meet the technical standards or functional equivalent, with or without reasonable accommodations, deemed essential functions for the care of patients. These abilities and skills, as determined by Georgetown University School of Medicine, are as follows:

1. **Perception:** Students enrolled in the M.D. degree program must be able to observe demonstrations and experiments required by the medical curriculum established by the medical faculty and be able to participate in such with adequate vision and other sensory modalities, including the senses of hearing and smell. A student must be able to observe a patient accurately at a distance and close at hand

2. **Communication:** Students must be able to skillfully (in English) communicate verbally and in written form to affect an adequate exchange of information with patients, family members, and other health professionals in order to fulfill academic requirements and to maintain accurate clinical records on patient care

3. **Motor:** Students must have sufficient motor function and tactile ability to meet the competencies required for graduation, as outlined by the Georgetown University School of Medicine, and to (1) attend (and participate in) classes, groups, and activities which are part of the curriculum; (2) communicate in a written format; (3) examine patients (including observation, auscultation, palpation, percussion, and other diagnostic maneuvers); (4) perform diagnostic procedures in addition to basic laboratory procedures and tests; and (5) provide general and emergency patient care in outpatient, inpatient, and surgical venues and perform in a reasonably independent and competent way in sometimes chaotic clinical environments

(continued)

Table 20.2 (continued)

4. **Intellectual-Conceptual, Integrative, and Quantitative Abilities:** Students must be able to demonstrate higher level cognitive abilities to meet the competencies required for graduation, as outlined by the Georgetown University School of Medicine, including an aptitude for timely problem-solving, capability to access and independently interpret medical files, evaluate physical examinations, and formulate a logical diagnosis and effective medical treatment plan. Students must possess good judgment in patient assessment, and the abilities to incorporate new information, comprehend three-dimensional relationships, and retain and recall pertinent information in a timely fashion

5. **Behavioral and Social Attributes:** Guided by the Jesuit tradition of *cura personalis*, care of the whole person, students must display compassion, sensitivity, and concern for others and maintain professional integrity at all times. In addition, students must develop mature, sensitive, and effective relationships: not only with patients but also with all members of the medical school community and healthcare teams. Students must also be able to promptly complete all assignments and responsibilities attendant to the diagnosis and care of patients (beginning with study in the first year). Students must tolerate physically, emotionally, and mentally demanding workloads and function effectively under stress. A student must be able to proactively make use of available resources to help maintain both physical and mental health. A student must display adaptability to changing environments, flexibility, and be able to learn in the face of uncertainty. All students enrolled in the M.D. degree program must take responsibility for themselves and their behaviors

Students enrolled in pursuit of an M.D. degree at Georgetown University School of Medicine are required to attest to these technical standards on an annual basis. The School of Medicine is committed to providing reasonable accommodations for students with disabilities. An applicant for the M.D. degree or an enrolled student seeking the M.D. degree with disabilities is encouraged to contact the Georgetown University Academic Resource Center as early as possible to begin a confidential conversation separate from an application or enrollment status, about what reasonable accommodations they may need to meet these standards

in its specifics but generally reflect the overall mission of educating students who can perform the essential functions for care of patients with or without reasonable accommodations. Reasonable accommodations at schools, based on their specific standards and available resources, can range

from allowing students extra time to take an exam due to learning disabilities to alternative clinical experiences during the COVID-19 pandemic for students who are immunocompromised and to supplying hearing-impaired students with specialized stethoscopes.

Student Financial Considerations

Remediation that requires an extension of time in medical school has financial implications for students in terms of additional tuition, fees, and associated costs of living. While some schools have instituted discounted tuition and fees for students who need to extend or decelerate their curriculum, the additional financial burden adds to the student stress of having to remediate. Other schools have worked to address the financial consequences by taking a "pay for degree" approach, where students pay a maximum of 4 years of tuition and fees and have up to a certain number of years (e.g., 7) to complete their medical degree. NYU, for example, prior to becoming a "tuition free" school, had already determined that the extra amount of tuition a very small number of students might contribute is ultimately administratively negligible. This "pay for degree" approach allows schools tremendous flexibility in placing students on a decelerated curriculum when needed to diagnose and address/remediate performance challenges.

Student Privacy Considerations

The Family Educational Rights and Privacy Act (FERPA)

The Family Educational Rights and Privacy Act (FERPA) [19] is a federal law that protects the privacy of student education records. The law applies to all schools that receive funds under an applicable program of the U.S. Department of Education. FERPA gives adult students certain rights with respect to their education records. Generally, schools must have written permission from the student to release any information from a student's education record and remind students of their rights annually. In certain cases (for example, to school officials with legitimate education interest), FERPA does allow schools to disclose those records without consent. *These rules, as well as concern for students' privacy, discourage extensive discussion across certain boundaries regarding challenging student cases.* Interpretation of these rules varies widely from school to school.

Forward Feeding of Information: Sensitive and Controversial

Schools vary greatly in their practice regarding whether information about students who struggle should be kept confidential or "fed forward," in other words, shared with those who will be working with the student. At some schools, only the dean's office is informed of a student's challenges, and only the dean's office can determine whether and which faculty members will be informed and to what level of detail, within the parameters of FERPA. Here, it is the dean's office or appropriate committee (e.g., committee on promotions or professionalism disciplinary committee) that reviews and makes remediation decisions, and student difficulties are often not disclosed or fed forward. At other schools, information on students who struggle may be fed forward by the dean's office, by a committee of course/clerkship directors, or by an individual course/clerkship director to the next course/clerkship director in order to allow the provision of additional support or identification of patterns of behavior. Sometimes, this information is further fed forward to the frontline faculty working directly with the student.

The practice of forward feeding is controversial, with only about half of US medical schools engaging in the practice. Few schools have written policies that make their practice clear to students and faculty [20, 21]. As noted in Chap. 2, there are advantages and disadvantages to feeding forward. As they move from one course to another, from the preclinical to clinical curriculum, or from one clerkship/specialty to another, it

is not unusual for students to stumble in one setting and then flourish in another. When information is fed forward, particularly when given to the faculty working directly with students, students can be unfairly branded, resulting in greater scrutiny of the student with expectations that they will struggle and explicit or implicit bias resulting in unfair treatment. On the other hand, when information is not fed forward, there are missed opportunities to work with and provide additional support to students who struggle. Often, patterns of difficulty or behavior may be overlooked, resulting in significant delays in identification and remediation of challenges [22].

Information-Sharing with Admissions

Medical schools also vary in their approaches to "feeding back" information to admissions offices and committees regarding students' medical school performance. Schools run the gamut from having admissions deans on promotions committees to having no communication to the admissions office regarding student performance once a student matriculates. The latter policy may hamper the admissions committee's ability to continuously improve upon their evaluations of future applicants. The former may introduce bias for or against certain student characteristics when making predictions based on the limited and unsystematic experience at one school, particularly given the paucity of research data available to guide admissions decisions.

Some dean's offices or promotions committees may routinely review the medical school application file of each student having difficulty to look for evidence of previous academic or behavioral difficulties. This review may provide insight into the nature of the issue, whether it is chronic or recurrent, and inform choice of remediation strategies. It can also identify and provide to admissions offices or committees retrospective "red flags" in application materials that could inform the admissions process. Some schools structure regular communications between the dean's office and the admissions committee to ensure information-sharing about curricular changes and feedback on support that is available for students after matriculation.

From time to time, the admissions office will "take a chance" on an applicant with an atypical or weaker academic history because of a particular experience or talent that suggests promise to become an outstanding physician. In these cases, *it is not clear whether giving proactive support to the student is beneficial or not.* Labeling a student as academically at risk may seriously hamper their self-confidence and cause undue anxiety (see also Chap. 3). Additionally, identifying at-risk students to faculty (see "forward feeding" section above) may unconsciously bias the faculty. Some schools offer elective academic support in advance of the start of medical school.

The Official Academic Record

The contents of the official academic record are specific to each school. At many schools, the official academic record consists of a student's transcript, student's duplicate record (transcript plus biographical information and USMLE scores), narrative evaluative comments from faculty, medical student performance evaluation ("MSPE," aka "Dean's Letter"), and, for a small number of students, a disciplinary report. The entire official academic record can be obtained by subpoena in a court of law.

> The American Association of Medical Colleges has guidelines regarding the medical student performance evaluation (MSPE), which include such issues as follows:
>
> - Inclusion of students' academic history including any extensions, leaves of absence, and gaps or breaks in a student's educational program
> - Information, based upon school-specific policies, of coursework that the student was required to repeat or otherwise remediate
> - Information, based on school-specific policies, of any adverse action(s) imposed on the student by the medical school or its parent institution
> - Information about students' academic performance and professional attributes in preclinical coursework, and clinical and elective coursework, including:
>   - Statement regarding a student's attainment of professional standards as defined by the school
>   - Graphic representation of a student's performance as compared to his or her peers
> - Narrative assessments of students from preclinical and clinical courses based upon summative faculty evaluations
> - Assessment of professional behavior:
>   - Information on citations for unprofessional behavior, including incident and remediation actions taken
>   - Information on commendations for exemplary professional behavior

Each state medical licensing board has its own requirements for documentation, which in some cases are quite extensive. For instance, California currently asks if a student has been on probation during medical school. Some schools have policies in which students are placed on probation for academic or professionalism reasons during medical school, with the agreement that the record will be "sealed" if the student does not have any repeat issues. However, this becomes an issue for students applying for licensure in select states that ask this question. The definition of probation is evolving and becoming more formalized and specific in response to this changing landscape. Some institutions are now reserving the term "probation" for use after the effectiveness of early stages of remediation can be assessed. In these cases, the terms "focused review" and "academic warning" are used to denote the early stages of remediation.

Credentialing services will contact medical schools on behalf of graduate programs and institutions to verify completion of medical education. Typically, they request information about interruptions in medical education, academic or disciplinary probation, unprofessional conduct or reports of negative behaviors, or questions of academic incompetence. Such reports should be completed based on the official academic record. Student data that are outside of the official academic record CANNOT be shared with outside parties, including residency programs and licensing boards. This includes oral or written "off-the-record" comments by faculty, peers, or others in the administration. Many dean's offices keep records of discussions with students. As long as their only purpose is to serve as the written "memory" of the dean, these records are private and not available at the time of subpoena.

What to Recommend to a Graduating Medical Student

Students who have undergone remediation in medical school may or may not be at risk for difficulties during postgraduate training. All students should be counseled to seek out training programs that best fit their goals, strengths, work styles, and personal requirements. Divulging remedial work that is not part of the student's record is the personal choice of the student and should be made carefully. Students should be encouraged to be honest and professional while understanding their own right to privacy. Generally, students who demonstrate insight, engage with enthusiasm, successfully complete, and grow from remediation programs are especially prepared for residency training and practice. In fact, the student may perform as well, or better, than their colleagues who did not struggle during school. Graduates can optimize their success by asking for feedback frequently from peers and supervisors and acting on the information gained. Graduates with disability accommodations in place should be encouraged to proactively bring documentation to their program director well in advance of needing the actual accommodations to ensure that appropriate supports are put in place. Students also need to be aware that accommodations within hospital systems can be particularly difficult to enact as patient care and patient privacy policies supersede their rights in some cases.

Dismissal of Medical Students

The percentage of medical students dismissed from school is strikingly small when compared to other professional schools such as law or business. Medical school faculty are more comfortable with their role in identifying and remediating students who need additional support than in determining when a student cannot meet milestones and must be dismissed. If dismissal from medical school is being seriously considered, the student must be informed. This discussion may be enough to motivate a student to be an active participant in successful remediation. It is also crucial to clearly outline, both verbally and in writing, the school's requirements, including exact deadlines, for the student to complete remediation activities that reflect the school's policies on student promotion and professional behavior. Legal counsel can be helpful with reviewing these documents, as policies may be subject to interpretation. Often, students are asked to meet with one of the deans when the school is considering dismissal. The dean's office can guide the student to prepare for an appearance before the promotions or professionalism disciplinary committees and give the student feedback on their written statements. Typically, students in this situation have already been told multiple times that they are at risk for dismissal and have undergone remediation unsuccessfully. Many schools have the appropriate committee deliberate and vote on recommending a student's dismissal to the dean, who makes the final decision. Students should have the right to appeal the decision within a defined time frame (see also Chap. 29).

The dismissal of a student is the most high-profile example of when the dean's office and the involved faculty must balance their advocacy for the student with their obligation to the medical school and society at large. In addition to following the institution's policies and procedures, the dean's office should consider the immediate needs and issues facing the dismissed student. Given the gravity of the situation, students should be encouraged to talk with a trusted friend or relative and referred to a mental health professional for support. The dean's office can also consider notifying the student health service in case the student contacts them for care. Once a student is officially dismissed, they need to leave school in a timely fashion. However, students do need time to move out of on-campus housing. If the school's policy allows it, refunding all or part of the semester's tuition is appreciated. A dismissed student may also appreciate and request that the dean's office explain the dismissal to a parent or spouse for them. The question of the next steps for a dismissed student, given the significant resources they have invested in medical training, is hotly debated and constitutes an area for continued investigation [23, 24].

References

1. Steinert Y. The "problem" junior: whose problem is it? BMJ. 2008;336:150–3.
2. Strand P, Edgren G, Borna P, Lindgren S, Wichmann-Hansen G, Stalmeijer RE. Conceptions of how a learning or teaching curriculum, workplace culture and agency of individuals shape medical student learning and supervisory practices in the clinical workplace. Adv Health Sci Educ. 2015;20:531–57.
3. McCabe DL, Trevino LT, Butterfield KD. Honor codes and other contextual influences on academic integrity: a replication and extension to modified honor code settings. Res High Educ. 2002;43:357–78.
4. Gill AC, Nelson EA, Mian AI, et al. Responding to moderate breaches in professionalism: an intervention for medical students. Med Teach. 2015;37:136–9.
5. Mak-van der Vossen MC, Teherani A, van Mook W, Croiset G, Kusurkar RA. How to identify, address and report students' unprofessional behaviour in medical school. Med Teach. 2020;42:372–9.
6. Bravata D, Watts SA, Keefer AL, et al. Prevalence, predictors, and treatment of impostor syndrome: a systematic review. J Gen Intern Med. 2020;35:1252–75.
7. Bullock JL, Seligman L, Lai CJ, O'Sullivan PS, Hauer KE. Moving toward mastery: changes in student perceptions of clerkship assessment with pass/fail grading and enhanced feedback. Teach Learn Med. 2021;20:1–11.
8. Goldman ML, Bernstein CA, Konopasek L, Arbuckle M, Mayer LES. An intervention framework for institutions to meet new ACGME common program requirements for physician well-being. Acad Psychiatry. 2018;42:542–7.
9. Lucey CR, Jones L, Eastburn A. A lethal hidden curriculum—death off a medical student from opioid use disorder. N Engl J Med. 2019;381:793–5.
10. Medical Society of the State of New York. MSSNY-CPH Mission. [Internet]. New York: Medical Society of the State of New York; c2011. https://www.mssny.org/get-help/committee-for-physician-health. Accessed 29 Dec 2022.
11. American Association of Medical Colleges. Graduation rates and attrition rates of U.S. medical students. https://www.aamc.org/media/48526/download. Accessed 29 Dec 2022.
12. Dong T, Gilliland WR, Cruess D, Hutchinson J, Morres L, Curtis J, Hewitt-Clarke GS, Durning SJ. A longitudinal study of commonly used admissions measures and disenrollment from medical school and graduate medical education probation or termination from training. Mil Med. 2018;183:e680–4.
13. Papadakis MA, Teherani A, Banach MA, Knettler TR, Rattner SL, Stern DT, Veloski JJ, Hodgson CS. Disciplinary action by medical boards and prior behavior in medical school. N Engl J Med. 2005;353:2673–82.
14. Ferguson E, James D, Madeley L. Factors associated with success in medical school: a systematic review of the literature. BMJ. 2002;324:952–7.
15. Patterson F, Knight A, Dowell J, Nicholson S, Cousans F, Cleland J. How effective are selection methods in medical education? A systematic review. Med Educ. 2016;50:36–60.
16. Eva KW, Reiter HI, Rosenfeld J, Trinh K, Wood TJ, Norman GR. Association between a medical school admission process using the multiple mini-interview and national licensing examination scores. JAMA. 2012;(308):2233–40.
17. Hosterman JA, Shannon DP, Sondheimer HM. Medical students with disabilities: resources to enhance accessibility. Washington, DC: Association of American Medical Colleges; 2010.
18. Georgetown University School of Medicine. Technical standards. https://som.georgetown.edu/admissions/prospectus/technicalstandards/ Accessed 29 Dec 2022.
19. Family Educational Rights and Privacy Act (FERPA), 20 U.S.C. § 1232g; 34 CFR Part 9. [Internet]. http://www.ed.gov/policy/gen/guid/fpco/ferpa/index.html. Accessed 29 Dec 2022.
20. Ziring D, Danoff D, Grosseman S, Langer D, Esposito A, Jan MK, Rosenzweig S, Novack D. How do medical schools identify and remediate professionalism lapses in medical students? A study of U.S. and Canadian medical schools. Acad Med. 2015;90:913–20.
21. Masangkay N, Adams J, Dwinell B, Hanson JT, Jain S, Tariq S. Revisiting feed forward: promoting a student-centered approach to education handoffs,

remediation, and clerkship success. Teach Learn Med. 2022:1–9. Epub ahead of print.

22. Chou CL, Kalet A, Costa MJ, Cleland J, Winston K. Guidelines: the dos, don'ts and don't knows of remediation in medical education. Perspect Med Educ. 2019;8:322–38.

23. Aagaard EM, Moscoso L. Practical implications of compassionate off-ramps for medical students. Acad Med. 2019;94:619–22.

24. Bellini LM, Kalet A, Englander R. Providing compassionate off-ramps for medical students is a moral imperative. Acad Med. 2019;94:656–8.

Commentary on Chapter 20: Perspective from a Brazilian Medical Professor

21

Suely Grosseman

I have been a medical professor for more than 25 years. In my office, located on the same floor where students from the first two semesters have classes, I was available, in an unofficial capacity, to any student who wanted to talk whenever possible. Often, they knocked on my door to open their hearts and showed gratitude for the opportunity to talk and cry with someone who listened and compassionately supported them. Their anxieties were caused by many issues: family or financial struggles, certainly, but mainly three: faculty who they felt oppressed them, peer relationships, and test performance. When I identified that they needed psychological support, I would accompany them to the on-demand support offered to all students by the psychology course. When I suspected that they might need psychiatric support, I would try to arrange an appointment with a psychiatrist, but his schedule was overloaded, and we often had to wait 2 weeks for an appointment. My many memories include a student who I encouraged to bring his mother in to mediate a problem he had with her; another student was kicked out of home after revealing his sexual orientation.

The undergraduate medical course in Brazil lasts for 6 years, the last two of which comprise the clerkship period. In 2020, there were a total of 335 Brazilian medical schools, with a total of 36,390 spots. A third of schools were tuition-free and administered by federal or state governments. The ratio of candidates per tuition-free spot may reach 120 to 1. Considering the principles of equity, a percentage of spots in tuition-free public schools are reserved for people whose family income is below 1.5 times the minimum wage, Indigenous Brazilians, people who self-declare as Black or mixed race, and people with disabilities.

Adaptation to medical school presents challenges even for students from privileged backgrounds. It may be additionally challenging for students who move to a new city, feel distant from their families, live alone, and/or have to adapt to new cultures and social perspectives. Thus, before thinking about remediation, it is essential to consider support during this transition to help students see medical schools as safe environments. This requires the development of a culture of respect, a collaborative teaching-learning process, and a comprehensive understanding of how people experience and view their social reality. This is also an important condition for effective teamwork, students' mental health, and quality of patient care. As one student memorably stated, in a qualitative study I conducted on how students learned phy-

S. Grosseman (✉)
Department of Pediatrics, Federal University of Santa Catarina, Florianopolis, Santa Catarina, Brazil

© The Author(s), under exclusive license to Springer Nature Switzerland AG 2023
A. Kalet, C. L. Chou (eds.), *Remediation in Medical Education*,
https://doi.org/10.1007/978-3-031-32404-8_21

sician-patient relationships, "The way the teacher treats us is the way we will treat our future patients" [1].

Regarding remediation, in Brazil, we call it "recovery." Both terms assume that mental health problems, unprofessional behaviors, or failure to pass factual or performance assessments are seen as illnesses. In my view, we should reframe it as coaching for catching up or a partnership for attaining better personal and professional development.

In schools that emphasize content-heavy, basic science-focused lectures early on, students who need recovery only get a single second chance at assessment, within a short timeframe. Sometimes, instead of supporting the student, this new assessment does not guide the student to master the content they failed to grasp and instead covers all subjects of the semester. In medical schools with small tutor-facilitated groups, it is easier to identify students who are struggling to learn or who have attitudinal limitations. Here, tutors are generally attentive, and there are many opportunities for self and peer assessment. Once a problem has been identified, tutors meet with students to listen to their explanations about what is happening with appreciative feedback, understand the problem's origin, and find the best way to provide support. Tutors may coach students with theoretical or practical assessment and/or recommend that they receive other forms of support.

Regardless of curriculum design, some Brazilian medical schools have well-developed support mechanisms: (1) offices comprising pedagogy, psychology, and psychiatry professionals who can support and follow students; (2) medical professors who are specifically dedicated to coaching students with difficulties; and/or (3) mentorship programs, which may be individual and conducted by faculty or near-peer students, or in small groups aimed at professional and/or personal development.

Dismissal of medical students, as in the USA, is rare in Brazil. It mainly occurs when a student does not complete the course within twice the expected timeframe (i.e., 12 years).

I see attitudinal problems as the main challenge in medical schools, since it is our responsibility to ensure that the physicians we certify not only have technical excellence, but also act with professionalism. Lecture-heavy schools lack opportunities to observe students' attitudes. Sometimes, we can identify students who cheat on tests or who plagiarize; other important professionalism problems are only identified during clerkships, though peers have known about them for a long time. The approach to unprofessionalism behaviors varies greatly, depending on attitudinal assessments and codes of conduct. Decisions regarding students with professionalism lapses are much the same as those in Chaps. 13 and 14.

Reference

1. Grosseman S, Stoll C. O ensino-aprendizagem da relação médico-paciente: estudo de caso com esudantes do último semestre do curso de medicina. [Teaching and learning the doctor-patient relationship: case-study with medical students in the last semester]. Revista Brasileira de Educação Médica. 2008;32(3):301–308.

22

Commentary on Chapter 20: Perspective from the University of Minnesota Bachelor of Science in Nursing (BSN) Program

Carol Flaten

Students entering our BSN program either have graduated from high school in the previous 4 months or may have transferred into the program, having met prerequisites and having had additional life/work experience. The application and admissions process is highly competitive. We utilize a holistic review and admission process, which results in diverse student cohorts.

In contrast to most medical students, our BSN students are in an earlier stage of adult development, experiencing many transitions including new living environments, new academic expectations, and increased individual accountability. Students experience concerns and challenges that include mental health needs, professional conduct expectations, clinical ability, academic requirements, and demands from family or community of origin.

Addressing the needs of students so they can be successful requires a wide range of interprofessional colleagues who are experts in their areas, including disability resources, health and wellness services, counseling services (including crisis), health advocacy, and centers for writing and academic support. Faculty may be the first to notice changes in performance or behavior in the classroom or clinical setting and will offer these resources to students. Collaboration and commu-

nication among faculty and the academic advisors are crucial to provide a comprehensive set of supports for the student, and yet, we must balance this with the need to maintain confidentiality. Our different roles influence what students choose to share with faculty, academic advisors, and other colleagues.

When students do not meet the academic or clinical requirements of a course, the course faculty meet with the student. The student and faculty collaborate on a written remediation plan ("Success Plan") that names specific actions the student is recommended to take to improve their performance, including, when appropriate, work with a tutor for individual remediation sessions, meeting with a disability resource counselor, etc; a timeline; and consequences if the plan is not achieved. The Success Plan is sent to the academic advisor and assistant dean. The student is highly encouraged to follow the steps of the Success Plan and is encouraged to reach out to faculty, academic advisors, and additional resources named therein. The academic advisor concurrently meets with the student to explore ways to support the Success Plan and offers additional pertinent resources. The majority of students successfully complete their plan and stay on

C. Flaten (✉)
University of Minnesota School of Nursing,
Minneapolis, MN, USA
e-mail: cflaten@umn.edu

track in the program. The Success Plan does not become part of the student's permanent record.

The assistant dean may play several roles in this process, including counseling faculty to write a Success Plan that names reasonable expectations of the student and aligns with school policies and syllabus requirements. In cases where a student has multiple Success Plans across several courses, the academic advisor and assistant dean may meet to specify potential student needs in greater detail. Discovery of a disability, for example, with the student's permission, leads to consultation with the school's disability resource center liaison. In highly complex situations, they meet as a group to review program technical standards and identify further supports and/or insurmountable limitations. Performance concerns may also lead to additional consultation with the clinical unit manager. If needed, we invite the student to these meetings to keep communication open and transparent about the standards they must meet and the pathways for meeting those requirements.

If the student does not meet the requirements specified in a Success Plan, the consequence is typically a failing grade in the course. This will likely change the student's academic progression and, in some cases, lead to a delayed gradu-ation. Anecdotally, we have noticed that students who fail a course or pause for a semester in the program often return and flourish in the BSN program.

Students who fail two courses in the program are subject to dismissal. Students may appeal, whereupon the academic advising team, assistant dean, and BSN co-director review the case. If the appeal is successful, the academic advisor may construct benchmarks that the student must meet, such as monthly meetings with the advisor. When a student repeats a course, we encourage the student and faculty to meet at the start of the course to discuss potential difficulties and/or share an official accommodation letter from the university disability office.

In summary, we have developed a student-centered process of meeting with the student, incorporating an interprofessional team approach that includes the student, and collaborating on a written Success Plan, which we are able to track through the semester. Each Success Plan is unique, designed to address the individual needs of the student and specific to the program requirements the student has not met. This tailored and interprofessional approach to remediation upholds our values of meeting students where they are and supporting them in their educational development process toward graduation.

Commentary on Chapter 20: Perspective from the Nell Hodgson Woodruff School of Nursing, Emory University

23

Melissa Owen

A key takeaway of the Institute of Medicine's Future of Nursing report centers on creating a diverse healthcare workforce to care for our population. As educators in healthcare fields, we have an obligation to the public to graduate safe and adequately skilled practitioners. We also have an obligation to support all students as much as possible, to allow them to successfully graduate and enter the health professions. Educators must also approach all students, including those experiencing suboptimal academic or clinical performance, with a positive, supportive demeanor. All students can learn, perhaps just not in the same way or on the same timeframe.

Engaging with students who need additional support must begin with a holistic approach and review of potential barriers to learning and opportunities for growth. At our institution, many individuals may be involved in this process. Students are encouraged to start conversations with course faculty directly. Program directors, the Assistant Dean for Prelicensure Programs or Graduate Clinical Programs, and the Assistant Dean for Student Affairs and Diversity Initiatives may also be involved for complicated situations. Our Office of Diversity, Equity, and Inclusion also serves as a safe space for students to share their concerns and receive additional support and resources.

Many factors related to academic success involve social determinants of learning: student characteristics that may benefit or hinder a student's academic success and progression. In nursing school, whether pre- or post-licensure, many students have outside obligations, such as employment or caregiving responsibilities, financial concerns, or food insecurity, any of which may interfere with academic requirements and performance. For success, students must have basic needs, such as housing, course materials including recommended resources, and adequate food resources, met. Our faculty and school leadership often explore these factors and refer students to available services as appropriate. Additionally, the chapter authors highlighted the ever-increasing challenges related to mental health in our students. Early identification and timely referral to campus resources are key to improve student well-being and to support academic performance.

Other factors related to academic performance may be related to preparation prior to program matriculation. As noted, study strategies that worked well previously may be insufficient for rigorous nursing school exams requiring knowledge application rather than merely recall (see Chap. 7). Therefore, students who have previously not required academic accommodations

M. Owen (✉)
Nell Hodgson Woodruff School of Nursing, Emory University, Atlanta, GA, USA

Seattle University, College of Nursing, Seattle, WA, USA
e-mail: mowen@seattleu.edu

may need referral for a learning assessment and require accessibility services. Additional helpful resources include peer tutoring, study groups, and writing centers.

After a holistic review and discussion of the student's situation, we set explicit plans and goals to help students stay on task and track approaches previously tried by the student. Documentation of the expectations for and the results of peer tutoring sessions, practice question resources, or additional simulation skill training hold the student accountable for academic progress and help the school measure the benefit of the suggested approaches on academic performance. Collaborative planning between the student, course faculty, and administration as appropriate should result in clearly enunciated consequences if goals are not achieved.

Although small in number, students who require remediation utilize a significant amount of faculty resources. Additionally, these students may be less likely to pass licensing exams. In 2021, 17.5% of all test takers did not pass the NCLEX-RN exam on the first attempt. We clearly have much more work to do to help our learners succeed. Improving identification of commonly occurring systemic factors that lead to a need for remediation would allow schools to implement preemptive programming. These may include programs for study and test-taking skills, pre-admission review courses, and well-being initiatives. Additionally, support for social determinants of learning such as food, housing, and transportation may increase equity, allowing all students the same opportunity to learn and be successful health professionals.

24

Commentary on Chapter 20: Perspective from the Purdue University College of Pharmacy

Kimberly Illingworth

Chapter 20 highlights all the major factors that arise in our dean's office. Like other health professions students, pharmacy students struggle for many reasons. Overall, these can be grouped into two main buckets: comprehension and application of content, and life circumstances. Students also commonly experience stress and mental health symptoms. We recognize that they will have challenges while in school and as future practitioners. Yet, there are also unanticipated life circumstances, such as students newly diagnosed with major chronic illness who think that they can continue without modifications or family members who become ill or die. Regardless of the stage of life, these circumstances weigh heavily on the minds of individuals, including students. Lastly, we do have a handful of students that have issues with professionalism, but this is uncommon.

In part, to help students address stress and normalize conversations about mental health, our college has created wellness-related initiatives. As a first step, we are trying to create formal opportunities to have authentic discussions with students about their challenges with a focus area in each professional year of the curricular sequence. In the first professional year, we review the symptoms of depression and anxiety and encourage students to seek help early. We outline a wide variety of mental health and wellness resources available on campus. Then, we introduce a problem-solving process, similar to the patient care process, to prevent or mediate individual stressors. Students create a wellness and mental action plan as deliverables for this activity. Students revisit their action plans in each year of the didactic curriculum. In the second year, we ask students to complete Question-Persuade-Refer (QPR) training, a national program to reduce suicidal behavior and save lives (https://qprinstitute.com/). As a part of this training, students participate in role-plays with cases that include peers and patients. This activity emphasizes reflective listening, motivational interviewing, and assessing suicidality as core communication skills. In the third professional year, as students think about their transition to their clinical experiences, we focus on imposter syndrome and strategies to support their wellness. In the final year, the college develops activities that focus on community, including a mobile phone wellness application.

Though we have instituted wellness initiatives and support mechanisms for when students experience challenges, we currently do not have a formal remediation policy to help students when they struggle with their academic performance. Currently, students repeat courses they have failed. Failure results in a loss of their cohort, payment of another year's tuition, and incurrence

K. Illingworth (✉)
Purdue University College of Pharmacy,
West Lafayette, IN, USA
e-mail: illingworth@purdue.edu

of an opportunity cost by keeping them out of the workforce. The COVID-19 pandemic has amplified our need for such a policy, because a higher number of students have failed exams and courses than in past years. With lower academic performance, there is concern that license exam scores will drop and fewer students will pass. Our college is not alone with these concerns. Anecdotally, others in pharmacy education have expressed similar issues. As we try to thoughtfully put together a policy, we are considering how to promote student success with curricular changes (e.g., more frequent assessments) and adjustments to when we trigger academic alerts (e.g., missing a certain number of classes or failing an exam). The primary goal is to support students so they are academically successful and do not fail a course. However, if they do fail a course, we are considering strategies to help them "recover" by remediating and allowing them to remain on track. Finally, we are trying to find ways to incentivize students who are struggling to change their behaviors with the hope of supporting their success not only to pass an exam but also to succeed in future courses and on clinical rotations.

Commentary on Chapter 20: Perspective from the School of Physical Therapy, University of California, San Francisco

25

Amber Fitzsimmons, Kai Kennedy, Theresa Jaramillo, and Andrew Lui

The International Classification of Functioning, Disability, and Health (ICF) is the World Health Organization's framework for measuring health and disability at individual and population levels. Given its biopsychosocial foundations, the ICF model is central to physical therapy education and focuses on the domains of health conditions; body structures and functions (including impairments), and their impact on individuals' activities; and effects on societal roles, e.g., in their family or occupation. These domains depend on environmental and personal factors that either facilitate or hinder optimal functioning. In many ways, the ICF model for patient care parallels the approach needed for learner success, especially as we begin to destigmatize the concept of remediation and modernize our instructional processes to de-emphasize learner deficits and instead focus on learners' strengths and holistic plans for success.

In our 3-year physical therapy program, we prioritize our learner-centered success efforts before learners even enter the program. When students apply, sometimes directly out of college, and sometimes with work experience or advanced degrees, our holistic admissions process provides all students with specific expectations and resources to prepare them for the academic rigor, pace, and learning environment in our program. We explain our cohort-based approach and encourage them to recognize and appreciate the diversity of lived experiences represented in their learning community.

Once students enroll, we endeavor to help them adapt to their life transitions as they enter graduate education and to consider how to develop the accountability to be independent and self-directed in their learning. For example, we administer a Learning and Study Strategies Inventory (LASSI) to help them reflect on their attitudes toward and habits of learning and studying and to facilitate a growth mindset during their development into a healthcare professional. Additionally, we incorporate content from learning specialists who help normalize the emotions associated with graduate-level study and provide students with evidence-based study strategies. We also facilitate deep learning around professionalism by defining competencies and milestones in five domains: compassion, humility, accountability, social responsibility, and excellence. In these domains, we embed self-care,

A. Fitzsimmons (✉) · K. Kennedy
T. Jaramillo · A. Lui
Department of Physical Therapy and Rehabilitation Science, University of California, San Francisco, CA, USA
e-mail: amber.fitzsimmons@ucsf.edu;
kai.kennedy@ucsf.edu; theresa.jaramillo@ucsf.edu;
andrewj.lui@ucsf.edu

mental health, study strategies, working across differences, and self-reflection.

Structurally, our proactive approach to student success includes assigning all students a faculty advisor, who meets with the student regularly to offer support. Advisors and learners collaboratively review standard progress assessments and self- and faculty-generated professionalism assessments. Faculty advisors also check in with their advisees about academic, financial, and mental health as they navigate the complexities of healthcare education and delivery. Finally, we utilize a quarterly "observation tracker" system to provide course directors a mechanism to notify program administration of specific learners' needs, whether housing or food insecurity, learning-related, stress management or health, communication, participation, motivation, or other personal or professional needs.

Operationally, students in our program are expected to maintain a minimum B average; if a student receives a C or below in a course, which happens with a small number (i.e., 3–4 students) in each cohort, they may undergo a formal "learner success" process to improve their grade. This process includes having the student meet with an Academic Review Committee, the student's faculty advisor, course directors, and program directors. The resulting learner success plan is monitored and reassessed by the student's faculty advisor, and if appropriate, the Academic Review Committee, to determine progress, potential modifications, milestones, and ultimate success of the plan. Very occasionally, perhaps once every other year, prolonging their program to a fourth year is needed.

Dismissal is a very sensitive and challenging topic in our field. At our institution, dismissals occur infrequently, perhaps once every 3–4 years; more commonly, learners who struggle with the curriculum realize that a career in physical therapy is not their best choice. When these situations arise, we center our discussions around our professional core values to train healthcare professionals who are competent and safe and will provide the highest quality of physical therapy services to the public.

We continue to discuss how the context of the different learner and societal needs brought forth by the COVID-19 pandemic impacts dismissal. While we tend to focus learner success plans on support of the individual learner, we are keenly aware that our program must evolve to meet the needs of learners in the twenty-first century; our program, policies, and faculty need to evolve simultaneously. Our evolution will use a systemic approach to balance multiple factors, including representation of diverse identities, educational cost, external resources, and other structures for support and quality assurance.

Part V

Systems, Legal, and Ethical Considerations: Graduate Medical Education

The View from the Office of the Designated Institutional Officer (DIO), Washington University in St. Louis

26

Rebecca McAlister, Paul Wise, Erica Traxel, Andrew White, and Eva Aagaard

A Bad Day in the Life of the Designated Institution Officer (DIO)

It was a beautiful fall day, and I was looking forward to the weekend when I saw an email from one of our brand-new program directors (PDs), Dr. P. She was struggling with a resident and wanted to speak with me. I called and asked how I could help.

Dr. P: *Thanks for calling me back. I have been dealing with one of our senior residents with some serious patient care issues on his services. Many of our attendings believe that this has been in part due to his poor team management skills. I really do not see how he can be allowed to stay in the program. I am thinking we need to terminate him. Can you even do that to a senior resident?*

DIO: *Well, that is distressing. Have you had challenges with him prior to this?*

Dr. P: *Oh, he was never a strong resident, scored low on the in-service exams, that sort of thing. I know that the prior PD was reluctant to promote him last spring, but the Clinical Competency Committee (CCC) determined that he had improved, so he was promoted. However, it is becoming clear that he really can't put it all together. His patient care plans are sloppy, junior residents don't get clear direction, and things are being missed. The attendings on his first rotation as a chief tell me that they couldn't trust him to manage*

R. McAlister
Department of Obstetrics and Gynecology,
Washington University School of Medicine,
St. Louis, MO, USA
e-mail: mcalisterr@wustl.edu

P. Wise
Department of Surgery, Washington University
School of Medicine, St. Louis, MO, USA
e-mail: wisepe@wustl.edu

E. Traxel
Division of Urology Surgery, Department of Surgery,
Washington University School of Medicine,
St. Louis, MO, USA
e-mail: traxele@wustl.edu

A. White
Department of Pediatrics, Washington University
School of Medicine, St. Louis, MO, USA

Department of Pediatrics, Saint Louis University
School of Medicine, St. Louis, USA
e-mail: white_a@wustl.edu

E. Aagaard (✉)
Washington University School of Medicine,
St. Louis, MO, USA
e-mail: aagaarde@wustl.edu

© The Author(s), under exclusive license to Springer Nature Switzerland AG 2023
A. Kalet, C. L. Chou (eds.), *Remediation in Medical Education*,
https://doi.org/10.1007/978-3-031-32404-8_26

their patients. After that rotation, I told him that he was going to have to do a better job running his services. Things really didn't get better; attendings had to check up on him all the time and often found problems. Now, on his third month-long service rotation as Chief Resident, a patient with a large ovarian mass underwent a right oophorectomy and was doing poorly in the recovery room. The nurses asked him to come and see the patient, but he sent the intern instead. The intern reported back that the patient was tachycardic and the hourly urine output was low, but the estimated blood loss on the case was only 300 cc. The intern asked the chief to come and see the patient, but he said that he was busy and told the intern to just give the patient a fluid bolus. He promised to come see her soon. Two hours later after two fluid boluses, the nurses called the attending physician to tell her that the patient was still tachycardic, not making adequate urine, and the chief resident had not come to see her. The attending showed up immediately to find the patient's abdomen distended and rigid. Stat labs documented a 5 gm drop in hemoglobin from preoperative values. The patient went to the operating room immediately where a 1000 cc hemoperitoneum was evacuated and a bleeding ovarian pedicle was ligated, and hemostasis was achieved. The patient received two units of packed red cells intraoperatively and subsequently received another unit. The attending had paged the chief twice with no response. Later that evening, the chief resident answered the page, explaining that his phone battery had been dead earlier. After hearing about what had happened with the patient, he asked if she wanted him to come in or just see the patient in the morning. The attending said, "Don't bother. You won't be taking care of my patients anymore."

I got an earful from that attending and promised her to assign a different chief to her patient and deal with this guy. I really think we have to terminate.

DIO: *Yes, that is all very serious. Let me back up a few steps. Had the resident ever had a written remediation plan, been on probation, or been told that he could be terminated if his performance didn't improve? Did you document your discussion after the first rotation?*

Dr. P: *There is no written remediation plan in his file. I had always heard to start with a verbal warning so didn't document my talk with him, and now I think that it can't wait until then. There is an informal note from the 6-month evaluation last spring that said that he needs to improve his fund of knowledge, but there is no definite plan. The former PD didn't like to "label" residents; he was worried it might hurt them down the road.*

DIO: *Can you send me your program's policies on evaluation, promotion, and disciplinary action? Where do you think you are in that process?*

Dr. P: *I can ask the coordinator to find it. I haven't had time to look at it. I only took over in July, you know.*

DIO: *Several other questions come to mind. You noted that he had low scores earlier. Are there any threshold scores for the in-training exam? How has he done on his milestones? Are there any standards for those in your program?*

Dr. P: *I am really not sure. I will have to look at it. We will send a copy of it all to you.*

DIO: *Have you had any behavioral concerns? Has he been facing any personal challenges?*

Dr. P: *He seemed fine when I brought him in earlier about his performance. He never said anything about personal challenges. He was surprised he wasn't doing well, since he had been promoted.*

DIO: *Where is the resident now?*

Dr. P: *Well, it's Thursday afternoon. He is likely about to sign out. I can ask the backup chief to cover for him Friday, and then he is scheduled to go on vacation for the week. I guess I need to call him in and let him know we are reviewing all of this.*

DIO: *Yes, I think that would be best. I think you should bring him in and tell him you are taking all of this seriously. Patient care must be protected, so he will be on administrative leave for Friday. Then let him know that you will sort things out and be in touch with him next week about next steps. It's never a bad idea to acknowledge that all of this is probably very stressful for him. You should give him the contact information for the counseling folks. And be sure to document all of that in his record.*

Dr. P: *Oh, what a mess. I will send you his file and our policies, and I will see you tomorrow.*

DIO: *Indeed. Once we hang up, I am going to write the hospital legal folks a note about all of this. They are going to want to be part of the review. See you tomorrow.*

Introduction

Up to 18% of residents will require some form of remediation during their training [1, 2]. Causes for remediation vary widely among programs and specialties with common deficits including substandard performance in medical knowledge, clinical reasoning, efficiency or organization, communication skills, and professionalism ([1–5]; see Chaps. 7, 9, 11–14). Residency and fellowship training programs invest a significant amount of time, energy, and resources to provide underperforming high-risk learners with remediation [3, 6]. Despite best efforts, not all trainees can be remediated, and some residents will go on to probation or termination [3, 7]. Being placed on probation during residency training is associated with poor career outcomes, including low graduation rates, low board pass rates, and unusually high rates of citation by the state medical boards [2]. Termination is more common in residents with multiple deficiencies and in those with significant professionalism violations [1, 8].

Remediation of residents and fellows should include clear goals and identify targeted skills to be practiced with close monitoring and ongoing feedback. Remediation ideally should conclude with a reassessment to ensure that the gaps have closed and that the learner is qualified to return to supervised practice and ultimately progress to independent practice [9–12]. However, specific remedial processes such as this are rarely used in graduate medical education [13]. Predominant remedial interventions include repeated exposure to rotations without new learning strategies or changes to organizational aspects of residency, like reducing workload [14, 15]. While a recent study highlighted that surgical residency programs with low attrition were more likely to provide resident remediation, there remain limited data on systematic or individual interventions that are associated with improved career outcomes [3, 16–18]. A few studies have utilized centralized resources with an established framework to diagnose areas of learner deficiency and to build remediation plans that incorporated deliberate practice with specific individualized feedback and reflection [17, 18]. These studies have demonstrated significant improvement in learner performance and sustained improvements in graduation rates over time.

While the vast majority of physicians in residencies and fellowships successfully complete their programs, it is always problematic when a trainee fails to meet expectations. Institutional leadership, in the form of program directors (PDs) and the designated institutional official (DIO), must provide strong support for remediation. PDs are charged with developing robust educational programs, ensuring timely and effective assessment of trainees, and identifying those who need additional support. In Accreditation Council for Graduate Medical Education (ACGME)-accredited programs, the DIO plays a key role in supporting the work of the PDs (see text box for definitions). The DIO collaborates with a governing body inclusive of PDs, called the Graduate Medical Education Committee (GMEC), to ensure substantial compliance with the applicable program requirements. (The authors of this chapter include a long-standing DIO and Associate Dean for GME, three experienced PDs, and a Senior Associate Dean for Education and Associate Vice Chancellor with oversight of GME at Washington University in St. Louis School of Medicine. Together, these authors represent a broad array of specialties and subspecialties and have extensive experience in both successful and unsuccessful remediation.)

ACGME Definitions

Sponsoring Institution (SI): An SI is an entity (medical school, hospital system, or consortium of these organizations) that oversees, supports, and administers a certain set of ACGME-accredited residency/fellowship programs. An SI's organizational chart(s) should illustrate the ultimate authority of a single governing body and its relationships with a DIO, GMEC, and other components of GME in the SI (e.g., program directors, participating sites). While a variety of organizational structures can be found among ACGME-accredited SIs, a substantially compliant SI has a DIO who collaborates with a GMEC under a singular governing body in overseeing GME at all of an SI's participating sites.

Designated Institutional Official (DIO): A designated institutional official (DIO) collaborates with a Graduate Medical Education Committee (GMEC) to ensure an SI's and its programs' substantial compliance with the applicable ACGME institutional, common, and specialty/subspecialty-specific program requirements. The Institutional Requirements do not specify qualifications of a DIO. An SI must identify a DIO positioned in the organizational structure to have authority and

responsibility for overseeing the SI's ACGME-accredited programs. While it is currently acceptable for one individual to serve as DIO for more than one SI, each SI must define the financial support and protected time committed to the DIO for his/her responsibilities relating to oversight, education, administration, and leadership in that SI only.

A DIO may be a faculty member or an administrative staff member with expertise in GME who has specific protected time and resources provided by the SI to meet these needs. The DIO provides institutional support, including onboarding new PDs, consulting with PDs as problems arise, reviewing policies and documentation, and working with institutional legal counsel and human resources (HR) to assure that all trainees have access to appropriate institutional review of the program's disciplinary actions.

Program Director (PD): The program director is responsible for implementing and ensuring compliance with policies and procedures for grievance and due process, duty hours, selection, evaluation and promotion of residents, disciplinary action, and supervision of residents within a given residency program. PD qualifications vary by specialty: https://www.acgme.org/Portals/0/PDFs/Specialty-specific%20Requirement%20Topics/DIO-PD_Qualifications.pdf.

Graduate Medical Education Council (GMEC): As specified in Institutional Requirements I.B.4.-I.B.6., a GMEC has responsibilities that include (1) oversight of institutional and program accreditation and (2) review and approval of various actions. "Oversight" includes routine monitoring of program and institutional accreditation as well as the formalized Annual Institutional Review (AIR) and Special Review processes. There are activities that must be documented in GMEC meeting minutes at least annually. These include (1) oversight of program and institutional accreditation outcomes; (2) oversight of Annual Program Evaluations and Self-Studies (I.B.4.a) (4); (3) review and approval of recommendations to the SI's administration regarding stipends and benefits (I.B.4.b) (2); and (4) oversight of the AIR and resulting action plans (I.B.5, I.B.5.b) (2). The GMEC includes the DIO, a representative sample of program directors (minimum of two) from its ACGME-accredited programs, a minimum of two peer-selected residents/fellows from its ACGME-accredited programs, and a quality improvement or patient safety officer or designee.

Clinical Competency Committee (CCC): The PD must appoint the CCC and provide a written description of its responsibilities, including its responsibility to the SI and the PD. It must participate actively in reviewing all resident evaluations by all evaluators and make recommendations to the PD for resident progress, including promotion remediation and dismissal. The CC should be composed of members of the program faculty.

Typically, many factors combine to complicate the implementation of academic disciplinary actions. Despite these administrative issues, it is the societal expectation that high academic standards be met by all graduates. In the above scenario, complicating factors included the reluctance of PDs and faculty to take actions that could adversely affect the future careers of trainees [19, 20], and turnover in PDs that increases administrative handoffs for training programs. The PD, DIO, and legal counsel felt that patient safety concerns for this resident were significant and warranted dismissal from the program. The program's disciplinary policy was reviewed and found to have been appropriately followed. Documentation of prior counseling and failed remediation attempts were sufficient to move forward with

this action. The resident was advised of the decision and given access to the institutional appeal for due process, which is an ACGME requirement for sponsoring institutions (SIs). Although the resident appealed the disciplinary action, it was reviewed by the SI and sustained.

Early Identification of the Trainee Who Struggles: Role of Evaluations, Milestones, and Competency Committees

This unfortunate case illustrates what studies across several disciplines have documented: the failure of post-rotation evaluations to identify at-risk trainees early in training. These failures have been attributed to grade inflation, attending physicians' lack of willingness to document poor performance, and lack of knowledge about how to document performance concerns [21–23]. In a study of internal medicine residents, PDs found that emails, hallway conversations, and phone calls from faculty members or chief residents were the more common means of identifying residents who struggle [24]. Notably, when deficits are documented in evaluations, the comments section often does not correlate with the numeric ratings given for the corresponding ACGME competencies [23].

The ACGME introduced the Outcomes Project in 2002, wherein all residency programs were to train and assess residents and fellows in the six core competency domains: medical knowledge, patient care, interpersonal and communication skills, systems-based practice, practice-based learning, and professionalism. In 2012, the ACGME transitioned from the Outcomes Project to the Next Accreditation System [25], which requires programs to report learner progress using specialty-specific milestones [26]. These milestones are intended to portray a developmental progression of trainee behaviors in each of the six ACGME competency domains [27], ultimately to help trainees and faculty provide criterion-based feedback leading to performance improvement. More recently, with independent development of milestones and resultant heterogeneity among related disciplines, the ACGME has launched a Milestones 2.0 project to refine and harmonize milestones where appropriate. Notwithstanding the challenges in implementation of the milestones [28], studies have suggested that they are a valid means of assessing resident performance [29–34].

A strategy to effectively assess these milestones [35] ideally involves a variety of tools, including global assessment and more specific approaches, including direct observation of clinical skills, simulation, observed structured clinical evaluations, multisource feedback, in-training exams, and medical record review. Individual assessments should be mapped to each competency domain and be used only in environments where those competencies can be assessed [32, 36–38]. The ACGME is compiling online learning resources for assessment, including remediation, which can be found at https://dl.acgme.org. When a program fully and richly implements this plan, a Clinical Competency Committee (CCC) reviews the compiled assessments [39–43]. The CCC also assigns milestone evaluations for each trainee on at least a biannual basis; identifies learners in need of potential remediation; makes recommendations regarding promotion, remediation, failure of promotion, probation, and dismissal; and reports their findings and recommendations to the PD [41–46]. Importantly, the CCC mechanism allows for data to be incorporated into the biannual milestones that comes from a myriad of sources, including those emails and hallway conversations that so often raise flags about trainees. Formal reports from the CCC are also sent to each trainee and generally reviewed through a meeting with the trainee and a faculty member or PD. Many believe that the milestones may aid with the early identification of the learner who struggles and specifically the linking of that information with detailed information about the deficit area(s) to enable effective remediation [27].

Remediation and Probation

To give clear direction to trainees and to determine when individuals are not meeting expectations, programs must develop policies for evaluation, promotion, and disciplinary action. This requires that standards for unsuccessful completion of rotations, projects, in-training exams, etc. be described in the program's policies and shared with faculty and trainees. The CCC and the PD can then apply these standards fairly and equitably with the goals of describing the areas of concern, developing specific goals for improvement, and providing needed support. When the deficit appears to be a single concern and not severe in nature, the PD often elects to have an informal discussion with the resident or fellow, describing the program's expectations and how the trainee has failed to meet them (see Chap. 6). It is best practice to document this conversation, and any similar conversations, for both the PD/program and the trainee.

Pediatric Residency Program Policy on Promotion and Graduation

Evaluation: Educational and professional progress and achievement are evaluated by the program director and program faculty (CCC) on a regular and periodic basis. The program director or designee shall have a meeting with you to discuss a written summary of all evaluations at least once in each 6-month period or more frequently if needed.

The evaluations are based on established milestones and competencies, within the following elements:

- Fund of medical knowledge and application of that knowledge
- Judgment
- Personal character traits displayed, interpersonal skills
- Clinical and technical skills
- Ability to assume increasing levels of responsibility for patient care

An evaluation file shall be maintained by the program director for each house officer and treated as confidential. The file may be reviewed by the house officer and by departmental faculty and staff with legitimate educational and administrative purposes. In addition, reviewers from the GME Consortium's standing committee on Program Evaluation may ask to review a representative set of house officer files as part of the internal review process set forth by the GME Consortium.

Promotion: Promotion to the next level of the program depends upon your performance as recommended by the Clinical Competency Committee to the program director, who shall have the final say. Decisions about promotion or reappointment by the program director will be communicated to you as soon as reasonably practicable. Decisions not to renew contracts will be communicated in writing no later than 4 months prior to the end of the contract term. In instances where the primary reason for nonrenewal occurs within the 4 months prior to the end of the contract, written notice will occur as soon as reasonably possible before the end of the contract period.

Completion of training: The requirements for satisfactory completion of the training program are defined by the program director with input from the Clinical Competency Committee and are consistent with the requirements of the ACGME and the Pediatric Residency Review Committee (RRC). Certificates are issued upon completion of the residency training program. At a minimum, the following criteria must be completed to achieve satisfactory completion of the residency program:

- Demonstrate a level of clinical and procedural competence to the satisfaction of the program director.
- Fulfill the department's scoring requirements on the resident's In-Training

Examination as used by the program and approved by the pertinent RRC.
- Fulfill the requirements of the American Board of Pediatrics for completion of approved training in the pediatric specialty.
- Demonstrate attitude, demeanor, and behavior appropriate to the pediatric specialty regarding how you relate to patients, other healthcare professionals, and colleagues.
- Completion of any other requirements of the pediatric residency program.

In addition to the requirements of the program, satisfactory completion requires that your medical records be in order and completed, that any financial obligations owed to the hospitals or school of medicine are paid or terms established for payment, that all hospital or school of medicine property issued solely for use during an academic year, including identification badges and pagers, must be returned or paid for, and that a forwarding mailing and email address be provided to the Residency Program Office.

When deficits are persistent or more severe, structured written remediation plans should be developed with the following elements:

1. Description of the deficiencies as compared to program standards for successful completion
2. Description of specific interventions for improvement
3. Description of how, when, and how often performance will be reevaluated
4. Description of potential consequences of failure to meet expectations
5. Proof of notification (trainee signature that they have reviewed and understood the document)

This written plan serves as a letter of warning to the trainee that improvement must occur to allow their continued progress in the program.

Many institutions require that the PD consult with the DIO and institutional legal counsel when such a letter of warning is issued. The purpose of this consult is to ensure consistency in communication and documentation across programs and provide any needed support about remediation planning.

Unfortunately, effective remediation can look quite inconsistent across programs. This variability reflects the resources and skills of individual program faculty and the priorities of the program and institution for retaining learners who struggle. To facilitate consistent decision-making regarding failure to progress, it is helpful to use the collective judgment of a well-trained CCC to review data that are expediently collected. A well-trained CCC understands the strengths and weaknesses to the system of assessment and the assessment instruments, including potential impacts of systemic and individual bias and racism. It brings an understanding of the policies that govern their decision-making and access resources effectively when entering unknown territory. Well-trained CCC members practice effective group dynamics by encouraging active listening, principled debate, and constructive conflict. During this remediation, decisions as to whether the trainee has satisfactorily resolved their deficits, whether to continue the remediation efforts, or whether to move to disciplinary action should be clearly documented and communicated in writing to the trainee. Lack of clarity in communication may give the trainee a false impression of success, as in our example.

Should the CCC or the PD find that the trainee has not made sufficient progress during the remediation, or if the severity of the deficit(s) worsens, the PD may elect to place the trainee on probation. PDs can reduce trainees' inevitable feelings that the process is highly subjective by clearly stating the criteria for success up front and providing frequent feedback regarding progression. Probation includes a formal written plan, like a remediation plan in structure, with the added caveat that if the trainee does not meet expectations within the planned period or the situation worsens, they risk adverse disciplinary action, as described below. The decision to proceed to probation should be made by the PD in consultation with the DIO and institutional legal counsel. Depending on the severity of the deficits, the PD is not required to place a trainee on probation prior to instituting a formal adverse disciplinary action; however, doing so generally reduces the risk of subsequent appeal and legal action. As in remediation, timely collection and review of evaluations of the trainee's performance inform decision-making for next steps, and trainees should be provided written notice of these decisions. All corrective action taken to this point is at the discretion of the PD in consultation with the CCC and should be consistent with the individual program's written policies. Residents may appeal all suspension, nonrenewal of contract, non-promotion, or dismissal decisions to the SI as part of due process required by the ACGME.

Placing a learner on probation has significant consequences to the learner. Specifically, probation generally must be disclosed on licensure and specialty board applications and may prohibit movement on to additional training. Probation generally follows trainees throughout their careers, and PDs are, therefore, often reluctant to move to this step. The DIO and CCC can be critical partners in helping the PD make these difficult decisions.

Policy on Disciplinary Action, Suspension, or Termination

Informal procedures: The program director is encouraged to use informal efforts to resolve minor instances of poor performance or misconduct. In any case in which a pattern of deficient performance has emerged, informal efforts by the program director shall include notifying the house officer in writing of the nature of the pattern of deficient performance and appropriate steps to be taken by the house officer as needed. If these informal efforts are unsuccessful, or where performance or misconduct is of a serious nature, the department chair or program director may impose formal disciplinary action.

Formal disciplinary action: Disciplinary action may be taken for due cause, including but not limited to any of the following:

- Failure to satisfy the academic or clinical requirements of the training program
- Professional incompetence, misconduct, or conduct that might be inconsistent with or harmful to patient care or safety
- Conduct that is detrimental to the professional
- Conduct that calls into question the professional qualifications, ethics, or judgment of the house officer, or conduct which could prove detrimental to the hospital's or school of medicine's patients, employees, staff, volunteers, or operations

Violation of the bylaws, rules, regulations, policies, or procedures of the GME Consortium, school of medicine, hospital, department, division, or training program, including violation of the responsibilities of house officers set forth above.

Specific procedures: If there are any instances of poor performance or questionable behavior, *intradepartmental proceedings* will be instituted. The first step is a meeting with the pediatric chief residents and the resident in question. The next level of escalation will include meeting with the associate PD and the chiefs. If the issues are not resolved, a meeting with the PD will occur and will be documented. Failure to resolve the issue will result in a meeting with the department chair and the PD and possibly the director of GME and the hospital president. Examples of issues that will trigger this recourse include failure to satisfy the academic or clinical requirements

of the training program, professional incompetence, misconduct, or conduct that might be inconsistent with or harmful to patient care or safety; conduct that is detrimental to the professional; conduct that calls into question the professional qualifications, ethics, or judgment of the house officer; or conduct which could prove detrimental to the hospital's or school of medicine's patients, employees, staff, volunteers, or operations.

If *intradepartmental procedure* is insufficient, then formal action may take place.

Formal disciplinary action includes (1) suspension, termination, or non-reappointment; (2) reduction, limitation, or restriction of the house officer's clinical responsibilities; (3) extension of the residency or denial of academic credit that has the effect of extending the residency; or (4) denial of certification of satisfactory completion of the residency program.

The program director or department chair shall notify the house officer in writing of the action taken and the reasons. A copy of the notification shall be furnished to the hospital's GME office and the Associate Dean for Medical Education (Graduate Medical Education). The notification should advise the house officer of their right to request a review of the action in accordance with the grievance procedure set forth below. In the case of a suspension, the written notification should precede the effective date of the suspension unless the program director or department chair determines in good faith that the continued appointment of the house officer places safety or health of hospital or school of medicine patients or personnel in jeopardy or when immediate suspension is required by law or necessary in order to prevent imminent or further disruption of hospital or school of medicine activities, in which case the notice shall be provided at the time of suspension.

Dismissal and Appeal Processes

The goal for all programs is to support and assist their trainees to provide safe patient care and, upon successful completion of their training, to ensure that they are prepared for independent practice. However, there are occasionally instances when the resident or fellow is not able to successfully meet the program's expectations. This results in the PD, in collaboration with the CCC, making the decision to render an adverse disciplinary action, defined as immediate termination, nonrenewal of contract, or extension of training by failure to promote or failure to graduate. PDs should make such decisions carefully and only in close consultation with the CCC, DIO, and institutional legal counsel. Such decisions should be based on having scrupulously documented compliance with the ACGME Common Program Requirements [47].

Trainees have the right to appeal disciplinary decisions, and institutions must provide due process. The United States Constitution delineates due process (see Chap. 29). Due process in appeals should establish at a minimum that the program utilized appropriate procedures and

V.A.d.3 Develop plans for trainees who fail to progress, following institutional policies and procedures

The ACGME Institutional Requirements [48] state that the SI must:

IV.C.1 Require each program to develop criteria for promotion

> IV.C.1.a Require the program to provide trainees written notice of an adverse disciplinary action
> IV.C.1.b Have a policy that provides due process to appeal these decisions

applied them fairly, that the trainee was given notice of their deficiencies, and that the trainee was given an opportunity to respond to the program's decision. To minimize any effect of personal bias or potential for biased application of standards, programmatic disciplinary decisions should be made by an unbiased decision maker or decision-making body, for example, a PD in consultation with trained members of the CCC. Decisions must not be arbitrary or capricious. Each SI may develop policies that best suit its educational environment so long as due process is provided [49]. It is important that all program- and institution-level evaluation and disciplinary policies be clearly defined and shared with PDs, faculty, and trainees to ensure that all have a clear understanding of the rules, roles, and responsibilities governing the educational and work environment.

ACGME Common Program Requirements

Programs must:

IV.A.2 Provide goals and objectives for each educational assignment

V.A.1.a Provide frequent feedback during each assignment

V.A.1.b Document evaluation at the end of each assignment or at least every 3 months

V.A.1.c Provide objective performance evaluation based on the competencies and the specialty-specific milestones

V.A.d.1 Provide semiannual evaluation of progress including milestone assessments

V.A.d.2 Assist trainees in development of individual learning plans

Trainees Are Both Learners and Employees

An additional complicating factor is that residents and fellows simultaneously inhabit the roles of learner and employee. This unique dichotomous role has been the subject of sometimes-conflicting decisions on trainees' employment status by the US National Labor Relations Board (NLRB).

Residents as Students: In 1976, the NLRB held that residents are students who are primarily engaged in an academic endeavor. As such, they were not eligible for employment benefits such as collective bargaining or forming unions and not subject to Social Security or Medicare taxes [50].

Residents as Employees: In 2011, the US Supreme Court ruled that residents were employees instead of students and so were subject to taxes for Social Security and Medicare paid by both the trainees and their employers [51]. The NLRB reversed its prior stance in 2014 and ruled that resident physicians are employees and can unionize [51].

Certainly, trainees sign contracts with their institutions and provide many hours of work in the form of patient care as they participate in the education provided by their programs. Employers such as hospitals and universities provide residents with wages and benefits and expect that their employment policies will apply to trainees. Some SIs allow all adverse disciplinary actions to be appealed under the required ACGME process; others carve out the appeals process to apply to only those concerns affecting academic achievement. Issues relating to misconduct such as dishonesty, inappropriate documentation, breach of code of conduct (e.g., HIPAA, sexual harassment), criminal behavior, or being "unfit for duty" are then designated as falling to employer policies and are not subject to the SI's appeals process.

Residents and the Americans with Disabilities Act (ADA): Those trainees who have a condition identified as protected under the ADA may request that the program make a reasonable accommodation to enable the trainee to be successful in meet-ing program expectations (see Chap. 17). PDs should consult with their institutional legal counsel and human resources (HR) department to determine the extent to which programs must accommodate these requests. Unless the disability is obvious or apparent, such conditions and requests for accommodation must be declared by the trainee before an adverse disciplinary action is given [52]. The PD, in consultation with legal counsel and HR, must determine whether the request directly affects the trainee's ability to perform their work responsibilities and would still allow the trainee to satisfactorily meet training goals. They must also consider whether the request would adversely affect the program or patient care. This may involve an assessment by the PD as to whether the trainee can meet the technical standards required to achieve the program's training goals in preparation for independent practice. For example, a surgical trainee must have adequate visual acuity to safely perform surgical procedures. This may be achieved through low vision aids but must still provide sufficient vision to perform surgery. Fellows in a Critical Care Medicine program must be able to manage multiple complex patients at any hour of the day. Should sleep disruptions from shift work adversely affect their existing sleep disorder and cognitive abilities to function at this very high level, it may not be felt reasonable to allow them to forego working night shifts, as these will likely be required in independent practice. Assigning those shifts to other trainees would also unfairly add to their colleagues' workload. Should an accommodation be made, the program standards for success should not be compromised. All evaluation and disciplinary policies must be applied fairly and consistently across trainees and programs.

Implications of Probation and Dismissal

Many PDs and faculty worry that trainees who have been disciplined will bring civil legal action against them in retaliation for poor evaluations or disciplinary actions. When the program and the institution establish fair policies compliant with ACGME regulations, document compliance with these scrupulously, and apply them equally to all trainees, it is very unlikely that such legal actions will succeed if institutions provide due process. Courts have consistently deferred to medical faculty in determining academic success [53] (see Chap. 29).

Additionally, many PDs hesitate to document the trainee's record of remediation, probation, or adverse disciplinary action because they are concerned about the adverse effect this will have on the resident's subsequent medical career. State medical boards, specialty boards, future credentialing bodies, or future training programs are likely to request a report of instances of probation and formal adverse action. Instances of remediation/corrective action that are successful should be reviewed with institutional legal counsel to determine if they are discoverable. In general, any training information may only be shared when the trainee has given written authorization. However, individuals seeking a training position or employment are expected to share this information, and refusal to do so is likely to be interpreted by future employers as a negative sign (see example case below). When asked to provide such information about instances of remediation/corrective action that have been successfully resolved, the description should include notation of satisfactory resolution. PDs should consult with institutional legal counsel when they receive requests for information on trainees who have struggled to assure that honest, non-prejudicial information based on documentation in the trainee's record is transmitted and that this occurs only after appropriate waivers are obtained.

Case Examples

Right This Ship: Probation and Successful Remediation

Early in Dr. A's (she/her) residency training, faculty members noted deficits in her medical knowledge. She regularly failed to recognize important components of the history, physical examination, or diagnostic testing when assessing patients and developed insufficient or inappropriate patient care plans. It was also noted that she was not receptive to feedback and would in turn criticize the plans of care that were developed by the faculty, which was interpreted by faculty as insubordination. Nurses reported that Dr. A would quickly become defensive when asked to clarify her orders and patient care plans. These concerns were documented in end-of-rotation evaluations, which were reviewed at the program's semiannual CCC meeting. The CCC identified deficiencies, documented in the ACGME milestones, across multiple competencies, including medical knowledge (MK), practice-based learning and improvement (PBLI), interpersonal and communication skills (ICS), and professionalism. The largest gaps were noted in MK and professionalism.

At approximately the same time, an outside institution where Dr. A had previously participated in research notified us that there had been an investigation into research misconduct, and Dr. A had admitted to falsifying research data. She had not disclosed this to our institution when applying for residency.

The PD conferred with the clinical division chief and department chair, as well as the office of the vice chancellor for research integrity and compliance, in-house legal counsel, and the DIO. Given the severity of the allegations, it was decided to place Dr. A on probation for the remainder of residency training and to bar her from participating in any research during residency. The terms of probation included regular meetings of PD with faculty, senior residents, and hospital staff to obtain feedback on Dr. A's performance; a regular and specific study program, including biweekly meetings with the PD to review subject matter and ongoing performance; and consultation and counseling with the Employee Assistance Program (EAP), which provides free and confidential counseling services to all hospital employees, including trainees, regarding professionalism. The terms of the probation were to be reviewed after the next semiannual CCC, and if her performance was not deemed satisfactory, then Dr. A was to be terminated. The PD formally presented the probation, including causes, terms, and timeline, in writing and in-person to Dr. A, and she signed the document, acknowledging receipt.

Dr. A sought continued counseling through the EAP and studied and met biweekly with the PD for management of learning plans and coaching on professionalism. However, her next annual in-service examination score was below the 20th percentile, which automatically activates academic probation/remediation based on our internal program polices that intend to identify residents who are at increased risk of failing the board examination. Evaluations suggested that there had been overall improvement in the domains of PBLI and ICS; however, the CCC was notified of an unprofessional and contentious interaction between Dr. A and a hospital staff member. This was discussed within the next CCC, and the decision was made to continue the probation with new terms, stipulating additional study requirements. An updated letter outlining the terms of the probation was presented to Dr. A for signature.

Over the remainder of Dr. A's training, there was gradual improvement in in-service examination scores to a level above the cutoff requiring remediation. Other faculty and staff also noted an increased willingness to accept feedback and incorporate constructive feedback. In ongoing meetings between the PD and Dr. A,

she was earnest in her desire for continued self-improvement and consistently actively sought to comply with terms of probation. This improvement was noted at subsequent CCC meetings and documented in the ACGME Milestones. Ultimately, the resident graduated the program in good standing. When training verification has since been requested for purposes of hospital credentialing and medical licensure, Dr. A's probation has been disclosed, as has her successful ability to comply with probation and to complete residency, capable of independent practice.

It Follows You

Dr. B (she/her), a pediatrics resident, was brought to the attention of the PD after multiple episodes of missing continuity clinic without notification. The clinic attending, as well as other residents in the clinic, had been covering by seeing her scheduled patients. The PD met with Dr. B to discuss the unprofessional behavior, the lack of commitment to her patients, and the downstream implications of increased work for the rest of the clinic. She expressed understanding and said that she would attend more reliably. Several months later, she once again was noted to be skipping clinic. The PD issued her a formal warning that with one more instance, she would be placed on formal probation. Dr. B had decided on a subspecialty career and told her PD that primary care was just "not her cup of tea" but that she would oblige and attend.

Once again, however, it became apparent that she was continuing to miss clinic, and she was formally placed on probation. A letter was written describing the reasons for probation, as well as potential future consequences, including termination, which she signed. The letter was placed in her file.

Her behavior improved, and she completed residency without any additional lapses, although her clinic attending resigned from supervising any future resident clinics because of the experience.

The resident went on to complete a fellowship in neonatology without any more professionalism issues. The neonatology program was aware of her probation but decided to rank her anyway, and they were pleased with her performance and professionalism throughout the 3 years.

She completed the fellowship and was offered a faculty position as an attending neonatologist. However, after she was hired, the credentialing process uncovered the probation, which was noted by the PD completing the credentialing forms. Dr. B, however, did not state on her own paperwork that she had ever been placed on probation, despite having signed the probationary letter. Her new department chair and the credentials committee contacted the PD for clarification, assistance, and discussion regarding her probationary status and her failure to disclose the probation, another violation of professionalism. She told the department chair and credentials committee that she did not know that the probation was "serious" and was not aware that it would follow her from one institution to the next. The decision was made to place her on probationary status as a new faculty member for 1 year. Any subsequent violations in professionalism would be cause for termination.

Time to Say Goodbye

A new intern, Dr. C (he/him), started a surgical program with a marginal application based on national licensing exam scores and medical school grades. Of note, his completed application was delayed beyond the usual ERAS application release date. Despite these potential "red flags," he had the support of several trainees at the residency institution who knew him, and the faculty at his medical school and their local residency program were positive about him. He had compelling stories of grit and resilience, and he interviewed well, which further made Dr. C's case for being selected. His start was delayed due to an incomplete assignment as a fourth-year medical student, which held up his final grade and medical school graduation. Once he started, there were frequent concerns about professionalism in completing administrative tasks (e.g., duty hours submissions, case logs), his knowledge base, technical skills, and clinical acumen. Dr. C was frequently given support by his colleagues on services who would help complete his patient care tasks (e.g., writing notes, entering orders), but he did seem to improve in efficiency and effectiveness over the first few months of residency. Nevertheless, the CCC found that he was deficient in professionalism, medical knowledge, and patient care competencies. The resultant remediation plan included frequent meetings with an associate PD and PD, regimented task completions, and clear consequences for delay or lack of completion (e.g., held from clinical duties or operating until tasks were complete) as well as frequently scheduled one-on-one technical training in the skills lab. While there were improvements in technical skills and some aspects of task completion and patient care efficiencies, the in-service exam results that year were below the remediation threshold and reflective of known knowledge deficiencies. At the end of the first year, the CCC recommended enhanced remediation given signs of improvement but failure to achieve set goals (including those determined in the earlier CCC). A more detailed written plan and schedule for remediation were developed and agreed to by Dr. C and the PD, with additional input from HR. The EAP was enlisted for counseling and coaching. Dr. C then remediated the first year of training with minimal progress through the first 6 months and continued deficiencies in multiple competencies despite the improvement plan and agreements. Ultimately after a multitude of discussions, counseling, coaching, and remediation plans, Dr. C progressed sufficiently to receive credit for completion of the PGY-1 but was not felt to meet the requirements necessary to progress in the program. His position was not renewed, and he elected not to appeal the decision and left the program thereafter. Assistance was offered for job placement, but he has been unsuccessful in obtaining another position in either another specialty or another surgical program.

Conclusion

PDs must provide trainees and faculty with transparent policies and procedures to document trainees' successful progression in the program and to identify trainees who struggle. Programs must clearly document the reasons, methods, and outcomes of remediation and communicate them to trainees to allow them to make corrections and progress. When programs document that trainees are not able to meet program expectations despite such remediation, it is essential that the programs work with the institution and DIO to determine whether adverse disciplinary actions are warranted. DIOs, institutional legal, and HR resources should be consulted by PDs early and frequently when significant deficits with trainees are identified to assist in the development of remediation plans, to assure that all policies are fairly applied and all remediation efforts, outcomes, and decisions are clearly documented. Courts have generally supported program assessments of trainee performance and usually focus on whether due process was provided rather than judging the competence of the trainee. Through transparent, fairly applied training standards and rigorous assessment and

feedback, GME programs meet the dual goals of preparing graduates for independent practice while maintaining the highest standards of patient safety in training hospitals. Further studies must define the training, background, and constitution necessary to support effective decision-making by a CCC.

References

1. Raman HS, Limbrick DD, Ray WZ, et al. Prevalence, management, and outcome of problem residents among neurosurgical training programs in the United States. J Neurosurg. 2018;130:322–6.
2. Guerrasio J, Brooks E, Rumack CM, Christensen A, Aagaard EM. Association of characteristics, deficits, and outcomes of residents placed on probation at one institution, 2002-2012. Acad Med. 2016;91:382–7.
3. Guerrasio J, Garrity MJ, Aagaard EM. Learner deficits and academic outcomes of medical students, residents, fellows, and attending physicians referred to a remediation program, 2006-2012. Acad Med. 2014;89:352–8.
4. Reamy BV, Harman JH. Residents in trouble: an in-depth assessment of the 25-year experience of a single family medicine residency. Fam Med. 2006;38:252–7.
5. Resnick AS, Mullen JL, Kaiser LR, Morris JB. Patterns and predictions of resident misbehavior—a 10-year retrospective look. Curr Surg. 2006;63:418–25.
6. Zbieranowski I, Takahashi SG, Verma S, Spadafora SM. Remediation of residents in difficulty: a retrospective 10-year review of the experience of a postgraduate board of examiners. Acad Med. 2013;88:111–6.
7. Shweikeh F, Schwed AC, Hsu CH, Nfonsam VN. Status of resident attrition from surgical residency in the past, present, and future outlook. J Surg Educ. 2018;75:254–62.
8. Riebschleger MP, Haftel HM. Remediation in the context of the competencies: a survey of pediatrics residency program directors. J Grad Med Educ. 2013;5:60–3.
9. Hauer KE, Ciccone A, Henzel TR, et al. Remediation of the deficiencies of physicians across the continuum from medical school to practice: a thematic review of the literature. Acad Med. 2009;84:1822–32.
10. Katz ED, Dahms R, Sadosty AT, Stahmer SA, Goyal D, CORD-EM Remediation Task Force. Guiding principles for resident remediation: recommendations of the CORD remediation task force. Acad Emerg Med. 2010;17(Suppl 2):S95–S103.
11. Lacasse M, Audetat MC, Boileau E, et al. Interventions for undergraduate and postgraduate medical learners with academic difficulties: a BEME systematic review: BEME guide no. 56. Med Teach. 2019;41:981–1001.

12. Shearer C, Bosma M, Bergin F, Sargeant J, Warren A. Remediation in Canadian medical residency programs: established and emerging best practices. Med Teach. 2019;41:28–35.

13. Cleland J, Leggett H, Sandars J, Costa MJ, Patel R, Moffat M. The remediation challenge: theoretical and methodological insights from a systematic review. Med Educ. 2013;47:242–51.

14. Audetat MC, Laurin S, Dory V. Remediation for struggling learners: putting an end to 'more of the same'. Med Educ. 2013;47:230–1.

15. Rosenblatt MA, Schartel SA. Evaluation, feedback, and remediation in anesthesiology residency training: a survey of 124 United States programs. J Clin Anesth. 1999;11:519–27.

16. Schwed AC, Lee SL, Salcedo ES, et al. Association of general surgery resident remediation and program director attitudes with resident attrition. JAMA Surg. 2017;152:1134–40.

17. Warburton KM, Goren E, Dine CJ. Comprehensive assessment of struggling learners referred to a graduate medical education remediation program. J Grad Med Educ. 2017;9:763–7.

18. Guerrasio J, Brooks E, Rumack CM, Aagaard EM. The evolution of resident remedial teaching at one institution. Acad Med. 2019;94:1891–4.

19. Burack JH, Irby DM, Carline JD, Root RK, Larson EB. Teaching compassion and respect. Attending physicians' responses to problematic behaviors. J Gen Intern Med. 1999;14:49–55.

20. Ziring D, Frankel RM, Danoff D, Isaacson JH, Lochnan H. Silent witnesses: faculty reluctance to report medical students' professionalism lapses. Acad Med. 2018;93:1700–6.

21. Guerrasio J, Cumbler E, Trosterman A, Wald H, Brandenburg S, Aagaard E. Determining need for remediation through postrotation evaluations. J Grad Med Educ. 2012;4:47–51.

22. Guerrasio J, Weissberg M. Unsigned: why anonymous evaluations in clinical settings are counterproductive. Med Educ. 2012;46:928–30.

23. Schwind CJ, Williams RG, Boehler ML, Dunnington GL. Do individual attendings' post-rotation performance ratings detect residents' clinical performance deficiencies? Acad Med. 2004;79:453–7.

24. Yao DC, Wright SM. National survey of internal medicine residency program directors regarding problem residents. JAMA. 2000;284:1099–104.

25. Nasca TJ, Philibert I, Brigham T, Flynn TC. The next GME accreditation system—rationale and benefits. N Engl J Med. 2012;366:1051–6.

26. Swing SR, Beeson MS, Carraccio C, et al. Educational milestone development in the first 7 specialties to enter the next accreditation system. J Grad Med Educ. 2013;5:98–106.

27. Green ML, Aagaard EM, Caverzagie KJ, et al. Charting the road to competence: developmental milestones for internal medicine residency training. J Grad Med Educ. 2009;1:5–20.

28. Hauer KE, Clauser J, Lipner RS, et al. The internal medicine reporting milestones: cross-sectional description of initial implementation in U.S. residency programs. Ann Intern Med. 2016;165:356–62.

29. Hauer KE, Vandergrift J, Hess B, et al. Correlations between ratings on the resident annual evaluation summary and the internal medicine milestones and association with ABIM certification examination scores among US internal medicine residents, 2013-2014. JAMA. 2016;316:2253–62.

30. Hauer KE, Vandergrift J, Lipner RS, Holmboe ES, Hood S, McDonald FS. National Internal Medicine milestone ratings: validity evidence from longitudinal three-year follow-up. Acad Med. 2018;93:1189–204.

31. Holmboe ES, Yamazaki K, Nasca TJ, Hamstra SJ. Using longitudinal milestones data and learning analytics to facilitate the professional development of residents: early lessons from three specialties. Acad Med. 2020;95:97–103.

32. Kinnear B, Bensman R, Held J, O'Toole J, Schauer D, Warm E. Critical deficiency ratings in milestone assessment: a review and case study. Acad Med. 2017;92:820–6.

33. Korte RC, Beeson MS, Russ CM, Carter WA, Emergency Medicine Milestones Working Group, Reisdorff EJ. The emergency medicine milestones: a validation study. Acad Emerg Med. 2013;20:730–5.

34. Turner TL, Bhavaraju VL, Luciw-Dubas UA, et al. Validity evidence from ratings of pediatric interns and subinterns on a subset of pediatric milestones. Acad Med. 2017;92:809–19.

35. Schumacher DJ, Spector ND, Calaman S, et al. Putting the pediatrics milestones into practice: a consensus roadmap and resource analysis. Pediatrics. 2014;133:898–906.

36. Easdown LJ, Wakefield ML, Shotwell MS, Sandison MR. A checklist to help faculty assess ACGME milestones in a video-recorded OSCE. J Grad Med Educ. 2017;9:605–10.

37. Gardner AK, Scott DJ, Choti MA, Mansour JC. Developing a comprehensive resident education evaluation system in the era of milestone assessment. J Surg Educ. 2015;72:618–24.

38. Kelleher M, Kinnear B, Wong SEP, O'Toole J, Warm E. Linking workplace-based assessment to ACGME milestones: a comparison of mapping strategies in two specialties. Teach Learn Med. 2020;32:194–203.

39. Conforti LN, Yaghmour NA, Hamstra SJ, et al. The effect and use of milestones in the assessment of neurological surgery residents and residency programs. J Surg Educ. 2018;75:147–55.

40. Ekpenyong A, Baker E, Harris I, et al. How do clinical competency committees use different sources of data to assess residents' performance on the internal medicine milestones? A mixed methods pilot study. Med Teach. 2017;39:1074–83.

41. Friedman KA, Raimo J, Spielmann K, Chaudhry S. Resident dashboards: helping your clinical competency committee visualize trainees' key performance indicators. Med Educ Online. 2016;21:29838.

42. Hauer KE, Chesluk B, Iobst W, et al. Reviewing residents' competence: a qualitative study of the role of clinical competency committees in performance assessment. Acad Med. 2015;90:1084–92.

43. Nabors C, Forman L, Peterson SJ, et al. Milestones: a rapid assessment method for the clinical competency committee. Arch Med Sci. 2017;13:201–9.

44. Ketteler ER, Auyang ED, Beard KE, et al. Competency champions in the clinical competency committee: a successful strategy to implement milestone evaluations and competency coaching. J Surg Educ. 2014;71:36–8.

45. Schumacher DJ, Michelson C, Poynter S, et al. Thresholds and interpretations: how clinical competency committees identify pediatric residents with performance concerns. Med Teach. 2018;40:70–9.

46. Schumacher DJ, Sectish TC, Vinci RJ. Optimizing clinical competency committee work through taking advantage of overlap across milestones. Acad Pediatr. 2014;14:436–8.

47. Common program requirements. https://acgme.org/What-We-Do/Accreditation/Common-Program-Requirements. Accessed 29 Dec 2022.

48. Institutional requirements. ACGME. https://acgme.org/Portals/0/PFAssets/InstitutionalRequirements/000InstitutionalRequirements2018.pdf?ver=2018-02-19-132236-600. Accessed 29 Dec 2022.

49. Conran RM, Elzie CA, Knollmann-Ritschel BE, Domen RE, Powell SZ. Due process in medical education: legal considerations. Acad Pathol. 2018;5:2374289518807460.

50. Mason MV. Are residents considered students or employees? JAMA. 1998;279:1668F.

51. https://www.jdsupra.com/legalnews/nlrb-rules-hospitals-resident-physician-05848/. Accessed 29 Dec 2022.

52. Lefebvre C, Williamson K, Moffett P, et al. Legal considerations in the remediation and dismissal of graduate medical trainees. J Grad Med Educ. 2018;10:253–7.

53. Board of Curators of University of Missouri vs. Horowitz 1978:89–91.

Commentary on Chapter 26: Perspective from the Oman Medical Specialty Board (OMSB)

27

Shaima Darwish, Raghdah Al-Bualy, and Siham Al Sinani

The OMSB is the national body responsible for supervising and accrediting residency and fellowship training programs in Oman with over 600 current residents and fellows. It is a sponsoring institution accredited by the Accreditation Council for Graduate Medical Education International (ACGME-I). It has 19 residency and 4 fellowship programs, of which 16 are ACGME-I accredited.

The structure of the OMSB is unique in that it is not a training site or hospital. It is an overseeing body that receives trainees from multiple sponsors/employers and distributes them to multiple training sites depending on clinical specialty. Clinical training occurs at various sites and is managed by assigned faculty contracted by the OMSB. Each program has an education committee which is responsible for managing educational activities at the training sites and reporting progress to the OMSB.

Despite the organizational and structural differences in Oman, we face many of the same issues identified in Chap. 26, reinforcing their commonality across national borders and cultures. Similarities can be categorized into four areas. These include failure to identify struggling trainees, faculty and trainee perceptions about remediation, lack of insight on the part of the trainee, and utilization of nonspecific remediation plans. The few differences are attributable to cultural, social, organizational, and legal issues specific to our region.

The average percentage of residents who undergo remediation in the OMSB programs is approximately 5%, considerably lower than the 18% quoted in Chap. 26. This difference is likely due to failure to identify struggling trainees, grade inflation, lack of willingness to document poor performance, and lack of understanding of resources and processes. We have recently introduced a framework to identify at-risk trainees and diagnose areas of deficiency and have experienced an increase in the number of residents being identified for remediation.

There may be cultural and sociological factors contributing to the low number of struggling trainees identified as needing remediation. Remediation is still generally perceived as a punishment rather than as an educational aid. Therefore, faculty may resist suggesting remediation, as they fear accusation of being overly harsh or having personal reasons influencing their actions. Trainees identified as requiring remediation are likely to feel ashamed and therefore refuse to accept the need for help.

Trainees commonly exhibit poor insight into their performance, especially in instances when medical school and internship scores were comparatively high. We see this most often when remediating for professional issues where, like

S. Darwish (✉) · R. Al-Bualy · S. Al Sinani
Oman Medical Specialty Board, Muscat, Oman
e-mail: raghdah.b@omsb.org; siham.s@omsb.org

Dr. P in the described case, trainees assume that since they have been promoted, all is well. They are then surprised when informed that they need help.

The most common deficits we encounter are poor performance in the areas of medical knowledge, patient care, and professionalism. These each require specific remedial interventions; however, historically, our remediation plans have been generic in content and across programs. Similar to those described in Chap. 26, plans have included repeated exposure to the same rotations with no new strategies to target the deficiency and no changes in trainee workload. These nonspecific interventions and delay in producing written remediation plans negatively influence the outcomes of remediation. Inconsistencies seen across programs are likely to reflect differences in the educator skills and experience of the faculty and members of the CCC, including monitoring of and feedback to trainees. We are addressing these issues through faculty training and development.

One of the changes recently introduced to tackle this misconception is changing the title of the plans from "remediation plans" to "academic improvement plans," in hopes that the plans will be perceived more positively. Work still needs to be done to better understand perceptions of remediation and current practices across our various programs. We also need to work with faculty and trainees to "normalize" remediation.

We often encounter inconsistency in implementing remediation and procedures attributable to organizational and legal issues specific to our context. There are marked differences between the probation and dismissal processes in Oman and those described in the chapter. For example, in Oman probation does not follow trainees throughout their career, and only rarely does the OMSB directly communicate about probation during training with future employers.

Historically, trainees had the right to appeal disciplinary decisions and took the matter to court, even when the OMSB's policy on grievances and appeals has been followed. Currently, Omani courts no longer accept academic-related matters and refer them back to their academic institutions. This process parallels the description in the chapter deputizing academic programs to enforce remediation and probation actions fairly.

In conclusion, our remediation and probation issues seem largely similar despite differing structures and geographic locations. Cultural, sociological, and legal factors may affect areas of remediation, probation, dismissal, and appeals. Encouraging international research collaboration in these areas would illuminate the impact of local contextual issues on remediation practices.

Commentary on Chapter 26: Perspective from the National Healthcare Group Family Medicine Residency, Singapore

28

Irwin Clement Alphon Chung, Darren Seah, and Jason Meng Huey Chan

In Singapore, undergraduates enter medical school soon after junior college, while males designated for national service in the military join 2 years later. A smaller number may opt to join the postgraduate Duke-National University of Singapore Medical School after obtaining a degree in another field. Facing a stressful medical undergraduate education system at a relatively young age, with perhaps fewer life experiences than medical students in other countries, the Singaporean medical student may struggle more.

At our residency in Singapore, faculty regularly undergo training workshops to identify common areas where at-risk trainees face difficulties, to increase awareness of possible interventions and available resources, and to direct learners to these resources. We have adopted the DICED framework: proper **D**ocumentation of the perspectives of faculty and residents, **I**dentifying the red flags, **C**larifying the facts and getting corroborative history, **E**xploring the causes of the issues, and finally **D**iagnosing and remedying behaviors.

At the microsystem level, resources have been provided for resident peers, core faculty, and pro-

gram directors to identify the warning signs of residents facing difficulty. After identifying such residents, clear plans for action and escalation are provided in a simple yet comprehensive way.

At the mesosystem level, the National Healthcare Group also established guidelines to identify and proactively address deficiencies noted during meetings of our Clinical Competency Committee (CCC). These guidelines define the discussions that should take place with the residents, the targets to be achieved, and the consequences of not meeting them. Typically, residents with difficulty in specific competency domains are brought up for discussion by faculty at CCC meetings, where further in-depth exploration of the concerns is thoroughly addressed. For example, when the CCC notes that a resident is faltering in medical knowledge, faculty would discuss the additional teaching sessions or assessments needed and the standards expected at the end of the remediation. Faculty members who directly work with the resident would also give specific input on deficiencies. After the CCC makes a decision for remediation, the resident meets with their main faculty supervisor to determine if there are other issues affecting them socially, to discuss options to maximize success (such as a lower caseload for a period of time), and to collaborate on a learning plan. We also work with external counselling organizations to provide struggling trainees with confidential counselling where needed.

I. C. A. Chung · D. Seah · J. M. H. Chan (✉)
National Healthcare Group Polyclinics,
Singapore, Singapore
e-mail: irwin_ca_chung@nhgp.com.sg;
darren_ej_seah@nhgp.com.sg;
jason_mh_chan@nhgp.com.sg

Even though our family medicine residency has not sought ACGME-I accreditation since July 2021, we will continue using the DICED framework in our remediation efforts. Our residents have uniformly received this program as helpful, and after initial disappointment, they have enthusiastically and successfully participated. We have had no residents pursue further legal action.

Part VI

Systems, Legal, and Ethical Considerations: Preparing for Dismissal

When the Prognosis Is Poor: Documentation, the Law, and When and How to Give Up

29

Jeannette Guerrasio, Calvin L. Chou, Sara Tariq, and Lee Jones

Previous chapters in this volume have addressed the need for structured approaches to remediating trainees who struggle, including an institutional emphasis on clear policies, expectations for excellence, robust and fair assessments, compassionate and firm remediation practices, respect for due process and privacy with detailed documentation of deficits and outcomes of remediation plans (Chaps. 2, 20, and 26), and attention to bias and conflicts of interest in assessment (Chaps. 2 and 3). This chapter describes zones of remediation, specific approaches to documentation, legal considerations, and approaches to a learner on probation or requiring dismissal.

J. Guerrasio
Medicine Within Reach, PLLC, Denver, CO, USA
e-mail: jeannette@coloradocme.com

C. L. Chou
Department of Medicine, University of California, San Francisco, CA, USA

Veterans Affairs Healthcare System, San Francisco, CA, USA
e-mail: calvin.chou@ucsf.edu

S. Tariq
University of Arkansas for Medical Sciences School of Medicine, Little Rock, AR, USA
e-mail: tariqsarag@uams.edu

L. Jones (✉)
Georgetown University School of Medicine, Washington, DC, USA
e-mail: lj485@georgetown.edu

Not all students who start health professions training *should* graduate. Graduating incompetent health professionals betrays our social contract with patients, our colleagues, and our professions. Medical schools in the United States graduate more than 95% of entering students by 6 years after admission [1]. In 2020–2021, of 153,843 residents in the United States, 1036 (0.67%) withdrew, were dismissed, or failed to complete their programs [2]. Although these statistics may reflect high admissions standards, diligent trainees, and good education practices, they have not changed measurably since implementation of competency-based evaluations. This "failure to fail" paradigm extends across health professions and continents [3, 4] and arises from numerous factors, including faculty time and effort, emotional and professional tolls on faculty and learners, insufficient resources including faculty development, incomplete institutional support for decisions to fail, and a high need for physicians in underserved areas [4]. Notably, medical school failure rates internationally have historically been significantly higher: the medical school failure rate is 17% in the Netherlands [5], 18% in India [6], 21% in Italy [7], and 60% in Iran [8]. There are also broad differences in graduation rates across health professions schools.

The assessment phase of remediation (Chap. 6) requires an ultimate determination of whether the trainee has successfully completed remediation and is back on course. The criteria should be twofold: achieving minimum competency *and* demonstrating sustained improvement over time. As previously discussed, it is optimal if academic and performance standards committees make critical promotion decisions (Chaps. 20 and 26). With the right composition of experts who have sufficient experience with learner training, such committees can assimilate and evaluate disparate and often conflicting data, perspectives, and potential biases, on a trainee's progress. While an arduous task, it is essential that our graduates have earned their respective degrees. Making a fair competence determination is ultimately a judgment call that requires experience and courage (see Chap. 19).

Limits to Remediation

The educational costs to train health professionals commonly outweigh tuition; finding additional resources to remediate learners who struggle may prove challenging in many training settings. Therefore, limits to remediation vary based on institutional culture and resources, patient safety risks, and the trainee's efforts and abilities [9]. An institution with a mission that emphasizes assisting all students to reach their maximal potential may prioritize investment in remediation and make allowances (for example, subsidizing faculty development and programs to support remediation, schedule changes, contract extensions, and specialized communication or professionalism training programs for learners). Other institutions, based on size, resource limitations, or prior costly experiences with poor remediation outcomes, may be less able or willing to support remediation.

While there are no specific legal requirements to provide remediation, we believe that all trainees who have made the investment to enter health professions training and yet find themselves struggling deserve reasonable access to effective remediation. In fact, for some institutions, supporting historically marginalized and minoritized trainees who struggle is regarded as an ethical imperative. Additional research is needed to describe the full range of institutional perspectives on remediation. In general, in the US medical context, institutions consider dismissal only if reasonable attempts at remediation fail, patient safety is at imminent risk, or a crime has been committed.

Zones of Remediation

The model in Fig. 29.1 depicts sequenced "zones" with different rules of engagement depending on the learner's length and degree of struggle [10, 11]. On identification of a deficit in one or more milestones or competencies, Learner A enters Zone 2 (sometimes described as informal remediation, focused review, or academic warning), in which the documentation process begins (see below).

If corrective action succeeds, the learner returns to the "normal curriculum," and no further disclosure is necessary.

If a learner does not correct an identified deficiency within a specified period, or if the deficiency is serious, they enter Zone 3 (Learner B in Fig. 29.1). Zone 3 indicates the institution of formal remediation practices, including review of documentation of previously unsuccessful informal corrections, and presentation of a formal action plan with clear outcomes, expected timelines, and consequences. Learners in Zone 3 require disclosure to institutional overseers (e.g., Graduate Medical Education office or student affairs dean). For such learners, regardless of ultimate trajectory, it is also prudent to consult institutional legal counsel early and frequently.

A learner who does not successfully complete the formal remediation action plan enters probation, Zone 4 (Learner C in Fig. 29.1), with an updated action plan and consequences, formal disclosure to overseers, and disclosure in letters of recommendation and final training certification.

Learner D, in Zone 5, has failed the probation terms of Zone 4 or has committed an egregious act warranting immediate removal. Documentation

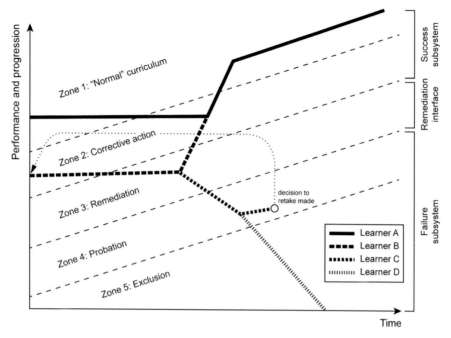

Fig. 29.1 A model depicting five "zones" of remediation with different rules of engagement depending on the length and degree of a learner's struggle. See text for details [10]

continues, and ongoing consultation with institutional overseers, legal counsel, and, if applicable, human resources professionals is necessary to ensure due process.

Standards for Decision-Making

For institutions to successfully defend decisions to change a learner's status (e.g., to probation or dismissal), institutions must have and follow very clear guidelines that set expectations for competent performance. These expectations should be explicit to learners on matriculation and include goals and objectives for courses and clinical experiences, defined performance targets, academic and professionalism standards, expectations for communication (e.g., regular checking of e-mail), grading and assessment policies, and consequences for failure to meet expectations, which must also include an outline of the procedures for remediation, probation, and dismissal [9, 12] (see also Chaps. 2, 20, and 26). Competency-based

Table 29.1 Characteristics of at-risk trainees

- Recurrent unprofessional behavior—when a cause cannot be elucidated and remediated [13]
- Egregious unprofessional behavior (first strike, you are out)
- Poor insight into deficits (e.g., inability to acknowledge failure to progress despite multiple warnings, direct feedback, and attempts to help illuminate the situation)
- Failure to progress at a pace that will allow the student to graduate in a reasonable length of time—because of mental health disorders, physical health diseases, disability despite access to treatment or accommodations, or insufficient ability) [9, 14, 15]
- Refusal to participate in remediation

assessment milestones and entrustable professional activities can act as a robust basis for these standards.

Table 29.1 lists some characteristics of trainees at risk for dismissal. Such cases are significant and warrant discussion; however, they make up less than 2% of all learners referred for remediation [16].

Legal Considerations

Documentation

Prior chapters in the book have emphasized—and we strongly reiterate—the importance of documentation. Clear, detailed, and accurate documentation not only is necessary to communicate with and convince a trainee that they have a deficit [17] but also gives the remediation team a foundation to build a remediation strategy and can be used to justify assessments, remedial actions, and, if necessary, dismissal. Such documentation also protects individuals and institutions from becoming the target of legal action, against which documentation provides necessary evidentiary support.

Even if the learner has only a minor deficit to remediate, thorough documentation remains crucial, since it is impossible to predict who will not succeed, choose to challenge or appeal an academic decision, or file a lawsuit.

> Steve (he/him) is a second-year student who failed two major preclinical courses after doing well his first year. Per school policy, as part of a remediation protocol, the promotion committee allowed him to repeat the second year and continue to take the board exam provided that he received no lower than a C grade in all second-year courses. The policy also stated that failure in any course would lead to dismissal.
>
> When explored further, he noted that he was on medications for attention deficit disorder (see Chap. 17) during his first year, but his parents insisted he stop taking medications once they learned that he was on them. He has struggled with mental health and shame since then. With this additional information, he was required to meet with the student success center and to check in with available mental health professionals regularly. However, he did not comply with either stipulation.
>
> Having failed a second-year course for the second time, dismissal proceeded, with opportunity to appeal per school policy.

To document a learner's deficits and initiate a *formative* remediation plan, course or program directors should compile verbal comments, e-mail communications, and written evaluations, as well as assessments from multiple sources, and place them into the trainee's academic record. *Documentation of comments regarding a learner's performance is as valid for making academic decisions as formal written evaluations.*

Each document should include the date of observation or identification of deficit(s), identification of who made the observations, specific examples of objective behaviors or actions that highlight the deficits, and content of feedback conversations with the learner. If concern about a learner's poor performance leads to considering a change in status, for instance to probation or dismissal, proof of a feedback conversation with the learner is important. This should be accomplished with a follow-up e-mail after verbal feedback, with written feedback, or by having a witness (e.g., a chief resident) present during verbal feedback.

Subjective impressions of the learner's behaviors and actions should also be documented. However, in writing their impressions, observers must be careful to distinguish between subjective interpretations and relatively objective descriptions of learner behavior. Furthermore, care should be taken to express respect for the learner as a person and avoid suggesting malicious intent [18]. Program or course directors can also use informal networks to collect information. Written summaries of meetings in which the learner's academic progress was discussed should include the meeting date and time, list of attendees, any decisions made, plans to "feed forward" performance difficulties, reasoning behind all decisions, and if the learner was notified [19]. Minutes should be taken and retained for all promotions committee meetings discussing the trainee of concern.

It is critical to communicate to the learner in writing any remediation action plans with timelines, proposed outcomes, consequences for failure to achieve improvement, and the process by which the learner will acknowledge receipt

Table 29.2 Components of a letter informing a learner of change in academic status

- Promotions committee meeting date(s) when decision was made to change academic status from good to focused review
- Date that the status change will take effect
- Clear descriptions of deficit(s) or competencies to be remedied
- Summary of the information that led to the decision, including source of information, assessment technique, and format (such as written or verbal)
- Date when the learner's status will be reassessed
- Performance or actions required to reverse the change in academic status, and how they will be measured
- Consequences for achieving or failing the reassessment

of the notification (Table 29.2). We have included examples of such letters (see Figs. 29.2, 29.3, and 29.4); others are available [20, 21]. Even if the learner refuses to sign the letter, proof of receipt or a witness to attest that the information was given serves as confirmation of notification. We emphasize that expectations regarding communications should be established upon entrance to a program. For example, a school should collect students' acknowledgements of receipt of a student handbook that clearly outlines expectations that students are responsible for checking e-mail and any other form of official communication.

When developing a remediation plan, we recommend, at a minimum, that clear documentation of the following elements be included:

- The deficit or competency being addressed
- A specific description of the behaviors or actions of concern
- The time frame for remediation
- The specific plan
- The objective measures that will be used to assess the deficit post-remediation
- The date the plan was communicated to the learner
- Written evidence or contemporaneous written statement of a witness to a verbal conversation attesting that the plan was communicated to the learner [9]

Due Process

Most of the information below is based on legal precedent in the United States. Clear differences will exist in other settings and across jurisdictions. We intend the following three sections as an overview of precedents and practices to assuage anxiety about litigation. They by no means replace close relationships and early consultation with lawyers at your institution.

Trainees have increasingly appealed to grievance committees and the judicial system [22–24]. Of those who sued their medical schools, 96% did so because of dismissal, denial of admission, cheating, and mandating repeating coursework [23, 24]. Faculty and institutions should be prepared to defend their professional judgment [9, 25, 26]. Although legal threats can feel chilling, being informed about the legal system, principles, and precedent can help faculty participate more confidently in remediation with integrity and transparency.

The US Constitution provides for "due process," which protects individuals' rights of liberty and property from federal or state governmental action. In health professions education contexts, some courts have ruled that education is a trainee's property [27] and that programmatic decisions that inhibit a trainee's academic progress are subject to due process [28]. Due process comprises two types: *procedural*, where individuals being deprived of rights receive notice and can be heard, and *substantive*, providing safeguards that decisions made are not arbitrary or capricious. The documentation practices outlined above support both procedural and substantive due process.

In addition, accreditation standards for both undergraduate (Liaison Committee on Medical Education standard 9.9) and graduate medical education (Accreditation Council on Graduate Medical Education standard IV.C.) require that institutions have "fair and formal" processes in all decisions from promotion to dismissal, essentially reflecting due process [29, 30]. Because clinical performance depends on some subjective evaluation, convening faculty review committees (Chaps. 20 and 26) that collectively arrive at

University School of Medicine
Remediation Program

Sent by certified mail:

Dear Michael Miller,   Date: 7/17/2022

Based on review of your entire academic record, you were referred for remediation of interpersonal skills and professionalism, which were determined to be below expectations. Specifically, your deficits included interrupting the learning of others, demeaning comments to peers about assignments, confronting supervisors about decisions regarding patient care, providing patients with incorrect information, using jargon with patients, and not respecting others' roles.

Per the program director, you will have 4 weeks to complete the remediation plan. As per our discussion, the remediation plan will include:

- Assigned reading on clinical and team based communication skills.
- 2 written assignments, no less than 500 words with 5 literature references, describing how interpersonal communication skills and collaboration can facilitate or hinder patient care.
- Weekly, 1-hour sessions with the coach assigned to you to discuss and analyze past and present examples of your behavior on clinical teams, comparing perspectives and perceptions of each party involved and listing alternative methods of handling the situation.
- 2, 2-hour sessions in the simulation lab practicing communication tasks with actors playing other team members or patients, reviewing video recordings and feedback from actor and nurse trainer, and repeated exercises incorporating feedback.
- Submit the videotapes from those sessions.
- Discuss, with program director the short term and long term consequences of confrontational and disrespectful behaviors on clinical teams.

At the conclusion of the 4-week period, you will be placed on a 2-week rotation with a team that is unaware of your prior deficits and need for remediation. At the end of the rotation, you must meet the expectation for competent performance on multisource evaluations from faculty, residents, nurses, and patients, pass an observed structured clinical examination in the simulation lab, and pass two mini-clinical examinations conducted by your clinical attending.

If you meet this benchmark, you will pass the rotation and be allowed to proceed with your remaining intern year. At anytime during the remediation process or reassessment, this plan may be altered, your remediation and reassessment interrupted, or you may be referred to the promotions committee. If you do not meet these benchmarks, you may be required to repeat the rotation or be dismissed from the residency program.

It is our hope that you will make the necessary changes to be successful in our course.

Sincerely,
Jon Jones, MD
Program Director
Adam Addisons, MD
Assistant Program Director
Remediation Team

Fig. 29.2 Example letter documenting notification of deficits and details of remediation plan

University School of Medicine
Remediation Program

Dear Michael Miller;   Date 8/7/2022

The remediation team is now concerned that you are struggling with clinical reasoning. This was identified during direct observation of your interpersonal skills and participation on rounds and confirmed on chart review. This was discussed with you and your course director.

As per the remediation team, the plan addresses your interpersonal skills and professionalism deficits and incorporates some introductory remediation steps to help with your clinical reasoning, such as teaching you a framework for building a differential diagnosis. The team reports that you have not been making progress in any of these areas.

The remediation team would strongly recommend that you undergo neuropsychiatric testing to help you and us, determine if your recent head injury is impacting your ability to learn new skills. We are also recommending to the institution that you undergo alcohol and drug monitoring as this can also impair performance.

Our recommendations have been cc'd to the Dean of Graduate Medical Education.

Sincerely,
Sarah Smith, MD
James Jackson, MD
Lynn Lyons, MD
Carol Crabtree, PsyD
Remediation Team

cc. Steven Stone MD, Program Director, Linus Li, MD, Chair of the Residency Review and Education and members of the Residency Review and Education Committee

Fig. 29.3 Example letter documenting new concerns of competence and new expectations for the remediation plan

decisions to assess trainee performance can mitigate substantive due process claims [31].

US laws about student evaluation vary slightly between public and private (defined as receiving no federal or state subsidy support or influence) institutions. Public institutions must provide formal constitutional due process, as their students are protected under the 14th Amendment of the US Constitution. Accordingly, such institutions must notify the learner of their deficiencies, warn of potential consequences, and give adequate time to prepare for any hearing to air grievances. The date and time of the hearing are usually provided upon notification of such deficiency. While learners should be allowed to have a witness present for the hearing, attorneys may be denied access to these proceedings.

Conversely, private institutions may create and follow their own rules and policies. They are only required to provide adequate notice of charges and an opportunity for the student to respond. Private institutions are not required to hold a hearing, and the student's response can be in writing [32]. Institutional policies should reflect these requirements.

Regardless of private or public institutional status, due process can provide trainees with the opportunity to defend themselves and/or summon legal counsel [33–35], but an appeals process is not required.

Furthermore, court precedent may be unique to specific circumstances. For example, in 1982, Heisler v. New York Medical College held that a student was permitted to repeat the first year of medical school after three other first-year students with equally poor academic records were permitted by the college to do so [36]. Yet, faculty members and institutions may dismiss a student even if students in past years have not been dismissed for similar deficits [37]. In addition,

University School of Medicine
Remediation Program

Dear Michael Miller;,   Date: 9/17/2022

On 9/1/2022, you were reported to the Residency Review and Education Committee. After reviewing your entire academic record, you were invited to appear before the committee. You were given an opportunity to contest the results of the outcome of the remediation and comment on why you have refused neuropsychiatric testing and alcohol and drug monitoring.

This letter serves as an official notification that your academic status has changed from good standing to probation, effective 9/17/2022. You are being placed on probation because of serious concerns related to interpersonal skills, professionalism and clinical reasoning. This action is based on interrupting the learning of others, obstructing patient care, providing patients with incorrect information, in appropriately confronting residents and attending about patient care judgments, continuing to use jargon with patients, demonstrating poor clinical reasoning on rounds and in your notes. This information was collected from your evaluations, chart review, direct observation, e-mails and verbal conversations with supervising faculty.

The following conditions must be met for your status to return to "good academic standing"
- Continue working with the remediation team to remedy these deficits in interpersonal skills, professionalism, and clinical reasoning. Their recommendations may include changes in your schedule, repeating courses, additional reading, additional assignments, practice time in the simulation lab, direct observation, increased supervision, and frequent feedback.
- Be evaluated by the Physician's Health Program, which will include alcohol and drug monitoring, AND sign a release of information for them to communicate their findings to the Residency Review and Education Committee.
- Repeat the rotation you failed, and achieve a passing score on all components.
- Maintain passing grades in all subsequent assignments.
- Return a signed copy of this letter to your program director and the Chair of the Residency Review and Education Committee

In 90 days from your change in status, the Residency Review and Education Committee will re-evaluate your performance and determine whether to return you to good academic standing, continue your probationary status or dismiss you from medical school. Failure to meet all of the above requirements by the time of re-evaluation by the Promotions Committee may result in dismissal. The Promotions Committee reserves the right to re-evaluation your progress and/or change your status prior to 90 days. Please see the medical school policies manual for additional details about the process.

It is also my duty to inform you that in the future you must inform licensing boards, credentialing agencies and malpractice insurance organizations of your probationary status. This is part of your official academic record.
- You are not permitted to attend away electives or to moonlight while on probation.
- It is our genuine hope that you complete the actions required of you as stated above and return to good standing and a positive learning environment.

Sincerely,
Steven Stone MD
Program Director
Linus Li, MD
Chair of the Residency Review and Education   Alejandra Garcia, MD
Alejandra Garcia, MD   Vlad Levin, PhD
Vlad Levin, PhD   Mario Martelli PhD
Mario Martelli PhD   Residency Review and Education
Residency Review and Education Committee   Committee Members

I have received a copy of this document. I understand the actions required of me.

Signature _____   Date: _____

Fig. 29.4 Example letter informing of a change in academic status and the requirements of probation

the courts have not consistently mandated that all students be treated exactly alike [22]. This became apparent during the COVID-19 pandemic when students who would have been summarily dismissed because of their inability to schedule board examinations were given some leniency due to closure of test centers and ensuring heightened anxiety. Also, faculty members are allowed to evaluate underperforming students in greater depth than other students, can modify their training as needed, and can alert future faculty that the student is struggling to enhance remediation efforts [33, 38] (Chap. 2, Goal 2B).

Tara (she/her) is a third-year medical student who passed all courses in the first 2 years with some difficulty. She has intermittently accessed the school's student success team to help her. She has little family, social, or economic support and grew up in an impoverished rural community.

She failed the first board exam and had to take 3 months off to study. The school subsidized her board review course. While awaiting her score on the exam retake, she started her clinical rotations. During her first clerkship, she struggled to keep up and failed. School policy clearly stated that failure of a third-year clerkship is grounds for dismissal.

She appealed to the promotions committee, stating that she received little support from the school and suffered mistreatment in the toxic work culture during the clinical rotation she failed. However, because the school regularly followed up with documentation delineating her subpar performance, the steps taken to support her, and the policies and ramifications of failure, her appeal was denied, and she was dismissed.

Judicial Deference

The US Supreme Court has repeatedly held that academic institutions have the best perspective to determine a profession's requirements [27, 35]. Courts cannot fairly evaluate academic performance as they lack the appropriate professional judgment and therefore should defer to faculty ("judicial deference"). Regardless of the correctness of the decision, if it is reasoned, then courts will uphold the decision.

Therefore, to prevail in a challenge, the student must demonstrate both that decision makers disregarded the facts in their academic record and that the decision was irrational and unreasonable [19, 22]. The rare exceptions are with concerns that an institution did not allow for due process, did not follow its own rules, or made a decision that lacked professional judgment. Therefore, in the absence of evidence that an institutional decision is arbitrary and capricious, it is generally upheld. If the decision is nonacademic, i.e., disciplinary in nature, then a hearing is required, with potential involvement of law enforcement. Comprehensive descriptions of cases and their decisions validate these principles [27, 34].

Other Legal Issues

Employment Considerations. Because residents are both trainees and employees, contract law applies to the resident's employment. Courts have treated dismissals of residents for academic reasons similarly to those of students in degree-granting institutions since postgraduate education programs require successful completion of goals to achieve certification (see Chap. 26). Therefore, as long as institutions adhere to policies and due process, they should not be in breach of contract when choosing not to grant certification to an unsuccessful learner [18]. Many residency programs offer renewable yearly contracts as they facilitate terminating employment if a trainee fails to achieve educational benchmarks: it is more straightforward not to renew a contract than to "buy it out" early [24].

Resignation in Lieu of Disciplinary Action. To avoid the potential consequences of formal disciplinary action, a resident might seek instead to resign preemptively. While this might seem a reasonable option from the perspective of a learner or employee, especially in cases involving personal hardship or career change, program leaders should consider that allowing a trainee who has demonstrated egregious or unethical conduct to resign may interfere with establishing documentation that potential future employers will need to protect patient safety [34].

Evaluation Libel. Trainees have also sued faculty members for libel, arguing the negative impact an unflattering evaluation may have on their reputations. However, if the potentially concerning documentation is accessible only to involved parties, and the statements made are relevant and truthful, courts have found that negative evaluations are not defamatory. Furthermore, courts have noted that trainees give implied consent for their program to evaluate them when they enter an academic institution [39].

Failure to Educate. While a graduate could accuse a program of perceived failure to provide "sufficient" education, courts to date have not recognized the tort of "educational malpractice" [18].

Fitness for Duty

Healthcare institutions must monitor their trainees and can be held liable for their behavior [40]. If an institution reasonably believes that a trainee's lack of ability becomes a threat to themselves or others, it may act immediately by suspending the trainee, pending a fair determination of competency and fitness for duty, usually by a medical professional [32]. Trainees may be deemed unfit for duty if they:

- Cannot continue caring for patients' safety
- Appear not capable of learning given the circumstances
- Are a danger to themselves or others
- Greatly impede the learning environment for other trainees
- Cannot continue to effectively teach their peers and students, if that is part of their role

Programs may not force learners to undergo treatment but may require them to be evaluated and determined fit for duty. If found to be unfit, the learner is responsible for seeking treatment to restore fitness for duty [18]. Programs can strongly suggest a leave of absence or make it a condition of contract renewal.

For cases of established disability in the United States, the Americans with Disabilities Act (ADA) applies. Though requests for accommodations cannot be made retroactively, institutions must address reasonable requests under the ADA, which may include modified schedules, job restructuring, and possible reassignment. However, if such accommodation requests prove an undue hardship to the program, it is not obligated to provide them (see Chap. 17).

When a Trainee Commits a Crime

In any large academic medical center, while rare, trainees and physicians unfortunately do commit crimes, including vandalism, theft, assault, rape, offenses involving illegal substances (e.g., buying, selling, or using), "drunk and disorderly" behavior, and carrying or using firearms that do not meet the standard of the law or violate institutional policy.

Criminal activity does not fall under the jurisdiction of the educational remediation team and should be referred to law enforcement. Occasionally, especially when program directors are inexperienced, they may unintentionally delay distinguishing between an unprofessional and a criminal act (see Chap. 14). If any criminal activity is suspected, and in the absence of an imminent threat to safety (which should trigger an appropriate response, including the involvement of law enforcement), program directors should seek institutional legal counsel, which may refer such matters to outside counsel or recommend other appropriate avenues of response. Additionally, if trainees are licensed to practice, the institution may have a duty to report any criminal activity to the state licensing board.

Pat Smith (she/her) was in the MD/PhD track throughout medical school. Between her pre-clerkship and clinical years, she spent 8 years earning her PhD in immunology. When she subsequently rotated on the clinical services as a clerkship student, she routinely called nurses, introduced herself as "Doctor" Smith, and gave verbal patient care or medication orders for patients. When confronted, she also admitted to intentionally standing behind counters to obscure her student-length short white coat and portraying herself as a licensed physician to patients, nurses, and some consultants. She felt justified in doing these things because, "After all, I am Dr. Smith."

> Pat not only threatened patient safety and behaved unethically by lying and deceiving, but she also committed a crime by impersonating a physician and practicing medicine without a license [40].
>
> After further investigation of her behavior, the university and hospital lawyers met with the School of Medicine deans and hospital risk management professionals. The decision was to immediately dismiss her, and she was subsequently charged with a crime.

In summary, we encourage legal consultation for any learner entering the remediation, probation, or dismissal stages; whenever changes are made to institutional handbooks or other remediation processes, so that language can be vetted and due process upheld; for learners needing disability review or undergoing psychiatric or substance use treatment; or whenever the situation does not appear to be straightforward.

Dismissal and the Exit Interview

For the small minority of cases where a trainee is to be dismissed, the dean, program director, and competency committee must review academic policies and all documentation, and legal counsel and ancillary personnel (e.g., designated institutional officer, medical education dean) should conduct an independent review.

Suggestions for the exit interview include preparing thoroughly (including re-reviewing documentation, reconsulting legal counsel, and rehearsing what to say during the encounter), interacting respectfully throughout, having a witness present, delivering the dismissal news succinctly and factually, and providing means for the trainee to avoid embarrassment (e.g., allowing the trainee to collect personal items after hours). Legal counsel can further assist by providing language to avoid potential defamation. It is important to maintain privacy about the terms of the dismissal and to document what happened [34]. Concerns about possible trainee responses to dismissal, including mental health issues and violence, must be addressed with the appropriate institutional resources.

Handling Lawsuits

If a trainee does take legal action against you or your institution, it is natural for emotions to run high. It is therefore important to first acknowledge, reflect on, and manage your own feelings about the circumstances. Second, seek institutional and/or personal legal counsel, and accept that a lawsuit will require time and energy to address. Seeking the advice of institutional legal counsel should occur immediately once the lawsuit is served. Table 29.3 lists some suggested preparation and behavioral steps during legal proceedings.

Table 29.3 Advice for educators called to testify in a hearing or trial or to give a deposition [41]

- Arrive prepared, both cognitively (having read all the evidence) and physically (rested, adequately nourished, and as distraction-free as possible)
- Know the strengths and weaknesses of the program's remediation decision-making processes, and be prepared to address them
- Preserve without alteration any documentation or evidence, including e-mails, file, letters, recordings, etc.
- Represent yourself and the institution with moral integrity, be prepared to defend your professional judgment, and continue to reinforce the mission of excellent training and patient and public safety, understanding that the tone of the proceedings will almost certainly be adversarial and should not be taken personally
- Tell the truth directly, and do not alter your responses based on a desired outcome
- Do not guess or speculate
- Be sure that you understand the question being asked, asking for clarification if needed
- Answer only the question that is asked and do so concisely without unneeded embellishment, particularly if "yes" or "no" is sufficient
- Acceptable responses can be "I don't know" and "I don't remember," if accurate
- Speak to your audience (lawyers and judges) as you would speak to your patients, as they are not clinically trained and likely not familiar with clinical education and terminology
- Discuss only one issue at a time
- Maintain your credibility as a professional in your dress, responses, and actions as attempts may be made to discredit you

Aftermath of a Dismissal

For the Learner

Ideally, institutions would provide redirection toward appropriate careers better suited to the trainee's competence and skills. For residents, this may take the form of another residency program, even in a different specialty. Optimal methods for students not having completed a degree remain elusive, especially as failed training will likely be viewed as a blemish on the learner's record. One possibility is offering academic credit for completed work and to work with any subsequent institution to have such credit accepted [42, 43]. Providing reasonable resources and potential next steps to trainees allows for a compassionate stance in what are almost always adversarial conditions.

Alternative healthcare-adjacent careers:

Policy and government
Nonprofit organizations
Journalism
Informatics
Finance and consulting for industry
Biotechnology
Websites for alternative careers:
https://www.aamc.org/cim/explore-options/settings-and-environments
https://lookforzebras.com/start-here/
https://www.docjobs.com/jobs/list/
http://medicalsuccess.net

For Peers and Faculty

Dismissal of a peer will reverberate throughout the program. The broadest range of emotions can arise in the context of the loss, including happiness, relief, anger, frustration, confusion, and survivor guilt. It is important to provide a formal forum to allow for expressions of grief and to reassure that dismissal of one trainee does not mean that someone else is necessarily next. Without revealing details about the dismissal, such a meeting or gathering can be leveraged as an opportunity to reinforce program expectations, framing them not as a warning but as a commitment to the well-being of learners and faculty through applying due process [34].

Institutional administrators are routinely accused of targeting trainees with marginalized identities for dismissal proceedings. There are data suggesting that ongoing microaggressions against such students lead to poorer mental health and decreased satisfaction with training [44, 45]. At the same time, institutions must uphold standards that guarantee that graduates are competent to practice. Trustworthiness in faculty and administration, including a willingness to acknowledge and self-reflect on the potential for bias and a history of building strong relationships with students, can help to mitigate some of the inflammatory optics that may ensue. Specifically, explicitly stating and upholding institutional standards of excellence, a strong commitment to success and diversity, using "location of self" narratives by administrators (see Chap. 3), and flattening perceived hierarchy by involving learners in programmatic governance can build psychological safety [46] and trust.

For the Program/Institution

Any dismissal or close call represents an opportunity to review all processes of assessment, remediation, and decision-making about probation and termination. Because it is natural to quickly desire closure after an arduous process, this exercise for quality improvement takes courage and humility. Maintaining a supportive community of practice in remediation, and within resource constraints, optimizing remediation practices as outlined in Chap. 2, will ultimately strengthen a program's ability to appropriately serve its learners.

Conclusion

In summary, clinical training programs will occasionally need to dismiss trainees, typically after a carefully documented and rigorous attempt at remediation, a detailed summary example of which is presented below.

Michael (he/him) aced his first 2 years of medical school, receiving honors in every course. Unfortunately, this success fueled his arrogant confrontational personality.

Despite repeated feedback from faculty and peers, his behavior did not change. While his reputation for challenging interpersonal interactions worsened throughout the clerkship years, these concerns never appeared in his written evaluations. Ultimately, he graduated and matched into a residency program.

Very early in internship, while on his way home from work, he sustained a closed head injury from a bike accident. After 1 week in the hospital, he recovered from the acute injuries and resumed clinical duties. However, because of repeated episodes of unprofessional behavior and poor interpersonal skills, he was referred for remediation. During the process, the remediation team additionally noticed that he had difficulty processing information, leading to questions about whether the deficit predated the head injury.

Michael underwent 4 weeks of remediation of his unprofessional behavior and poor interpersonal skills, involving frequent meetings with skilled coaches who used case-based materials and direct observation to help Michael. Unfortunately, he showed little improvement, and attempts to remediate his clinical reasoning also failed (see Figs. 29.2 and 29.3). Neuropsychiatric and drug and alcohol testing was recommended, but he refused both, insisting that he had made progress. In a Clinical Competency Committee (CCC) meeting, the remediation team, program director, and designated institutional official jointly decided that they needed to reassess his skills to document whether he indeed had made progress.

After his next rotation, he received evaluations from faculty, residents, nurses, and patients; an observed structured clin-ical examination in the simulation lab; and two mini-clinical examinations conducted by his clinical attending. All evaluation methods identified impulsive, unprofessional behavior, poor interpersonal skills, and poor clinical reasoning. He received a poor evaluation for the rotation.

Michael's professional file includes the following:

- Documentation that all residents (including Michael) received instruction on how to access expectations for competent performance for each rotation and postgraduate year.
- A dated e-mail from a faculty member reporting that Michael's interpersonal skills and professionalism were poor, which included, "Michael often brags about his skills in front of other residents. During case conferences with other residents, he often interrupts conversations to shout out an answer and follows with a comment about how easy the cases are ... This behavior continues despite two breakfast conversations with me during which I gave him respectful but direct feedback and strongly suggested that he stop."
- A dated e-mail from another faculty member reporting that Michael "didn't let his simulation lab partner participate," because, as he stated, he "can do a better job."
- Notes documenting unsolicited feedback by the resident's clinic preceptor. In these notes, the preceptor expressed that Michael continues to interrupt her while she is speaking with patients to provide advice that is often incorrect, confronts her about patient care decisions in front of patients, uses inappropriate jargon, and shows condescending language with patients, often talking to them as if they

are children, e.g., "You are supposed to exercise. Do you know what that means?"

- Summaries of four meetings with Michael and his advisor, dated and documented by the advisor with follow-up e-mails, describing ongoing difficulties. The e-mails also contained a list of recommended resources to assist with improving and addressing these skills. This included that on request, Michael acknowledged having received each summary e-mail.
- A letter from Michael requesting an excused absence to recover from his bicycle accident.
- A letter granting his request.
- A documented conversation the Dean of Graduate Medical Education and one of Michael's peers initiated by the peer who reported that Michael has been drinking alcohol excessively outside of work.
- Two additional e-mails from a rotation attending describing Michael's inability to work with other residents and students on his team. "Michael often interrupts the other intern's presentation with additional information or with the plan." "He consistently interrupts other residents and volunteers to help with tasks because he can get the work done faster."

A dated e-mail referring him to the remediation team, letting Michael know that they will be given access to his entire academic record.

After 4 weeks of coaching and remediation efforts that were carefully documented, and following the policies and procedures of the institution, the promotions committee determined that Michael failed his reassessment, decided to skip a focused review, and placed him directly on probation because of his rotation failure, general failure to progress, and his refusal to undergo neuropsychiatric testing and alcohol and drug monitoring (see Fig. 29.4).

The CCC then reviewed his entire academic record and offered Michael the opportunity to appear before the committee to present his grievances. As an outcome of that hearing, Michael was evaluated by a medical professional. While he finally completed the alcohol and drug monitoring program without incident and was deemed fit for duty, he refused their recommendations for psychotherapy. He did not acknowledge that he had interpersonal skill problems, struggles with professionalism, or poor clinical reasoning. He continued to maintain that he was a leader among his peers. Overall, he failed to progress. After much debate and consultation with legal counsel, the CCC decided not to renew his yearly contract.

Despite an initial fear of litigation, Michael never sought legal action. Two years later, he requested a letter of recommendation from the residency program director, so that he could apply for another residency position. With the support of the CCC and institutional counsel, the program director wrote a very honest and frank letter about his strengths and weaknesses, including why his contract had not been renewed.

When due process has been followed and the institution's policies are applied without discrimination, trainees rarely win lawsuits. Public institutions must provide constitutional due process, while private institutions may create and follow their own rules and policies. The US Supreme Court has ruled on multiple occasions that it will defer to academic decisions made by institutions of higher education. US courts have repeatedly upheld academic and disciplinary decisions made by clinical faculty, but the same deference is not provided for disciplinary decisions. Lastly, universities and hospitals have historically not been harmed by detailed evaluations of learner's deficiencies. There is much still to be learned about the societal and sociocultural influences and implications that lead to failure of remediation efforts, and the different institutional approaches to dismissal.

Acknowledgments The authors are deeply grateful to Cynthia Irvine and Craig Kliger for reviewing an earlier version of this draft.

References

1. https://www.aamc.org/system/files/reports/1/graduationratesandattritionratesofu.s.medicalstudents.pdf.
2. https://www.acgme.org/globalassets/pfassets/publicationsbooks/2021-2022_acgme__databook_document.pdf.
3. Guraya SY, van Mook WNKA, Khoshhal KI. Failure of faculty to fail failing medical students: fiction or an actual erosion of professional standards? J Taibah Univ Med Sci. 2019;14:103–9.
4. Yepes-Rios M, Dudek N, Duboyce R, Curtis J, Allard RJ, Varpio L. The failure to fail underperforming trainees in health professions education: a BEME systematic review: BEME guide no. 42. Med Teach. 2016;38:1092–9.
5. Schmidt HG, Cohen-Schtnus J, Arends LR. Impact of problem-based, active learning on graduation rates for 10 generations of Dutch medical students. Med Educ. 2009;43:211–8.
6. Reem AR, Ramnarayan K, George BM, Adiga I, Kumari GR, Suvarna N, Devi V, et al. Effects of problem-based learning along with other active learning strategies on short-term learning outcomes of students in an Indian medical school. Int J Health Allied Sci. 2012;1:98.
7. Curtoni S, Cavallo F. International perspective. Basic Sci Educ. 1998;9:22.
8. Mohammadi A. National educational stratification of medical schools in Iran. J Med Educ. 2009;9:55–61.
9. Katz ED, Dahms R, Sadosty AT, Stahmer SA, Goyal D, on behalf of the CORD-EM Remediation Task Force. Guiding principles for resident remediation: recommendations of the CORD remediation task force. Acad Emerg Med. 2012;17:S95–S103.
10. Ellaway RH, Chou CL, Kalet A. Situating remediation: accommodating success and failure in medical education systems. Acad Med. 2018;93:391–8.
11. Smith JL, Lypson M, Silverberg M, Weizberg M, Murano T, Lukela M, Santen SA. Defining uniform processes for remediation, probation, and termination in residency training. West J Emerg Med. 2017;18:110–3.
12. Tulgan H, Cohen S, Kinne K. How a teaching hospital implemented its termination policies for disruptive residents. Acad Med. 2001;76:1107–12.
13. Papadakis MA, Teherani A, Banach MA, Knettler TR, et al. Disciplinary action by medical boards and prior behavior in medical school. N Engl J Med. 2005;353:2673–82.
14. Lupien SJ. Yearbook of science and technology. New York: McGraw Hill; 2003.
15. Lupien SJ, McEwen BS. The acute effects of corticosteroids on cognition: integration of animal and human model studies. Brain Res. 1997;24:1–27.
16. Guerrasio J, Garrity MJ, Aagaard EM. Learner deficits and academic outcomes of medical students, residents, fellows, and attending physicians referred to a remediation program, 2006-2012. Acad Med. 2014;89:352–8.
17. Yao DC, Wright SM. A national survey of internal medicine residency program directors regarding problem residents. JAMA. 2000;284:1099–104.
18. Lefebvre C, Williamson K, Moffett P, Cummings A, Gianopulos B, Winters E, Sokolosky M. Legal considerations in the remediation and dismissal of graduate medical trainees. J Grad Med Educ. 2018;10:253–7.
19. Irby DM, Milam S. The legal context for evaluating and dismissing medical students and residents. Acad Med. 1989;64:639–43.
20. Moffett P, Lefebvre C, Williamson K. Standardized letters of concern and remediation contracts: templates for program directors. J Grad Med Educ. 2019;11:606–10.
21. Schultz K, Risk A, Newton L, Snider N. Formal remediation and probation (part 2 of 3): when residents shouldn't become clinicians: getting a grip on fair and defensible processes for termination of training. Can Med Educ J. 2021;12:121–6.
22. Wren KR, Wren TL. Legal implications of evaluation procedures for students in healthcare professions. AANA J. 1999;67:73–8.
23. Minicucci RF, Lewis BF. Trouble in academia: ten years of litigation in medical education. Acad Med. 2003;78:S13–5.
24. Helms LB, Helms CM. Forty years of litigation involving medical students and their education: I. General educational issues. Acad Med. 1991;66:1–7.
25. Short JP. The importance of strong evaluation standards and procedures in training residents. Acad Med. 1993;68:522–5.
26. Bellocq JA. Student dismissal: part I—how much documentation is enough? J Prof Nurs. 1988;4:147, 230.
27. Conran RM, Elzie CA, Knollman-Ritschel BE, Domen RE, Powell SZ. Due process in medical education: legal considerations. Acad Pathol. 2018; 5:1–21.
28. Smith MH, McKoy YD, Richardson J. Legal issues related to dismissing students for clinical deficiencies. Nurse Educ. 2001;26:33–8.
29. Liaison Committee on Medical Education. Accreditation standards. https://lcme.org/wp-content/uploads/filebase/standards/2021-22_Functions-and-Structure_2021-04-16.docx. Accessed 11 Jan 2022.
30. American College of Graduate Medical Education. Institutional requirements. https://acgme.org/

Portals/0/PFAssets/InstitutionalRequirements/000In stitutionalRequirements2018.pdf?ver=2018-02-19-132236-600. Accessed 11 Jan 2022.

31. Schultz K, Risk A, Newton L, Snider N. Program foundations and beginning of concerns (part 1 of 3): when residents shouldn't become clinicians: getting a grip on fair and defensible processes for termination of training. Can Med Educ J. 2021;12:116–20.

32. Grieger CH, Shemonsky NK, Driscoll RE 3rd. Graduate medical education and the law. J Med Educ. 1984;59:643–8.

33. Shuffer v. Board of Trustees, 67 Cal. App. 3d 208,220, 136 Cal. Rptr. 527,534. 1977.

34. Schenarts PJ, Langenfeld S. The fundamentals of resident dismissal. Am Surg. 2017;83:119–26.

35. Pabian PS, Neely L. The legal foundation of student dismissal in professional education programs. J Allied Health. 2021;50:321–7.

36. Levinson H, Rosenthal S. CEO corporate leadership in action. New York: Basic Books; 1984.

37. Ewing v. University of Michigan, 1985; 514–515.

38. Masangkay N, Adams J, Dwinnell B, Hanson JT, Jain S, Tariq S. Revisiting feed forward: promoting a student-centered approach to education handoffs, remediation, and clerkship success, Teach Learn Med, 2022;1–9. Epub ahead of print).

39. Kraft v. William Alanson White Psychiatric Foundation, 498 A.2d 1145, 1149 D.C. App. 1985.

40. Capozzi JD, Rhodes R. Decisions regarding resident advancement and dismissal. J Bone Joint Surg. 2005;87:2353–5.

41. Schultz K, Risk A, Newton L, Snider N. The appeal process and beyond (part 3 of 3): when residents shouldn't become clinicians: getting a grip on fair and defensible processes for termination of training. Can Med Educ J. 2021;12:127–31.

42. Bellini LM, Kalet A, Englander R. Providing compassionate off-ramps for medical students is a moral imperative. Acad Med. 2019;94:656–8.

43. Aagaard E, Moscoso L. Practical implications off compassionate off-ramps for medical students. Acad Med. 2019;94:619–22.

44. Ackerman-Barger K, Jacobs NN. The microaggressions triangle model: a humanistic approach to navigating microaggressions in health professions schools. Acad Med. 2020;95:S28–32.

45. Anderson N, Lett E, Asabor EN, Hernandez AL, Nguemeni Tiako MJ, Johnson C, Montenegro RE, Rizzo TM, Latimore D, Nunez-Smith M, Boatright D. The association of microaggressions with depressive symptoms and institutional satisfaction among a national cohort of medical students. J Gen Intern Med. 2022;37:298–307.

46. Tsuei SH, Lee D, Ho C, Regehr G, Nimmon L. Exploring the construct of psychological safety in medical education. Acad Med. 2019;94:S28–35.

Epilogue: A Student's Perspective on Remediation

Jameze James

As a medical student, I encountered a bump in the road, which in retrospect was just a bigger jolt on a path that had been bumpy for a long time.

When doing any patient presentation, I learned that context matters: the full H & P for every patient is required before moving on to an assessment and plan. Case in point: when you hear that I did not pass Step 2 of the Boards, you may make immediate judgments about me. So, I think I need to start earlier, as a person of color, the first generation in my family ever to go to grad school.

I grew up in a single-parent household. My mom is Filipino, and my dad is African American. I did not know my father until I was in high school, when I met him briefly. When I was 3, my mom married my younger brother's dad, who is African American as well, but they got divorced when I was in middle school. So, I grew up as a latchkey kid. I pretty much stayed out of trouble because I was a big nerd, and I learned to be responsible to take care of a lot of our financial holes growing up. My mom, who has diabetes, had a hard time keeping employment after the Great Recession. So, in high school, I worked part time in high school at Round Table Pizza, and even though I got a scholarship at Berkeley, I worked my way through college as well, because I knew that my mom and my younger brother, who has bipolar disease, needed financial support. I felt obligated to be the caregiver, the mature one who never put my needs above any-

one else's. My mom always meant well but never really put in the work, so I was always the one to fill in the gaps. I learned to armor up and carry myself in a way to not appear vulnerable, to not let people know about my own personal stress, mental health, or family business.

After college, I held a job as a research associate and coordinator for 5 years and then applied to medical school. My mom had moved to Hawaii to live with my elderly grandparents. I did fine in the pre-clerkship period and during most of my clerkships, though I did struggle on two shelf exams. In retrospect, one of them was at the time my mom was hospitalized with hyperosmolar coma, and the other was when my brother was also hospitalized for a manic episode. But in medical school, I did not really think about mental health breaks or personal time. I felt I just had to plug through. Medicine trains us all to think about the context of other people but not ourselves, and for someone who was always the caregiver for others, it reinforced my own bad habit growing up, which was to just push through and not really think about the personal chaos.

After clerkships, I decided to take a year to do an MPH, because my wife and I were about to have our first kid. We were planning what to do when she went back to work after maternity leave, and I thought about my mom. Because my mom was needing to transition her living situation, I reasoned that she needed someplace to stay, we needed childcare, and I could be a good son, provide for my mother, and give her a chance to redeem her lack of action in my life previously. It seemed like a great idea at the time.

J. James
Department of Pediatrics, Kaiser Permanente Medical Center, Oakland, CA, USA

A. Kalet, C. L. Chou (eds.), *Remediation in Medical Education*,
https://doi.org/10.1007/978-3-031-32404-8

What I really did not take into account was that my mom suffered from undiagnosed mental illness: monopolar depression with an underlying personality disorder. So, when she came to live with us, she quickly became our second dependent, someone with decompensated chronic illnesses of diabetes and hypertension. She would lie about her blood glucose numbers and sneak carbs. Soon after she arrived, she was so ill that we had to take her to the emergency room twice—this is when my wife was eight and nine months pregnant. I remember thinking, what am I doing? But being brought up in Filipino culture, and now as the eldest son (my older brother had passed away while I was a research associate), I felt obligated to take care of her. This dynamic continued through my MPH, and then I went back to sub-internships. I then started developing headaches for the first time in my life, terrible migraines that were concerning to the neurologists for brain lesions. Fortunately, I had a negative CT scan. Then I was completing applications for residency programs and preparing for the Boards. Right before my exam, my mom had a mental breakdown, where she got really defensive about her behavior and living in our home, and she attempted to strike my wife. Luckily, she missed, but she fell to the ground, and it was just chaos. I felt I had no recourse, and of course my modus operandi was just to keep it to myself, so I just took the Boards exam the following day and did not focus.

When I found out that I did not pass, I was horrified. It completely derailed my application process. I had just accepted invitations to interview for all these great places, and now I was told I had to retake my Boards in a limited time period and to make sure that it showed some improvement.

And so, even though it is a call most students would loathe to receive, I was very fortunate that the dean reached out to me. He gave me the space to share. I told him that what was happening with me was more than just not preparing for exam, being confused by the material, or just not taking it seriously. He really heard me, and he recommended first that I take a leave of absence, and second that I get a coach. He recommended Dr. Phillips.

When I first met with her, I told her my story. I remember her saying, "Wow, I would've never imagined that was the story behind you. You hold yourself so well." Well, thanks, I thought, that is a good thing and a bad thing.

But as she spent time with me, I found I could really trust her with my story and off-load that huge burden I was carrying. She could really see me as a parent with a young kid and empathize with my situation. It was not easy to talk about, but she stuck with me. She gave me some great study advice that really fit into my parenting schedule and even gave me advice on what to do with my situation with my mom. I also reached out to another mentor, Dr. Miller, who in fact had been my pediatrician growing up. She told me, "You know when you fly, they tell parents to put on your own oxygen mask before putting one on their kids. That's what you need to do." She knew the context of everything and really told me straight out that I needed to really take care of this family stuff before thinking about anything else. She noted that if I did not, it would be even harder to get back on the right track after a leave of absence. And she was right! Through those words, and through therapy, I am becoming a more empathetic caregiver, because I am more empathetic to myself. I finally really got that I cannot provide the care for other people unless I care for myself. Taking the time off, I was really able to focus and then develop deeper insight into what I could do academically to really get myself to that next level.

So, in my leave of absence, I got busy. I got a job as an adjunct instructor at Merritt College teaching human anatomy to premeds and nursing students. I had an opportunity to be a grader for the clinical skills exam at the UCSF. I worked as an Outdoor Recreation Leader for the San Francisco Recreation and Parks Department, guiding free weekly walks to promote benefits of exercise, maintaining a diet, environmental stewardship, and socialization among diverse community members. It was important to really reanchor myself and have people who supported that decision, instead of saying, "Hey, you got to finish, you got to do this, you got to do that, there's a plan in place."

Having this combination of support was important to me because I realized the importance of -not just the family I grew up with, but also this idea of found family, where you create a community around you of people who are supportive and people who are invested in seeing you follow through with your goals. And I think I really found that. I think it is what really made the difference coming back after the leave of absence, because my supporters were less focused on the outcome of one exam, and more on how I could set myself up for longer term success. This included creating a study schedule with goals in mind that also incorporated sleeping, childcare, and work. It felt really regimented, but the schedule flexibility was really helpful.

As for my mom, she ended up breaking her hip a few months after I failed the Boards, so she is now in a nursing home.

After my time off, I returned to my subinternships and actually received honors in them. I think the best compliment I got was when I was getting my evaluation at the end of my rotation at Kaiser, they told me I took care of everything and was already working at intern level, and then they noted I got an MPH and asked me when I did it. I told them that I had just returned from a year-and-a-half hiatus. It made me feel really good that I actually came back more prepared, even though my clinical clerkships were at that point rather remote.

And so far, I have used that in residency too. Just having that protected time and protected space was something I did not understand, grow-

ing up with someone with a personality disorder. It was always about how much more I could give and sacrifice, and that is what led to my burnout with everything. Now, creating this sustainable structure, even beyond helping me as a med student, I feel more prepared as a parent, as a medical professional, and as a person.

This work still requires support people. I still work with the therapist I met with during this entire process. I still love to give updates to all the mentors that I cultivated and hope to continue to send holiday cards. It is just an incredible opportunity. I think it is just one of those things where if I did not hit the speed bump in med school, I could have just blown through residency, not even recognizing a lot of the adversity I experienced growing up. I see how I normalized that because as the only person of color in a lot of AP classes in high school, my premed classes, my MCAT class, and even in my class in med school, I felt very alone. I did not think anyone would understand or have a similar experience. Trust comes from letting your guard down and starting a conversation. And I realize that I have to be the one to do that and then set the example. It is very freeing for everyone to just say I am human, and this is what I am going through. And I think it is a great example, especially for my patients and my future patients, just to say, "You can tell me anything, because I've been in your shoes. I've been there. I was the kid that experienced things like you, and now I'm the adult." I can be the example.

Index

© The Editor(s) (if applicable) and The Author(s), under exclusive license to Springer Nature Switzerland AG 2023
A. Kalet, C. L. Chou (eds.), *Remediation in Medical Education*,
https://doi.org/10.1007/978-3-031-32404-8

Printed in the United States
by Baker & Taylor Publisher Services